Synthesis, Characterization and Applications of Drug Delivery

Synthesis, Characterization and Applications of Drug Delivery

Editor: Laurence Denton

AMERICAN
MEDICAL PUBLISHERS
www.americanmedicalpublishers.com

AMERICAN
MEDICAL PUBLISHERS
www.americanmedicalpublishers.com

Cataloging-in-Publication Data

Synthesis, characterization and applications of drug delivery / edited by Laurence Denton.
p. cm.
Includes bibliographical references and index.
ISBN 979-8-88740-075-4
1. Drug delivery systems. 2. Drug delivery devices. 3. Pharmaceutical technology.
4. Drugs. I. Denton, Laurence.
RS199.5 .S96 2023
615.6--dc23

American Medical Publishers,
41 Flatbush Avenue,
1st Floor, New York,
NY 11217, USA

ISBN 979-8-88740-075-4 (Hardback)

Contents

Preface

This book has been a concerted effort by a group of academicians, researchers and scientists, who have contributed their research works for the realization of the book. This book has materialized in the wake of emerging advancements and innovations in this field. Therefore, the need of the hour was to compile all the required researches and disseminate the knowledge to a broad spectrum of people comprising of students, researchers and specialists of the field.

Drug delivery comprises formulations, approaches, manufacturing techniques, storage technologies and systems that are involved in the transportation of a pharmaceutical compound towards the targeted site in order to attain the required therapeutic response. It is focused on changing the specificity and pharmacokinetics of the drugs through the formulation of different medical devices, drug carriers and excipients. Furthermore, it places additional weight on enhancing the duration of action and bioavailability of drugs to enhance the therapeutic outcomes. Drug delivery encompasses targeted delivery, controlled-release formulations, drug carriers, 3D printing, nanomedicine, as well as delivery of biologic drugs. The principles associated with the preparation of drugs, route administration, toxicity, metabolism and site specific targeting help in the synthesis, characterization and applications of drug delivery. They are utilized for optimizing safety and efficacy for improvement of patient compliance and convenience. This book includes some of the vital pieces of work being conducted across the world, on various topics related to the synthesis, characterization and applications of drug delivery. It is a resource guide for experts as well as students.

At the end of the preface, I would like to thank the authors for their brilliant chapters and the publisher for guiding us all-through the making of the book till its final stage. Also, I would like to thank my family for providing the support and encouragement throughout my academic career and research projects.

Editor

1

Xylan-Based Hydrogels as a Potential Carrier for Drug Delivery: Effect of Pore-Forming Agents

Minmin Chang †, **Xinxin Liu** †, **Ling Meng, Xiaohui Wang and Junli Ren** *

State Key Laboratory of Pulp and Paper Engineering, South China University of Technology, 510640 Guangzhou, China; 17728109456@163.com (M.C.); lxx19910312@163.com (X.L.); mengling0117@163.com (L.M.); fewangxh@scut.edu.cn (X.W.)

* Correspondence: renjunli@scut.edu.cn

† These authors contributed equally to the work.

Abstract: Pore-forming agents have a significant influence on the pore structure of hydrogels. In this study, a porogenic technique was employed to investigate the preparation of macroporous hydrogels which were synthesized by radical copolymerization of carboxymethyl xylan with acrylamide and *N*-isopropylacrylamide under the function of a cross-linking agent. Six kinds of pore-forming agents were used: polyvinylpyrrolidone K30, polyethylene glycol 2000, carbamide, NaCl, $CaCO_3$, and $NaHCO_3$. The application of these hydrogels is also discussed. The results show that pore-forming agents had an important impact on the pore structure of the hydrogels and consequently affected properties of the hydrogels such as swelling ratio and mechanical strength, while little effect was noted on the thermal property of the hydrogels. 5-Fluorouracil was used as a model drug to study the drug release of the as-prepared hydrogels, and it was found that the drug release was substantially improved after using the $NaHCO_3$ pore-forming agent: a cumulative release rate of up to 71.05% was achieved.

Keywords: carboxymethyl xylan; hydrogel; pore-forming agents; drug delivery

1. Introduction

Hydrogels are three-dimensional networks composed of cross-linked polymers which are insoluble in water and can absorb a large amount of water [1]. Recently, hydrogels have attracted extensive interest in some biomedical fields such as drug delivery, tissue engineering, and artificial muscles [2–4]. However, most hydrogels have a low swelling rate and take a long time to reach their equilibrium swelling state, which limits the application of hydrogels. Hydrogels with porous structure have attracted lots of attention due to their large pore size and surface area [5]. A porogenic technique could produce desirable pore sizes within the hydrogel network. Pore-forming agents are added during the hydrogel preparation and removed after polymerization to form the pore structure and control the pore size of hydrogels [6,7]. For example, a kind of macroporous polyacrylamide (PAM) hydrogel for protein immobilization was developed using poly(ethylene glycol) (PEG) as a pore-forming agent. The results showed that PEG could enhance macromolecule diffusion into the interior of the hydrogel and that this hydrogel could be used in tissue engineering and protein arrays [8]. Stable alginate hydrogels were fabricated with controlled pore dimensions in the range of 5–50 μm by sacrificial $CaCO_3$ templates [9]. A kind of DNA–polymer hybrid hydrogel was prepared using PEG as the pore-forming agent [10]. It was found that the pore size of the hydrogel increased with increasing PEG content. The pore size distribution of the altered hydrogels could enhance the permeability of the materials, resulting in faster hydrogel equilibration. Accordingly, pore-forming agents could be used to control the pore size of hydrogels [11].

With the deterioration of the environment and the shortage of resources, natural polymers such as cellulose, chitosan, collagen, and hemicellulose have been used for the preparation of hydrogels [12–14]. The introduction of natural polymers endows hydrogels with biocompatibility and biodegradation [15]. Xylan is a kind of hemicellulose with a backbone of β-(1→4) linked D-xylosyl residues substituted with L-arabinofuranosyl, 4-*O*-methyl-D-glucuronopyranosyl, L-galactopyranosyl, or D-glucuronopyranosyl units at C-2 and/or C-3 of the main chain [16]. Xylan also possesses some medical properties such as immunological defense, anticancer, and antioxidant properties [17]. Due to the stability of xylan in human stomach and intestine, it has great potential as a drug release carrier [18]. A few studies have focused on xylan-based hydrogels. A xylan-based hydrogel was prepared by the cross-linking polymerization of xylan with *N*-isopropylacrylamide (NIPAm) and acrylic acid (AA) under UV irradiation [19]. This hydrogel was further used for acetylsalicylic acid release. The cumulative release rate of acetylsalicylic acid could reach up to 90.5% after sustained release for 5 h in simulated intestinal fluid. A new photoresponsive hydrogel was prepared by free radical copolymerization of xylan-type hemicellulose methacrylate with 4-[(4-acryloyloxyphenyl)azo]benzoic acid (AOPAB) [20]. These hydrogels showed responsive behavior to light, and vitamin-B12-loaded hydrogel showed a high drug cumulative release rate under UV irradiation. A simultaneous in situ formation of xylan nanohydrogels and encapsulation of horseradish peroxidase (HRP) was achieved through the selective hydrolysis of oat spelt xylan by recombinant α-L-arabinofuranosidase (AbfB) with polymeric xylan substrate specificity [21]. These hydrogels could release the encapsulated HRP in its active form over a period of 180 min, indicating that these hydrogels could potentially be used as an encapsulation matrix for the targeted delivery and slow release of bioactive substances. A new pH-sensitive and biodegradable hemicellulose-based hydrogel was prepared by grafting AA into hemicellulose [22]. The cumulative release rate of the hydrogels loaded with acetylsalicylic acid could reach up to 85% after 6 h. Therefore, xylan is promising for applications in drug delivery.

5-Fluorouracil (5-Fu) is a kind of hydrophilic anticancer drug used in clinics and is employed in systemic chemotherapy of solid tumors such as breast, colorectal, liver, and brain cancer [23]. 5-Fu inhibits the synthesis of DNA to a lesser extent over a longer period [24]. Continuous administration of 5-Fu maintains its therapeutic activity via metabolism. However, excessive concentrations of 5-Fu would cause a toxic effect. Thus, it is necessary to control a low concentration and sustained release [25].

The pore structure of hydrogels has an important influence on their properties such as their swelling ratio and mechanical properties which would affect their application. Porogenic techniques are an effective method to produce different pore structures in hydrogels and are suitable for different applications such as a culture medium for marine bacteria or drug release. Some reagents have been used as pore-forming agents, including organic reagents and inorganic reagents such as PEG and $CaCO_3$ mentioned above. Very important for the selection of pore-forming agents is that the agents should have a good pore-forming effect and have no negative impact on the material properties. However, few studies have focused on the impact of different pore-forming agents on hydrogels, especially for xylan-based hydrogels. In this work, six different organic and inorganic pore-making agents with various molecular weights were applied to study their influence on the properties of xylan-based hydrogels such as the pore structure, swelling ratio, mechanical properties, and thermal stability. The preparation of xylan-based hydrogels was conducted by radical copolymerization of carboxymethyl xylan (CMX) with acrylamide (AM) and NIPAm under the function of cross-linking agents. During the preparation of hydrogels, six kinds of pore-forming agents were used: polyvinylpyrrolidone K30 (PVP), polyethylene glycol 2000 (PEG2000), carbamide, NaCl, $CaCO_3$, and $NaHCO_3$. These hydrogels were characterized by Fourier transform infrared (FTIR), scanning electron microscopy (SEM), and thermogravimetric analysis (TGA). The application of the as-prepared hydrogels as drug carriers for 5-Fu delivery was also investigated.

2. Materials and Methods

2.1. Reagent and Apparatus

Sodium chloroacetate (>99.6%) was purchased from Aladdin (Shanghai, China). Bagasse xylan (M_w of 49,000 g·mol^{-1}, xylose > 85%) was purchased from Yuanye (Shanghai, China). NaOH, carbamide, absolute ethyl alcohol, and glacial acetic acid were purchased from Jinhuada Chemical Reagent Factory (Guangzhou, China). AM, ammonium persulfate (APS), *N,N′*-Methylenebis(2-propenamide) (MBA), and $ZnCl_2$ were purchased from Fuchen Chemical Reagent Factory (Tianjin, China). NIPAm, *N,N,N,N*-tetramethylethylenediamine (TEMED), PEG2000, phosphate buffer (PBS, pH = 7.4), and 5-Fu were purchased from MACKLIN (Shanghai, China). Hydrochloric acid, NaCl, $CaCO_3$, and $NaHCO_3$ were purchased from Guangzhou Chemical Reagent Factory (Guangzhou, China). Polyvinyl pyrrolidone (PVP, M_w of 40,000) was purchased from Richjiont (Shanghai, China). Ultra-water was used in the preparation of hydrogels.

The thermostatic oscillator was used in drug release (TH7-C, Taicang Experimental Equipment Factory, Jiangsu, China). Microwave catalytic synthesizer was used to synthesize carboxymethyl xylan (XH-300UL, Beijing Xianghu Science and Technology Development Co. LTD, Beijing, China). Analytical balance was purchased from Sartorius Scientific Instruments (Beijing) Co. LTD (BSA224S-CW, Beijing, China). Heating agitator was used to control the reaction temperature (RCT basic, IKA, Staufen, Germany). UV spectrophotometer was used to detect the absorbance (UV-1800, Shimadzu, Kyoto, Japan). Vacuum drying chamber was purchased from Shanghai Yiheng Scientific Instrument Co. LTD (BPZ, Shanghai, China). Freeze-drying machine was purchased from Virtis (FM25XL-70, SP Scientific, Warminster, PA, USA).

2.2. Synthesis of Carboxymethyl Xylan (CMX)

CMX was synthesized under microwave irradiation according to our previous work [26]. Briefly, 6.6 g of xylan was added to 25 mL of ultra-pure water and was heated and stirred in an 80 °C oil bath. After 70 min, the xylan was completely dissolved. After the xylan solution cooled down to room temperature, 1.0 g of sodium hydroxide dissolved in 2 mL ultra-pure water was added. After 20 min, 11.648 g sodium chloroacetate (dissolved in 11 mL ultra-pure water) and 1.0 g sodium hydroxide (dissolved in 2 mL ultra-pure water) were added to the reaction system for 20 min. Then, the reaction was transferred to a microwave reactor at a power of 300 W and a temperature of 65 °C for 20 min. After the reaction was over, the system was cooled down and neutralized using acetic acid. The dialysis was conducted for one week at room temperature. At last, the sample was freeze-dried to get the sample powder and put into the dryer. The obtained CMX had a substituting degree of 0.14. The calculation method was obtained from the literature [27].

2.3. Peparation of Hydrogels

Xylan-based hydrogel was prepared by the following steps: Quantities of 0.5 g of prepared CMX, 4.5 g of AM, and 0.1 g of NIPAm were dissolved in 40 mL of ultra-pure water with a magnetic stirrer at 1 °C for 15 min. N_2 was bubbled into the system to remove oxygen during this process. Quantities of 0.05 g each of MBA and APS were added, and then 0.25 g of the pore-forming agent was added as well as 50 μL TEMDA. Subsequently, the homogeneous solution was poured into two molds (with a diameter of 30 mm and a height of 15 mm). After forming the gels, the mold was transferred to the refrigerator for 24 h for further reaction. Then, the hydrogels were immersed in $ZnCl_2$ solution (0.05 mol/L) for one day to enhance the hydrogels' strength by metal coordination bonding, and different methods were applied to remove the pore-forming agents and unreacted chemicals; these are shown in Table 1. Some of the samples were cut into slices (about 8 mm length, 5 mm width, and 3mm thickness) and dried in a freeze-dryer. The dried samples were stored in a dryer, and the wet untreated samples were put in the refrigerator before testing.

Table 1. Preparation conditions of hydrogels with different pore-forming agents.

Sample	Pore-Forming Agent	Washing Method
gel-1	—	Soaked with ultra-pure water for one week
gel-2	PEG2000	Soaked with ethanol for three days then ultra-pure water for four days
gel-3	NaCl	Soaked with ultra-pure water for one week
gel-4	$CaCO_3$	Soaked with HCl solution for three days then ultra-pure water for four days
gel-5	$NaHCO_3$	Soaked with HCl solution for three days then ultra-pure water for four days
gel-6	carbamide	Soaked with ultra-pure water for one week
gel-7	PVP	Soaked with ultra-pure water for one week

2.4. Characterization of Hydrogels

Hydrogels were characterized by their FTIR spectra (TENSOR27, Bruker, Germany). These spectra were collected from KBr-based discs. Each spectrum was obtained in the range of 4000–400 cm^{-1} at a resolution of 4 cm^{-1} and recorded for a total of 32 scans. Before testing, hydrogels were ground into powder with a mortar. Then, the 1% finely ground hydrogels were mixed with KBr to be pressed into a plate for measurement.

The mechanical properties of the hydrogels were measured at room temperature using a universal testing machine (INSTRON 5565, Instron Corpration, Boston, MA, USA). As-prepared hydrogels with a cylindrical shape were placed at the center of the lower compression plate. The upper plate then compressed the samples at a velocity of 3 $mm{\cdot}min^{-1}$ until the hydrogels were broken.

A thermal gravimetric analyzer (TA Q500, TA Instruments, Newcastle, DE, USA) was used to evaluate the thermostability of the hydrogels prepared by different pore-forming agents. Samples of 8–10 mg of the hydrogels were transferred to a Pd plate. The temperature was increased from room temperature to 700 °C at a 10 °C/min heating rate in an open Pd plate. The thermal analyses were conducted under a dry nitrogen atmosphere with a flow rate of 25.0 mL/min.

SEM (EVO 18, Carl Zeiss Jena, Germany) was used to observe the surface morphology of hydrogels at an acceleration voltage of 10 KV. Dried hydrogels were cut into thin sheets with a blade. Before testing, hydrogel samples were fixed on a metal stub and coated with gold to increase the conductivity of the samples.

Electronic probe energy-dispersive spectrometry (EDS) (EPMA-1600, Shimadzu, Kyoto, Japan) was used to confirm the presence of Zn^{2+} in hydrogels. The dry sheet sample was sprayed with gold before testing.

An atomic absorption spectrometer (Z-2000, Hitachi, Tokyo, Japan) was used to detect the content of zinc in the hydrogels. A certain weight of dry hydrogel was transferred to 0.5 mol/L HCl solution (10 mL), and the mixture was stirred at room temperature for 8 h. The zinc content of the eluent liquid was detected by atomic absorption spectrometry. The zinc content was expressed as percentage of mass, which was calculated using the following formula:

$$W = C \times V/M \times 100\% \quad (1)$$

where C is the mass concentration of zinc, V is the volume of solution, and M is the weight of the dry hydrogel.

2.5. Swelling Behavior Studies of Hydrogels

The swelling behavior of hydrogels was evaluated by the gravimetric method. The weight of the dry hydrogel was recorded firstly, and then the dry hydrogel was immersed in PBS solution at room temperature. After a fixed time, the swollen hydrogel was removed from water, dried with clean filter paper, and weighed. The swelling ratio (SR) and the equilibrium swelling ratio (Seq) were calculated using the following formulae [22]:

$$SR = (W_t - W_d)/W_d \quad (2)$$

$$S_{eq} = (W_{eq} - W_d)/W_d \quad (3)$$

where W_t is the weight of the swollen hydrogel, W_d is the initial weight of the dried hydrogel, and W_{eq} is the equilibrium weight of the swollen hydrogel.

2.6. Drug Release

2.6.1. Standard Curve of 5-Fu

For the method of drug release, we refer the reader to the published literature [28]. The standard curve of 5-Fu was obtained firstly. 5-Fu solution with a concentration of 0.233 mg/mL was accurately prepared. Then, 0.50, 1.00, 1.50, 2.00, 2.50, 3.00, or 3.50 mL of the solution was added to a 50.00 mL volumetric flask. The absorbance of these solutions was measured at 265 nm using an ultraviolet spectrophotometer. Finally, the standard working curve of 5-Fu was obtained ($A = 0.0527C - 0.0006$, $R^2 = 0.9995$).

2.6.2. Preparation of 5-Fu-Loaded Hydrogels

The aqueous solution of 5-Fu (0.8072 mg/mL) was prepared first. Dried hydrogels were placed in this 5-Fu solution at 20 °C. After 2 days, the hydrogels were removed from PBS, and the hydrogel surface was flushed with a small amount of deionized water to remove the unloaded drug. The volume of the mixture of residual liquid and flushing fluid was accurately measured. Then, the absorbance of the mixture was measured. According to the absorbance of the solution and standard curve, the weight of 5-Fu in the hydrogels was calculated. Finally, 5-Fu-loaded hydrogels were dried to a constant weight in a vacuum.

2.6.3. Drug Release of Hydrogels

Hydrogels loaded with 5-Fu were added to a PBS buffer solution (pH = 7.4) at 37 °C. Then, they were placed into a 37 °C thermostatic oscillator (100 r/min) and were sampled at regular intervals. The absorbance of the solution was determined by ultraviolet spectrophotometry at 265 nm. According to the standard working curve, the concentration of 5-Fu was calculated.

3. Results and Discussion

3.1. Pore-Making Mechanism for Hydrogels

The preparation process of the hydrogels is depicted in Scheme 1. The hydroxyl groups of CMX generated free radicals as the active site in the presence of APS, by which AM and NIPAm were grafted onto the CMX chain. AM and NIPAm could form polyacrylamide (PAM), polynitroisopropyl acrylamide (PNIPAm) and P(AM-co-NIPAm) under the function of APS. Then, the expected CMX-g-P(AM-co-NIPAm) hydrogels were formed under the function of MBA. Subsequently, the hydrogels were immersed in $ZnCl_2$ solution to further enhance the strength of the hydrogels by coordination bonds formed between Zn^{2+} and anionic groups such as $-COO^-$ [29]. During the process of hydrogel formation, the action of the pore-forming agents did not involve this chemical reaction. In view of the pore-forming agent type, different methods were used to remove pore-forming agents (Table 1). Thus, hydrogels with different pore sizes could be obtained.

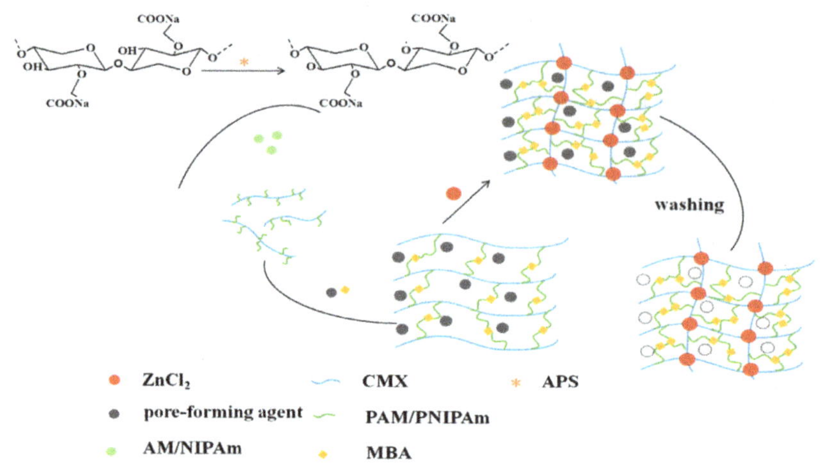

Scheme 1. The preparation process of hydrogels.

3.2. FTIR Analysis of Hydrogels

The FTIR spectra of CMX and CMX-based hydrogels with six kinds of pore-forming agents are illustrated in Figure 1. For the spectrum of CMX, the broad band at 3439 cm^{-1} is assigned to the –OH groups on xylan. The bands appearing at 1646, 1254, and 1170 cm^{-1} are the typical absorption bands of xylan [30]. The band at 2921 cm^{-1} is assigned to the C–H stretching vibration of the alkane on xylan. The band at 1051 cm^{-1} originates from the C–O–C stretching of the pyranoid ring of xylan [22]. The sharp peak appearing at 893 cm^{-1} is owing to the β-glucosidic bonds between the xylose units. The absorption peak appearing at 1468 cm^{-1} is associated with the –COO^- symmetric stretching vibration of CMX [19]. For the spectrum of the hydrogels, the band at 3268 cm^{-1} originates from the N–H asymmetric stretching vibration peak of the carbonyl in the amide group in PNIPAm and PAM [31]. A peak at 3204 cm^{-1} is attributable to –NH_2 stretching in PAM molecules [32]. The absorption peak at 1674 cm^{-1} is associated with the C=O stretching vibration peak of PAM and PNIPAm [33]. There is also an asymmetrical stretching band of carboxylate ions from 1468 cm^{-1} to 1457 cm^{-1} [34]. The FTIR spectra indicate that the monomers were grafted onto the structure of xylan. In addition, similar spectra of hydrogels with or without pore-forming agents were observed, indicating that organic pore-forming agents were completely removed during the elution stage and had no effects on the structure of the hydrogels.

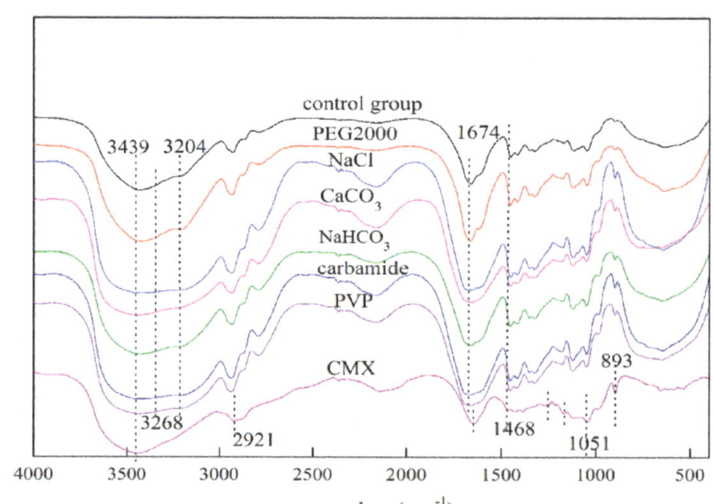

Figure 1. FTIR spectra of CMX and prepared hydrogels with or without six kinds of pore-forming agents.

3.3. Mechanical Properties Analysis of Hydrogels

Hydrogels should be endowed with suitable strength to broaden their applications. The compressive property was used to evaluate the mechanical properties of the hydrogels. Without the immersion of the hydrogels in $ZnCl_2$ solution, breakable hydrogels were obtained, and the testing of the mechanical properties of the hydrogels could not be conducted, limiting further applications. To substantially improve the strength of the hydrogels, $ZnCl_2$ was employed to facilitate the formation of strong cross-linked bonds (metal coordination bonds) between Zn^{2+} and $-COO^-$ groups in the hydrogels [29]. After immersion in $ZnCl_2$, the hydrogels had great elasticity and were not broken after pressing with fingers. The compressive strengths of the hydrogels with or without the six kinds of pore-forming agents are illustrated in Figure 2.

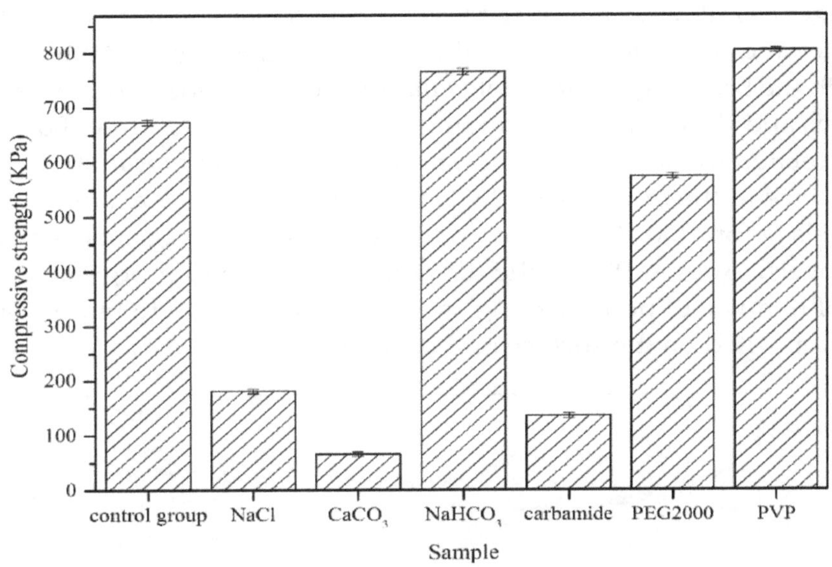

Figure 2. Compressive properties of hydrogels with or without six kinds of pore-forming agents.

The compressive strength of the CMXH hydrogels without pore-forming agents (control group) was about 673 KPa. Different compressive strengths were obtained for hydrogels with PVP, PEG2000, carbamide, NaCl, $CaCO_3$, and $NaHCO_3$. The highest achieved compressive strength of hydrogels was 803 KPa with PVP, followed by hydrogels with $NaHCO_3$, PEG2000, NaCl, carbamide, and $CaCO_3$ (765 KPa, 573 KPa, 181 KPa, 135 KPa, and 65 KPa, respectively). This difference was ascribed to the use of pore-forming agents during the formation of the hydrogels. For organic pore-forming agents, the compressive strength of hydrogels with PVP was highest due to the molecular weight and the chain length. The entanglement of PVP with CMX or other polymers increased the crosslinking density. However, the high crosslinking density limited the increase in the pore size. The compressive strength of the hydrogel with PEG2000 was lower than that of CMXH hydrogels. This might be related to pore shrinkage because ethanol was used during the process of removal of the pore-forming agents, resulting in low mechanical properties compared with the CMXH hydrogels (control group). The compressive strength of the hydrogel with carbamide was about 140 KPa. One possible explanation for this is that hydrogen bonds were formed between carbamide and monomers, which reduced the cross-linking density of the hydrogels.

The lowest compressive strength among the hydrogels was obtained by using $CaCO_3$ as the pore-forming agent. A possible reason for this is that the $CaCO_3$ was not dissolved in water, so $CaCO_3$ precipitate inhibited the effect of $ZnCl_2$ in cross-linking with the hydrogels. When the pore-forming agent was $NaHCO_3$, the compressive strength was relatively higher compared to the control group. $NaHCO_3$ is water soluble and was well distributed inside the hydrogels. During the removal of $NaHCO_3$ using HCl solution, no negative effect on the formation of crosslinking bands within the network of hydrogels was observed, unlike the situation for $CaCO_3$. The crimp phenomenon of CMX occurred in the salt solution, which weakened the effect of Zn^{2+} [35], so a lower compressive strength for the hydrogel with NaCl was observed. Therefore, the molecular weight and chain length of the pore-forming agents, the pore size of the hydrogels, and the methods of removal of pore-forming agents had an important influence on the compressive strength of the hydrogels.

3.4. TGA Analysis of Hydrogels

The thermogravimetric curves reflected the thermal stability of the materials as well as the structural changes to some extent. Figure 3 shows the thermogravimetric curves of different hydrogels, and Figures S1–S7 show the thermogravimetric curves of the seven kinds of hydrogels. TGA analysis was used to evaluate the thermal stability of the hydrogels. The whole degradation process could be divided into three stages as follows. The weight loss process which occurred at 20–200 °C was ascribed to the loss of free water and the water of crystallization in the hydrogels. Weight loss between 200 °C and 400 °C was due to the breaking of intermolecular hydrogen bonds and the degradation of mainly CMX molecular chains and PAM and PNIPAm molecular chains [31]. After 400 °C, the weight of the samples was mainly related to the carbonization process of the polymer matrix. The residual carbon rate of the hydrogels was in the range of 10–18%. Obviously, there were similar thermogravimetric curves for all hydrogels before 400 °C, indicating that the pore-forming agents had little effect on the stability of the hydrogels. Above 400 °C, the difference was due to inorganic pore-forming agents. During the method of removal of pore-forming agents, it was difficult to remove all inorganic agents because they can be deposited on the surface of the hydrogels.

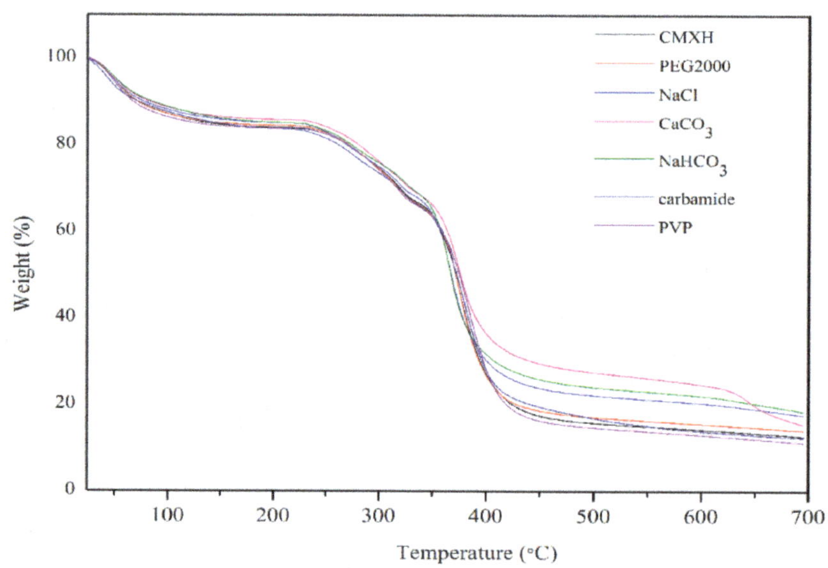

Figure 3. Thermogravimetric curves of the seven kinds of hydrogels.

3.5. SEM Analysis of Hydrogels

Figure 4 presents SEM images of the surface morphologies of the obtained hydrogels. Obvious network structures were observed for the hydrogels. The pore-forming agents had a remarkable influence on the pore sizes of the hydrogels. Hydrogels without a pore-forming agent (Figure 4a) had relatively small and nonuniform pores. Hydrogels with PEG2000 exhibited a smaller pore size in the range of 15–20 μm, which may be attributed to the PEG increasing the crosslink density [36]. Ethanol was used to dissolve PEG2000. The shrinkage of hydrogels in ethanol reduced the pore size and damaged the pore structure, which resulted in the low mechanical properties and swelling behavior compared with the CMXH hydrogels (control group). The pore size of the hydrogel with carbamide was in the range of 90–110 μm. One possible reason for this is that the carbamide decreased the cross-linking density by forming hydrogen bonds with reactive substances, which led to the relatively large pore size of the hydrogels after the removal of carbamide. The pore size of the hydrogels with PVP was about 60–90 μm. The high molecular mass of PVP increased the molecular entanglement. When the PVP was removed by water, pores were formed. For hydrogels with NaCl, the pore size was about 90–100 μm. One possible reason for this is that carboxymethyl xylan curled up in the salt solution, which decreased the crosslinking density. The pore size of the hydrogels with $CaCO_3$ was similar to that of the hydrogels with $NaHCO_3$ and was in the range of 100–130 μm. When hydrogels were soaked in the HCl solution, the CO_2 produced by $CaCO_3$ and $NaHCO_3$ increased the pore size [37].

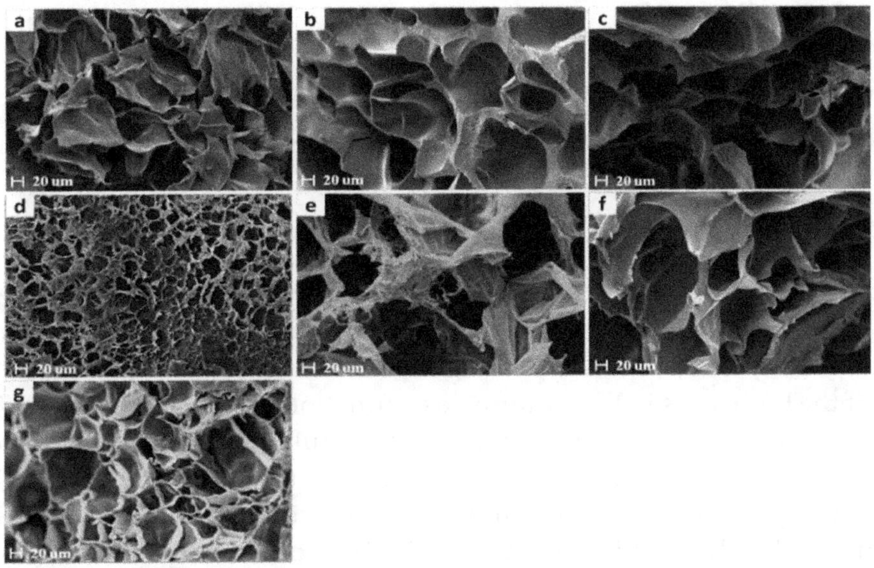

Figure 4. SEM images of hydrogels with (**a**) NaCl, (**b**) $CaCO_3$, (**c**) $NaHCO_3$, (**d**) PEG2000, (**e**) carbamide, (**f**) PVP, or (**g**) no pore-forming agents.

3.6. Zn^{2+} Analysis of Hydrogels

Zinc is a highly essential element for humans and has a good biocompatibility, so it can be applied in biomedical applications [38]. $ZnCl_2$ was used to increase the mechanical strength of hydrogels by interacting with carboxyl groups on CMX. An electron microprobe was used to confirm the presence of Zn^{2+} in hydrogels. Figure 5 showed the EDS of hydrogels without pore-forming agents. The EDS spectrum showed a Zn peak, indicating the existence of Zn in hydrogels. Table 2 shows the zinc content of the different hydrogels. The range of zinc contents in the hydrogels was about 0.09–0.3%, and the difference was cause by the pore-forming agents. The different contents were caused by pore-forming agents, suggesting that pore-forming agents had an impact on the metal coordination bonds between Zn^{2+} and $-COO^-$ groups in the hydrogels.

Table 2. Zinc content in the different hydrogels.

Sample	gel-1	gel-2	gel-3	gel-4	gel-5	gel-6	gel-7
Hydrogel Weight (mg)	33.80	50.80	71.50	43.40	63.90	43.60	51.50
Zinc Concentration (mg/L)	7.18	15.02	14.44	4.17	11.32	5.78	14.28
Weight Percent of Zinc (%)	0.21	0.29	0.20	0.09	0.18	0.13	0.27

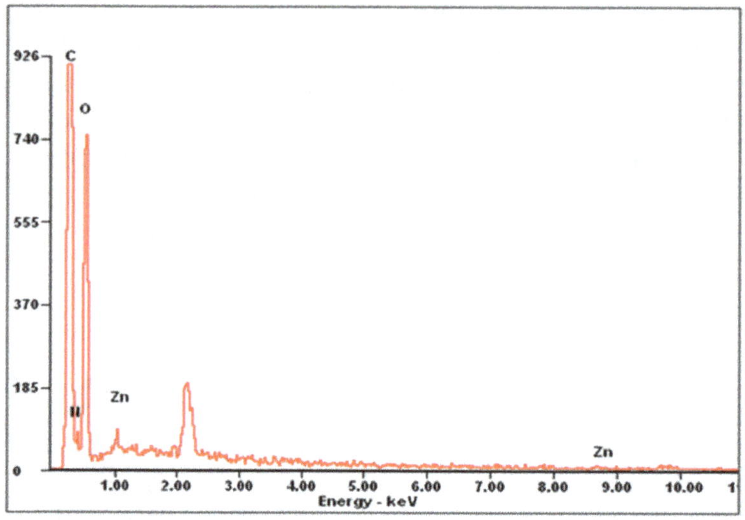

Figure 5. EDS spectrum of hydrogels without pore-forming agents.

3.7. Swelling Behavior Studies of Hydrogels

The swelling capacity of hydrogels is important to their application. The swelling rate of hydrogels is related to their pore size [39]. Large pores in hydrogels are conducive to the diffusion of water molecules into the hydrogels [40]. Thus, hydrogels with larger pores had the faster swelling rate. The swelling ratio of the hydrogels in PBS solution as a function of time is shown in Figure 6. Hydrogels without any pore-forming agents did not reach swelling equilibrium after 24 h. In contrast, hydrogels with $CaCO_3$ and $NaHCO_3$ reached swelling equilibrium after 6 h, while hydrogels with PVP and NaCl reached swelling equilibrium within 24 h. Hydrogels with carbamide did not reach the swelling equilibrium within 24 h but had a higher SR than the hydrogels without any pore-forming agents. Hydrogels with PEG2000 could not reach the swelling equilibrium after 24 h and had a lower SR than the hydrogels without any pore-forming agents. According to the swelling rate of hydrogels in the PBS solution, hydrogels with $CaCO_3$ and $NaHCO_3$ had the biggest pore size. Hydrogels with PVP, carbamide, and NaCl had bigger pore size and hydrogels with PEG2000 had smaller pore size than hydrogels made without any pore-forming agents. These results correspond to the SEM results.

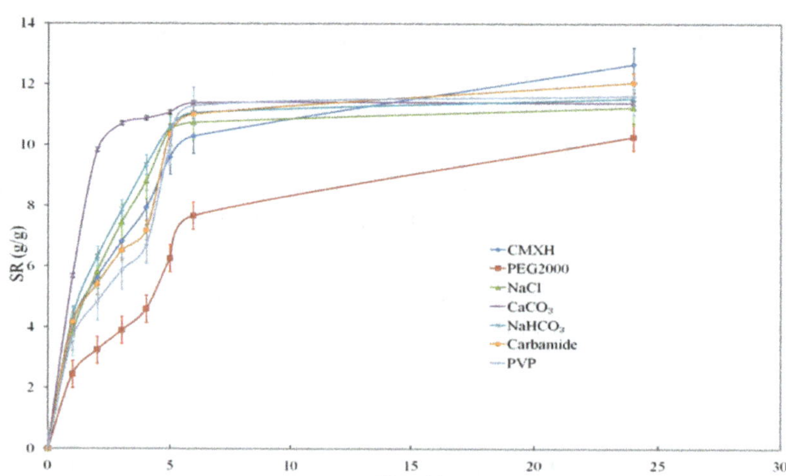

Figure 6. The swelling rates of hydrogels with or without six kinds of pore-forming agents in PBS.

3.8. Drug Release of the Hydrogel Made with $NaHCO_3$ Pore-Forming Agent

5-Fu, which has been investigated as an antitumor agent used for treating solid tumors, was chosen as the drug model in this work. In this work, hydrogels with or without six kinds of pore-forming were applied to study the 5-Fu drug release performance, which is shown in Figure 7. Obviously, for all the hydrogels, the cumulative drug release rate increased rapidly over the first hour, and the cumulative drug release then increased slowly. After 4 h, the cumulative release remained constant. The drug release of hydrogels with $NaHCO_3$ could reach up to 71.05% after 4 h, while the drug release of hydrogels with $CaCO_3$ was 42.28% and the drug release of hydrogels without pore-forming agents only reached 22.57%. The drug release of the other hydrogels was about 21–41%. These results imply that hydrogels made with $NaHCO_3$ have the high release rate for 5-Fu. Thus, the drug release properties of a hydrogel prepared using pore-forming agents could be significantly improved compared to a hydrogel without pore-forming agents. Suitable pore-forming agents gave rise to the enhancement of the drug release properties of the hydrogels due to the introduction of desirable pores within the network of the hydrogels. As shown in Figure 7, drug release balance was achieved after four hours in simulated intestinal fluid (pH = 7.4), and the maximum cumulative release rate achieved was 71.05%, implying that this hydrogel would have potential applications as a drug carrier.

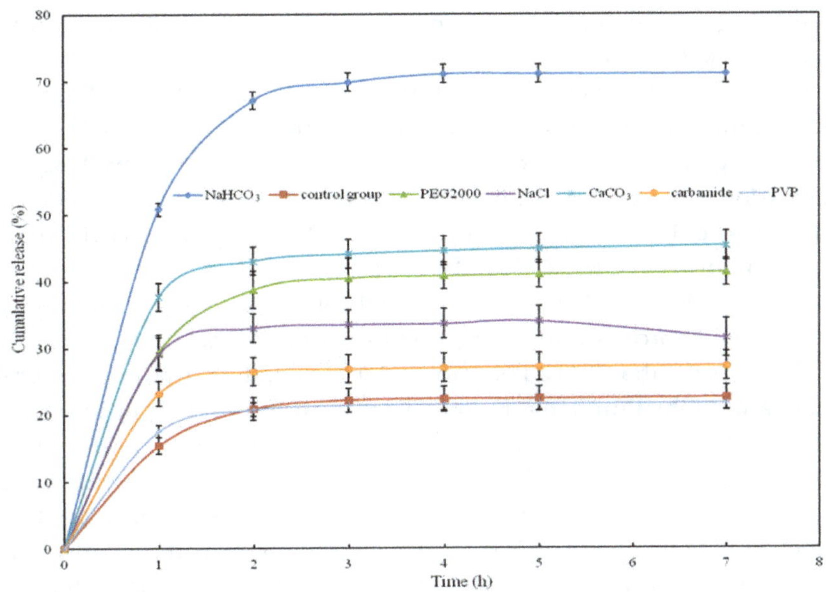

Figure 7. In vitro cumulative drug release from hydrogels in PBS solution (pH 7.4) at 37 °C.

4. Conclusions

In this work, CMX-based hydrogels with macroporous structure were prepared, and different inorganic or organic pore-forming agents were applied to study their influence on the pore size of the hydrogels. For organic pore-forming agents (PEG2000, carbmmide, PVP), the molecular weight and the chain length had an important influence on the pore size, the compressive strength, and the swelling ratio. For inorganic pore-forming agents (NaCl, $CaCO_3$, $NaHCO_3$), hydrogels with $NaHCO_3$ displayed great performance in terms of the pore size of the hydrogels, mechanical properties, and drug release. Moreover, the pore-forming agents had little influence on the thermal stability of the hydrogels. The cumulative drug release for 5-Fu-loaded hydrogels made with $NaHCO_3$ could reach up to 71.05%, which suggests that these hydrogels with macroporous structure have potential applications in the field of drug release. In the follow-up experiment, we will focus on the influence of different amounts of $NaHCO_3$ on the properties of xylan-based hydrogels, as well as their applications to drug delivery.

Author Contributions: Conceptualization, X.L.; Data curation, M.C.; Formal analysis, M.C.; Methodology, X.L.; Resources, L.M.; Writing—original draft, M.C.; Writing—review & editing, X.W. and J.R.

References

1. Rang, K.A.; Lee, S.L.; Park, S.N. Properties and in vitro drug release of pH- and temperature-sensitive double cross-linked interpenetrating polymer network hydrogels based on hyaluronic acid/poly(*N*-isopropylacrylamide) for transdermal delivery of luteolin. *Int. J. Biol. Macromol.* **2018**, *118*, 731–740. [CrossRef]
2. Benavidez, T.E.; Baruzzi, A.M. Comparative behavior of glucose oxidase and oxalate oxidase immobilized in mucin/chitosan hydrogels for biosensors applications. *Polymer* **2012**, *53*, 438–444. [CrossRef]
3. Seliktar, D. Designing cell-compatible hydrogels for biomedical applications. *Science* **2012**, *336*, 1124–1128. [CrossRef] [PubMed]
4. Iamsaard, S.; Aßhoff, S.J.; Matt, B.; Kudernac, T.; Cornelissen, J.J.L.M.; Fletcher, S.P. Conversion of light into macroscopic helical motion. *Nat. Chem.* **2014**, *6*, 229–235. [CrossRef] [PubMed]
5. Yuan, H.; Kurashina, K.; Bruijn, J.D.D. A preliminary study on osteoinduction of two kinds of calcium phosphate ceramics. *Biomaterials* **1999**, *20*, 1799–1806. [CrossRef]
6. Dey, A.; Bera, B.; Bera, R. Influence of diethylene glycol as a porogen in a glyoxal crosslinked polyvinyl alcohol hydrogel. *RSC Adv.* **2014**, *4*, 42260–42270. [CrossRef]
7. Badiger, M.V.; Mcneill, M.E.; Graham, N.B. Porogens in the preparation of microporous hydrogels based on poly(ethylene oxides). *Biomaterials* **1993**, *14*, 1059–1063. [CrossRef]
8. Lee, A.G.; Arena, C.P.; Beebe, D.J. Development of macroporous poly(ethylene glycol) hydrogel arrays within microfluidic channels. *Biomacromolecules* **2010**, *11*, 3316–3324. [CrossRef]
9. Sergeeva, A.; Feoktistova, N.; Prokopovic, V. Design of porous alginate hydrogels by sacrificial $CaCO_3$ templates: Pore formation mechanism. *Adv. Mater. Interfaces* **2016**, *2*, 1500386–1500395. [CrossRef]
10. Gao, M.; Gawel, K.; Stokke, B. Swelling dynamics of a DNA-polymer hybrid hydrogel prepared using polyethylene glycol as a porogen. *Gels* **2015**, *1*, 219–234. [CrossRef]
11. Kabiri, K.; Omidian, H.; Hashemi, S.A. Concise synthesis of fast-swelling superabsorbent hydrogels: Effect of initiator concentration on porosity and absorption rate. *Eur. Polym. J.* **2003**, *39*, 1341–1348. [CrossRef]
12. Kamoun, E.A.; Fahmy, A.; Taha, T.H. Thermo-and pH-sensitive hydrogel membranes composed of poly(N-isopropylacrylamide)-hyaluronan for biomedical applications: Influence of hyaluronan incorporation on the membrane properties. *Int. J. Biol. Macromol.* **2018**, *106*, 158–167. [CrossRef] [PubMed]
13. Sole, I.; Vilchez, S.; Miras, J.; Montanya, N. DHA and L-carnitine loaded chitosan hydrogels as delivery systems for topical applications. *Colloids Surf. A Physicochem. Eng. Asp.* **2017**, *525*, 85–92. [CrossRef]
14. Deng, C.; Li, F.; Hackett, J.M.; Chaudhry, S.H.; Toll, F.N. Collagen and glycopolymer based hydrogel for potential corneal application. *Acta Biomater.* **2010**, *6*, 187–194. [CrossRef] [PubMed]
15. Takei, Y.G.; Aoki, T.; Sanui, K.; Ogata, N.; Okano, T.; Sakurai, Y. Temperature responsive bioconjugates. 2. Molecular design for temperature-modulated bioseparations. *Bioconjug. Chem.* **1993**, *4*, 341–346. [CrossRef]
16. Wilkie, K.C.B. The hemicelluloses of grasses and cereals gramineae. *Adv. Carbohydr. Chem. Biochem.* **1979**, *36*, 215–264. [CrossRef]
17. Oliveira, E.E.; Silva, A.E.; Junior, T.N.; Gomes, M.C.S.; Aguiar, L.M. Xylan from corn cobs, a promising polymer for drug delivery: Production and characterization. *Bioresour. Technol.* **2010**, *101*, 5402–5406. [CrossRef]
18. Gao, C.; Ren, J.; Zhao, C. Xylan-based temperature/pH sensitive hydrogels for drug controlled release. *Carbohydr. Polym.* **2016**, *151*, 189–197. [CrossRef]
19. Kong, W.Q.; Gao, C.D.; Hu, S.F. Xylan-modified-based hydrogels with temperature/pH dual sensitivity and controllable drug delivery behavior. *Materials* **2017**, *10*, 304. [CrossRef]
20. Cao, X.; Peng, X.; Zhong, L. Multiresponsive hydrogels based on xylan-type hemicelluloses and photoisomerized azobenzene copolymer as drug delivery carrier. *J. Agric. Food Chem.* **2014**, *62*, 10000–10007. [CrossRef]
21. Chimphango, A.F.A.; Zyl, W.H.V.; Görgens, J.F. In situ enzymatic aided formation of xylan hydrogels and encapsulation of horse radish peroxidase for slow release. *Carbohydr. Polym.* **2012**, *88*, 1109–1117. [CrossRef]
22. Sun, X.F.; Wang, H.H.; Jing, Z.X.; Mohanathas, R. Hemicellulose-based pH-sensitive and biodegradable hydrogel for controlled drug delivery. *Carbohydr. Polym.* **2013**, *92*, 1357–1366. [CrossRef] [PubMed]
23. Kouvaraki, M.A.; Ajani, J.P.; Wolff, R. Fluorouracil, doxorubicin, and streptozocin in the treatment of patients

with locally advanced and metastatic pancreatic endocrine carcinomas. *J. Clin. Oncol.* **2004**, *22*, 4762–4771. [CrossRef] [PubMed]

24. Gardiner, S.J.; Begg, E.J.; Robinson, B.A. The effect of dihydropyrimidine dehydrogenase deficiency on outcomes with fluorouracil. *Advers. Drug React. Toxicol. Rev.* **2002**, *21*, 1–16. [CrossRef]
25. Singh, B.; Chauhan, N. Preliminary evaluation of molecular imprinting of 5-fluorouracil within hydrogels for use as drug delivery systems. *Acta Biomater.* **2008**, *4*, 1244–1254. [CrossRef] [PubMed]
26. Peng, X.W.; Ren, J.L.; Zhong, L.X. Microwave-induced synthesis of carboxymethyl hemicelluloses and their rheological properties. *J. Agric. Food. Chem.* **2011**, *59*, 570–576. [CrossRef] [PubMed]
27. Kwon, K.; Auh, J.H.; Kim, J.W. Physicochemical properties and functionality of highly carboxymethylated starch. *Starch Starke* **2010**, *49*, 499–505. [CrossRef]
28. Deng, C.; Han, X.; Li, R.; Zhang, Q. Preparation and in vitro drug release of 5-Fu in Poly(N-isopropylacrylamide-co-acrylate acid) hydrogel. *Acta Acad. Med. CPAF* **2010**, *19*, 695–697.
29. Kong, W.; Huang, D.; Xu, G. A new design strategy for graphene oxide/polyacrylamide/aluminium ion-crosslinked carboxymethyl hemicelluloses nanocomposite hydrogels with highly tough and elastic properties. *Chem. Asian J.* **2016**, *11*, 1697–1704. [CrossRef]
30. Peng, X.W.; Ren, J.L.; Zhong, L.X.; Peng, F.; Sun, R.C. Xylan-rich hemicelluloses-graft-acrylic acid ionic hydrogels with rapid responses to pH, salt, and organic solvents. *J. Agric. Food. Chem.* **2011**, *59*, 8208–8215. [CrossRef]
31. Gao, C.D.; Ren, J.L.; Kong, W.Q.; Sun, R.C.; Chen, Q.F. Comparative study on temperature/pH sensitive xylan-based hydrogels: Their properties and drug controlled release. *RSC Adv.* **2015**, *5*, 90671–90681. [CrossRef]
32. Wei, Q.B.; Fu, F.; Zhang, Y.Q. pH-responsive CMC/PAM/PVP semi-IPN hydrogels for theophylline drug release. *J. Polym. Res.* **2014**, *21*, 453–462. [CrossRef]
33. Patra, S.K.; Swain, S.K. Swelling study of superabsorbent PAA-co-PAM/clay nanohydrogel. *J. Appl. Polym. Sci.* **2011**, *120*, 533–1538. [CrossRef]
34. El-Mohdy, H.L.A. Water sorption behavior of CMC/PAM hydrogels prepared by γ-irradiation and release of potassium nitrate as agrochemical. *React. Funct. Polym.* **2007**, *67*, 1094–1102. [CrossRef]
35. Okay, O. Macroporous copolymer networks. *Prog. Polym. Sci.* **2000**, *25*, 711–779. [CrossRef]
36. Tang, Q.; Sun, X.; Li, Q. Preparation of porous polyacrylate/poly(ethylene glycol) interpenetrating network hydrogel and simplification of Flory theory. *J. Mater. Sci.* **2009**, *44*, 3712–3718. [CrossRef]
37. Ma, J.; Li, Z.; Zhen, L. Preparation and characterization of porous poly(N-isopropylacrylamide)/clay nanocomposite hydrogels. *Polym. Bull.* **2008**, *61*, 593–602. [CrossRef]
38. Zhang, E.; Yin, D.; Xu, L. Microstructure, mechanical and corrosion properties and biocompatibility of Mg-Zn-Mn alloys for biomedical application. *Mater. Sci. Eng. C* **2009**, *29*, 987–993. [CrossRef]
39. El-Din, H.M.N.; Alla, S.G.A.; El-Naggar, A.W.M. Swelling and drug release properties of acrylamide/carboxymethyl cellulose networks formed by gamma irradiation. *Radiat. Phys. Chem.* **2010**, *79*, 725–730. [CrossRef]
40. Sun, X.F.; Jing, Z.; Wang, G. Preparation and swelling behaviors of porous hemicellulose-g-polyacrylamide hydrogels. *J. Appl. Polym. Sci.* **2013**, *128*, 1861–1870. [CrossRef]

2

Synthesis, Structure–Activity Relationships and In Vitro Toxicity Profile of Lactose-Based Fatty Acid Monoesters as Possible Drug Permeability Enhancers

Simone Lucarini [1], Laura Fagioli [1], Robert Cavanagh [2], Wanling Liang [3], Diego Romano Perinelli [4], Mario Campana [5], Snjezana Stolnik [2], Jenny K. W. Lam [3], Luca Casettari [1,*] and Andrea Duranti [1]

1 Department of Biomolecular Sciences, School of Pharmacy, University of Urbino, 61029 Urbino (PU), Italy; simone.lucarini@uniurb.it (S.L.); laura.fagioli@uniurb.it (L.F.); andrea.duranti@uniurb.it (A.D.)
2 Drug Delivery and Tissue Engineering Division, School of Pharmacy, University of Nottingham, Nottingham NG7 2RD, UK; robert.cavanagh@nottingham.ac.uk (R.C.); Snow.Stolnik@nottingham.ac.uk (S.S.)
3 Department of Pharmacology & Pharmacy, The University of Hong Kong, 21 Sassoon Road, Pokfulam, Hong Kong, China; sophiawlliang@gmail.com (W.L.); jkwlam@hku.hk (J.K.W.L.)
4 School of Pharmacy, University of Camerino, 62032 Camerino (MC), Italy; diego.perinelli@unicam.it
5 Science and Technology Facilities Council (STFC), ISIS Neutron and Muon Source, Rutherford Appleton Laboratory, Didcot OX11 0QX, UK; mario.campana@stfc.ac.uk
* Correspondence: luca.casettari@uniurb.it

Abstract: Permeability enhancers are receiving increased attention arising from their ability to increase transepithelial permeability and thus, bioavailability of orally or pulmonary administered biopharmaceutics. Here we present the synthesis and the in vitro assaying of a series of lactose-based non-ionic surfactants, highlighting the relationship between their structure and biological effect. Using tensiometric measurements the critical micelle concentrations (CMCs) of the surfactants were determined and demonstrate that increasing hydrophobic chain length reduces surfactant CMC. In vitro testing on Caco-2 intestinal and Calu-3 airway epithelia revealed that cytotoxicity, assessed by 3-(4,5-dimethylthiazol-2-yl)-2,5-diphenyltetrazolium bromide (MTT) and lactate dehydrogenase (LDH) release assays, is presented for most of the surfactants at concentrations greater than their CMCs. Further biological study demonstrates that application of cytotoxic concentrations of the surfactants is associated with depolarizing mitochondrial membrane potential, increasing nuclear membrane permeability and activation of effector caspases. It is, therefore, proposed that when applied at cytotoxic levels, the surfactants are inducing apoptosis in both cell lines tested. Importantly, through the culture of epithelial monolayers on Transwell® supports, the surfactants demonstrate the ability to reversibly modulate transepithelial electrical resistance (TEER), and thus open tight junctions, at non-toxic concentrations, emphasizing their potential application as safe permeability enhancers in vivo.

Keywords: absorption enhancers; sugar-based surfactants; biocompatibility studies; transmucosal drug delivery

1. Introduction

Sugar-based fatty acid esters usually belong to the class of non-ionic surfactants and possess desirable characteristics suitable for different applications in food, cosmetic and pharmaceutical fields. They are constituted by a sugar moiety as hydrophilic head (polar) linked via an ester bond to a fatty acid chain as hydrophobic tail (non-polar). Various modifications, both on polar head or non-polar tail, have been rationally designed to obtain a broad class of sugar esters with different properties. Particularly, sugar-based fatty acid esters made up of carbohydrate moieties, including mono-, di- or tri-saccharides condensed with saturated or unsaturated fatty acids with different chain lengths have been synthesized to give products with various degree of esterification [1]. Constituted of natural substrates, easily available and therefore inexpensive and renewable, these products are considered ideal raw materials to be employed for a large variety of technological applications such as emulsification, stabilization of disperse systems, solubility or drug permeation enhancement [2–5].

Sugar-based fatty acid esters are receiving a growing attention due to the large demand for non-toxic, non-irritant and highly biocompatible and biodegradable amphiphilic compounds in different fields [6]. Many studies have recently reported the synthesis and possible applications of selective 6-*O*-sugar fatty acid monoesters, generally referred as sugar monoesters [7–9]. Several physico-chemical and biological properties have been studied [10,11], to develop advanced drug delivery systems, including skin penetration enhancing effect or transmucosal permeability enhancement [12–15]. The use of amphiphilic compounds as permeability enhancers (PEs) for transmucosal drug delivery represents one of the most promising application of surfactants in biopharmaceutics, able to provide a valid alternative (e.g., oral or pulmonary administration) to the conventional (e.g., injection) route of administrations of many therapeutic peptides [16–20].

Among the class of sugar monoesters, sorbitan and sucrose derivatives are those most easily available on the market. However, sugar-based surfactants bearing a different sugar moiety can also represent a valid alternative to the currently available amphiphilic compounds; particularly when industrial waste can be easily transformed in valued-added products. In this respect, the lactose monoester derivatives have been recently brought back into the spotlight, as promising eco-friendly emulsifier and antimicrobial compounds for pharmaceutical, food and cosmetic fields. These surfactants were synthesized for the first time in the 1970s [21], and, over the last decades, they have been proposed, including as excipients in drug formations, additives in the food industry and are being explored for their potential anticancer activity [22]. Despite being well-characterized in term of surface activity [23,24], and emulsifying properties [25], no detailed studies have been performed aimed at defining cytotoxicity profiles of these surfactants. Such information is required to broaden the potential applications of this class of sugar-based amphiphiles for pharmaceutical and cosmetic applications.

The aim of this work was to investigate the relationship between the structure and cytotoxicity of a series of lactose esters derivatives, enzymatically synthesized using saturated fatty acids with different chain lengths (C10; C12; C14; C16). The critical micelle concentration (CMC) was compared with cytotoxicity (IC_{50}) evaluated on two selected cell lines as models for the intestinal (Caco-2) and respiratory (Calu-3) epithelia, which are common route of drug administration. In addition, mitochondrial membrane potential, nuclear membrane permeability and effector caspase activation were studied on the same cell lines to deeper understand the mechanism upon cellular toxicity. Finally, transepithelial electrical resistance (TEER) measurements were performed to investigate the effect of saturated acyl chain lactose monoesters on the integrity of the cellular barrier and to provide a preliminary evidence of their transmucosal perturbance action, which is commonly exerted by surfactants acting as permeability enhancers across mucosa.

2. Materials and Methods

2.1. Materials

Decanoic, lauric, myristic and palmitic acids were purchased from TCI (Zwijndrecht, Belgium), lactose monohydrate from Carlo Erba (Milan, Italy), while Lipozyme® (immobilized from Mucor miehei), *p*-toluenesulfonic acid, 2,2-dimethoxypropane, tetrafluoroboric acid diethyl ether complex, carbonyl cyanide 4-(trifluoromethoxy) phenylhydrazone (FCCP) and all organic solvents used in this study were purchased from Sigma-Aldrich (Milan, Italy). Prior to use, acetonitrile was dried with molecular sieves with an effective pore diameter of 4 Å and toluene was saturated with water. CellEvent™ caspase-3/7 green detection reagent was purchased from Thermo Fisher Scientific (Waltham, MA, USA) and the CellTox™ green cytotoxicity assay acquired from Promega (Madison, WI, USA). The JC-1 probe (5,5′,6,6′-Tetrachloro-1,1′,3,3′-tetraethylbenzimidazolylcarbocyanine, iodide) was purchased from Biotium (Fremont, CA, USA).

2.2. Cell Culture Conditions

Caco-2 and Calu-3 cells were obtained from American Type Culture Collection. Caco-2 cells were cultured in advanced Dulbecco Modified Eagle Medium (DMEM) supplemented with 10% *v/v* Fetal Bovine Serum (FBS) and 1% *v/v* antibiotics-antimycotic. Calu-3 cells were cultured in DMEM F-12 supplemented with 10% *v/v* FBS and 1% *v/v* antibiotics-antimycotic. All cell lines were maintained at a 5% CO_2 in a humidified incubator at 37 °C. Caco-2 cells were used between passages 30–45 and Calu-3 cells between 25–40.

2.3. Synthesis of Lactose-Based Surfactants

The structures of compounds were unambiguously assessed by ^{1}H NMR and ^{13}C NMR recorded on a Bruker AC 400 or 100 (Milan, Italy), respectively, spectrometer and analyzed using the TopSpin software package (version 2.1). Chemical shifts were measured using the central peak of the solvent. Column chromatography purifications were performed under "flash" conditions using Merck 230–400 mesh silica gel. TLC was carried out on Merck silica gel 60 F254 plates, which were visualized by exposure to an aqueous solution of ceric ammonium molibdate.

2.3.1. General Procedure for the Synthesis of Lactose Tetra Acetal Monoesters

Lipozyme® (0.078 g) was added to a solution of the fatty acid (**1a–d**) (0.79 mmol) and 4-*O*-(3′,4′-*O*-isopropylidene-β-D-galactopyranosyl)-2,3:5,6-di-*O*-isopropylidene-1,1-di-*O*-methyl-D-glucopyranose (lactose tetra acetate, LTA) [26] (**2**) (0.402 g, 0.79 mmol) in water-saturated toluene at 25 °C [12,27]. The mixture was stirred at 75 °C for 12 h, cooled and diluted with acetone, then the enzyme was filtered, and the filtrate was concentrated. The purification of the residue by column chromatography (cyclohexane/EtOAc 8:2) gave **3a–d** as pale yellow oils. (Scheme 1).

[6′-O-Decanoyl-4-O-(3′,4′-O-isopropylidene-β-D-galactopyranosyl)-2,3:5,6-di-O-isopropylidene-1,1-di-O-methyl-D-glucopyranose] (**3a**) [27]. Yield: 53% (0.275 g). ^{1}H NMR (400 MHz, MeOD) δ: 0.92 (t, 3H, $J = 6.7$ Hz, CH_3), 1.32 (s, 6H, $2CH_3$), 1.33–1.37 [m, 12H, $(CH_2)_n$], 1.39 (s, 3H, CH_3), 1.41 (s, 3H, CH_3), 1.44 (s, 3H, CH_3), 1.49 (s, 3H, CH_3), 1.61–1.67 (m, 2H, CH_2CH_2COOR), 2.40 (t, 2H, $J = 7.0$ Hz, CH_2COOR), 3.46 (s, 6H, $2OCH_3$), 3.47 (dd, 1H, $J_{8-9} = 7.0$ Hz, $J_{8-7} = 8.0$ Hz, H^8), 3.91 (dd, 1H, $J_{4-3} = 1.2$ Hz, $J_{4-5} = 5.0$ Hz, H^4), 4.04 (ddd, 1H, $J_{11-12a} = 1.5$ Hz, $J_{11-10} = 2.1$ Hz, $J_{11-12b} = 6.8$ Hz, H^{11}), 4.05 (dd, 1H, $J_{6b-5} = 6.0$ Hz, $J_{6b-6a} = 8.7$ Hz, H^{6b}), 4.08 (dd, 1H, $J_{9-10} = 5.5$ Hz, $J_{9-8} = 7.0$ Hz, H^9), 4.14 (dd, 1H, $J_{3-4} = 1.2$ Hz, $J_{3-2} = 7.5$ Hz, H^3), 4.17 (dd, 1H, $J_{6a-5} = 6.0$ Hz, $J_{6a-6b} = 8.7$ Hz, H^{6a}), 4.22 (dd, 1H, $J_{10-11} = 2.1$ Hz, $J_{10-9} = 5.5$ Hz, H^{10}), 4.27 (dd, 1H, $J_{12b-11} = 6.8$ Hz, $J_{12b-12a} = 11.5$ Hz, H^{12b}), 4.30 (dd, 1H, $J_{12a-11} = 1.5$ Hz, $J_{12a-12b} = 11.5$ Hz, H^{12a}), 4.31 (ddd, 1H, $J_{5-4} = 5.0$ Hz, $J_{5-6a} \cong J_{5-6b} = 6.0$ Hz, H^5), 4.41 (d, 1H, $J_{1-2} = 6.2$ Hz, H^1), 4.51 (d, 1H, $J_{7-8} = 8.0$ Hz, H^7), 4.51 (dd, 1H, $J_{2-1} = 6.2$ Hz, $J_{2-3} = 7.5$ Hz, H^2) ppm. ^{13}C NMR (100 MHz, MeOD) δ: 13.0, 22.3, 24.2, 24.6, 25.1, 25.5, 25.6, 26.2, 27.0, 28.8, 29.00, 29.02, 29.2, 31.6, 33.5, 53.0, 55.1, 63.0, 65.5, 70.8, 73.3, 73.5, 75.4, 76.4, 76.8, 77.6, 79.4, 103.1, 105.7, 108.5, 109.7, 109.9, 173.8 ppm.

[6′-O-Dodecanoyl-4-O-(3′,4′-O-isopropylidene-β-D-galactopyranosyl)-2,3:5,6-di-O-isopropylidene-1,1-di-O-methyl-D-glucopyranose] (**3b**) [27]. Yield: 50% (0.274 g). ^{1}H NMR (400 MHz, MeOD) δ: 0.92 (t, 3H, $J = 6.7$ Hz, CH_3), 1.32 (s, 6H, $2CH_3$), 1.33–1.37 [m, 16H, $(CH_2)_n$], 1.39 (s, 3H, CH_3), 1.41 (s, 3H, CH_3), 1.44 (s, 3H, CH_3), 1.49 (s, 3H, CH_3), 1.62–1.67 (m, 2H, CH_2CH_2COOR), 2.40 (t, 2H, $J = 7.0$ Hz, CH_2COOR), 3.46 (s, 6H, $2OCH_3$), 3.47 (dd, 1H, $J_{8-9} = 7.1$ Hz, $J_{8-7} = 8.0$ Hz, H^8), 3.91 (dd, 1H, $J_{4-3} = 1.2$ Hz, $J_{4-5} = 5.0$ Hz, H^4), 4.05 (ddd, 1H, $J_{11-12a} = 1.2$ Hz, $J_{11-10} = 2.1$ Hz, $J_{11-12b} = 6.8$ Hz, H^{11}),

4.05 (dd, 1H, J_{6b-5} = 6.0 Hz, J_{6b-6a} = 8.7 Hz, H^{6b}), 4.08 (dd, 1H, J_{9-10} = 5.6 Hz, J_{9-8} = 7.1 Hz, H^9), 4.14 (dd, 1H, J_{3-4} = 1.2 Hz, J_{3-2} = 7.5 Hz, H^3), 4.17 (dd, 1H, J_{6a-5} = 6.0 Hz, J_{6a-6b} = 8.7 Hz, H^{6a}), 4.22 (dd, 1H, J_{10-11} = 2.1 Hz, J_{10-9} = 5.6 Hz, H^{10}), 4.27 (dd, 1H, J_{12b-11} = 6.8 Hz, $J_{12b-12a}$ = 11.5 Hz, H^{12b}), 4.30 (dd, 1H, J_{12a-11} = 1.2 Hz, $J_{12a-12b}$ = 11.5 Hz, H^{12a}), 4.31 (ddd, 1H, J_{5-4} = 5.0 Hz, $J_{5-6a} \cong J_{5-6b}$ = 6.0 Hz, H^5), 4.41 (d, 1H, J_{1-2} = 6.2 Hz, H^1), 4.51 (d, 1H, J_{7-8} = 8.0 Hz, H^7), 4.51 (dd, 1H, J_{2-1} = 6.2 Hz, J_{2-3} = 7.5 Hz, H^2) ppm. ^{13}C NMR (100 MHz, MeOD) δ: 13.0, 22.3, 24.2, 24.6, 25.1, 25.5, 25.7, 26.2, 27.0, 28.8, 29.0, 29.1, 29.2, 29.3, 31.7, 33.5, 53.0, 55.1, 63.1, 65.5, 70.8, 73.3, 73.5, 75.4, 76.4, 76.8, 77.6, 79.4, 103.1, 105.7, 108.5, 109.7, 109.9, 173.8 ppm.

[6′-O-Tetradecanoyl-4-O-(3′,4′-O-isopropylidene-β-D-galactopyranosyl)-2,3:5,6-di-O-isopropylidene-1,1-di-O-methyl-D-glucopyranose] (**3c**) [27]. Yield: 44% (0.248 g). ^{1}H NMR (400 MHz, MeOD) δ: 0.92 (t, 3H, J = 6.7 Hz, CH_3), 1.30–1.33 [m, 20H, $(CH_2)_n$], 1.35 (s, 6H, $2CH_3$), 1.39 (s, 3H, CH_3), 1.41 (s, 3H, CH_3), 1.44 (s, 3H, CH_3), 1.49 (s, 3H, CH_3), 1.61–1.67 (m, 2H, CH_2CH_2COOR), 2.40 (t, 2H, J = 7.0 Hz, CH_2COOR), 3.46 (s, 6H, $2OCH_3$), 3.47 (dd, 1H, J_{8-9} = 7.1 Hz, J_{8-7} = 8.0 Hz, H^8), 3.91 (dd, 1H, J_{4-3} = 1.2 Hz, J_{4-5} = 5.0 Hz, H^4), 4.04 (ddd, 1H, J_{11-12a} = 1.0 Hz, J_{11-10} = 2.2 Hz, J_{11-12b} = 6.8 Hz, H^{11}), 4.05 (dd, 1H, J_{6b-5} = 6.0 Hz, J_{6b-6a} = 8.7 Hz, H^{6b}), 4.08 (dd, 1H, J_{9-10} = 5.6 Hz, J_{9-8} = 7.1 Hz, H^9), 4.15 (dd, 1H, J_{3-4} = 1.2 Hz, J_{3-2} = 7.5 Hz, H^3), 4.17 (dd, 1H, J_{6a-5} = 6.0 Hz, J_{6a-6b} = 8.7 Hz, H^{6a}), 4.22 (dd, 1H, J_{10-11} = 2.2 Hz, J_{10-9} = 5.6 Hz, H^{10}), 4.27 (dd, 1H, J_{12b-11} = 6.8 Hz, $J_{12b-12a}$ = 11.5 Hz, H^{12b}), 4.30 (dd, 1H, J_{12a-11} = 1.0 Hz, $J_{12a-12b}$ = 11.5 Hz, H^{12a}), 4.31 (ddd, J_{5-4} = 5.0 Hz, $J_{5-6a} \cong J_{5-6b}$ = 6.0 Hz, H^5), 4.41 (d, 1H, J_{1-2} = 6.2 Hz, H^1), 4.51 (d, 1H, J_{7-8} = 8.0 Hz, H^7), 4.51 (dd, 1H, J_{2-1} = 6.2 Hz, J_{2-3} = 7.5 Hz, H^2) ppm. ^{13}C NMR (100 MHz, MeOD) δ: 13.0, 22.3, 24.2, 24.6, 25.1, 25.5, 25.6, 26.2, 27.0, 28.8, 29.0, 29.1, 29.2, 29.31, 29.34, 29.4, 31.7, 33.5, 53.0, 55.1, 63.1, 65.5, 70.8, 73.3, 73.6, 75.4, 76.4, 76.8, 77.6, 79.4, 103.1, 105.7, 108.5, 109.7, 109.9, 173.8 ppm.

[6′-O-Esadecanoyl-4-O-(3′,4′-O-isopropylidene-β-D-galactopyranosyl)-2,3:5,6-di-O-isopropylidene-1,1-di-O-methyl-D-glucopyranose] (**3d**) [27]. Yield: 34% (0.200 g). ^{1}H NMR (400 MHz, MeOD) δ: 0.92 (t, 3H, J = 6.7 Hz, CH_3), 1.30–1.33 [m, 24H, $(CH_2)_n$], 1.35 (s, 6H, $2CH_3$), 1.39 (s, 3H, CH_3), 1.41 (s, 3H, CH_3), 1.44 (s, 3H, CH_3), 1.49 (s, 3H, CH_3), 1.60–1.67 (m, 2H, CH_2CH_2COOR), 2.40 (t, 2H, J = 7.4 Hz, CH_2COOR), 3.46 (s, 6H, $2OCH_3$), 3.47 (dd, 1H, J_{8-9} = 7.1 Hz, J_{8-7} = 8.0 Hz, H^8), 3.91 (dd, 1H, J_{4-3} = 1.2 Hz, J_{4-5} = 5.0 Hz, H^4), 4.04 (ddd, 1H, J_{11-12a} = 1.5 Hz, J_{11-10} = 2.2 Hz, J_{11-12b} = 6.8 Hz, H^{11}), 4.05 (dd, 1H, J_{6b-5} = 6.0 Hz, J_{6b-6a} = 8.7 Hz, H^{6b}), 4.08 (dd, 1H, J_{9-10} = 5.5 Hz, J_{9-8} = 7.1 Hz, H^9), 4.14 (dd, 1H, J_{3-4} = 1.2 Hz, J_{3-2} = 7.5 Hz, H^3), 4.17 (dd, 1H, J_{6a-5} = 6.0 Hz, J_{6a-6b} = 8.7 Hz, H^{6a}), 4.22 (dd, 1H, J_{10-11} = 2.2 Hz, J_{10-9} = 5.5 Hz, H^{10}), 4.27 (dd, 1H, J_{12b-11} = 6.8 Hz, $J_{12b-12a}$ = 11.5 Hz, H^{12b}), 4.30 (dd, 1H, J_{12a-11} = 1.5 Hz, $J_{12a-12b}$ = 11.5 Hz, H^{12a}), 4.31 (ddd, 1H, J_{5-4} = 5.0 Hz, $J_{5-6a} \cong J_{5-6b}$ = 6.0 Hz, H^5), 4.41 (d, 1H, J_{1-2} = 6.2 Hz, H^1), 4.51 (d, 1H, J_{7-8} = 8.0 Hz, H^7), 4.51 (dd, 1H, J_{2-1} = 6.2 Hz, J_{2-3} = 7.5 Hz, H^2) ppm. ^{13}C NMR (100 MHz, MeOD) δ: 13.0, 22.3, 24.2, 24.6, 25.1, 25.7, 26.2, 27.0, 28.8, 29.1, 29.2, 29.4, 31.7, 33.5, 53.0, 55.1, 63.1, 65.5, 70.8, 73.3, 73.6, 75.4, 76.4, 76.9, 77.6, 79.4, 103.1, 105.7, 108.5, 109.7, 109.9, 173.8 ppm.

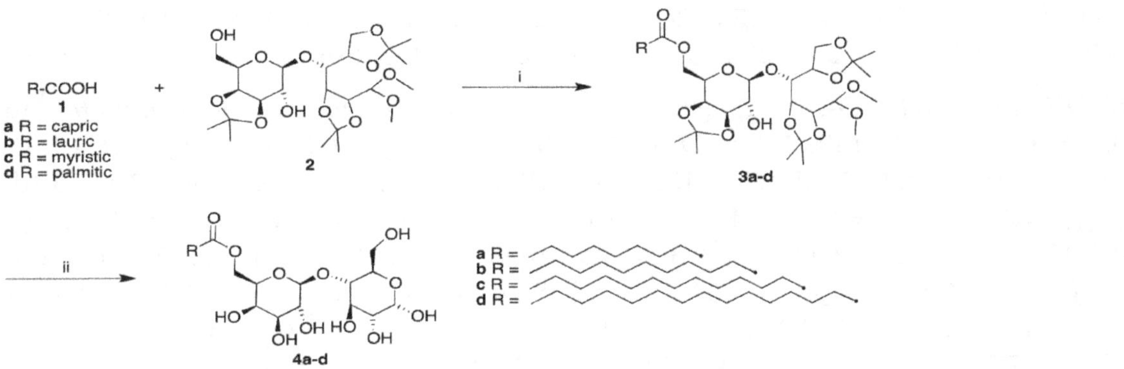

Scheme 1. Reagents and conditions: (**a**) toluene, 75 °C, 12 h; (**b**) HBF_4 Et_2O, CH_3CN, 30 °C, 3 h.

2.3.2. General Procedure for the Synthesis of Lactose Fatty Acid Monoesters

Compounds **3a–d** (0.25 mmol) were dissolved in tetrafluoroboric acid diethyl ether complex/water/acetonitrile (2.1 mL, 1:5:500) and the mixture was stirred at 30 °C for 3 h [12,27]. The white solids precipitated were then filtered, washed with acetonitrile and dried. The purification by recrystallization from methanol gave **4a–d** as white solids. (Scheme 1).

[6′-O-Decanoyl-4-O-(β-D-galactopyranosyl)-D-glucopyranose, lactose caprate] (**4a**) [27]. Yield: 75% (0.093 g). ^{1}H NMR (400 MHz, DMSO) δ: 0.86 (t, 3H, J = 6.6 Hz, CH_3), 1.20–1.32 [m, 12H, $(CH_2)_n$], 1.48–1.57 (m, 2H, CH_2CH_2COOR), 2.31 (t, 2H, J = 7.3 Hz, CH_2COOR), 3.17 (ddd, 1H, $J_{2\text{–}1}$ = 4.0 Hz, $J_{2\text{–OH2}}$ = 7.0 Hz, $J_{2\text{–}3}$ = 9.5 Hz, H^2), 3.27 (dd, 1H, $J_{4\text{–}3} \cong J_{4\text{–}5}$ = 9.5 Hz, H^4), 3.33–3.37 (m, 2H, H^8, H^9), 3.57 (dd, 1H, $J_{3\text{–}2} \cong J_{3\text{–}4}$ = 9.5 Hz, H^3), 3.60–3.67 (m, 3H, H^{6a}, H^{6b}, H^{10}), 3.68–3.76 (m, 2H, H^5, H^{11}), 4.09 (dd, 1H, $J_{12b\text{–}11}$ = 4.5 Hz, $J_{12b\text{–}12a}$ = 11.5 Hz, H^{12b}), 4.17 (dd, 1H, $J_{12a\text{–}11}$ = 8.5 Hz, $J_{12a\text{–}12b}$ = 11.5 Hz, H^{12a}), 4.20–4.25 (m, 2H, H^7, OH^3), 4.43 (dd, 1H, $J_{OH6\text{–}6a} \cong J_{OH6\text{–}6b}$ = 6.0 Hz, OH^6), 4.55 (d, 1H, $J_{OH2\text{–}2}$ = 7.0 Hz, OH^2), 4.78 (d, 1H, $J_{OH10\text{–}10}$ = 5.0 Hz, OH^{10}), 4.86 (d, 1H, J = 3.0 Hz, OH), 4.90 (dd, 1H, $J_{1\text{–OH1}} \cong J_{1\text{–}2}$ = 4.0 Hz, H^1), 5.15 (d, 1H, J = 3.0 Hz, OH), 6.33 (d, 1H, $J_{OH1\text{–}1}$ = 4.0 Hz, OH^1) ppm. ^{13}C NMR (100 MHz, DMSO) δ: 14.4, 22.6, 24.8, 28.9, 29.1, 29.2, 29.3, 31.7, 33.8, 60.9, 63.8, 68.7, 70.2, 70.8, 71.7, 72.7, 72.9, 73.3, 81.6, 92.5, 104.0, 173.4 ppm.

[6′-O-Dodecanoyl-4-O-(β-D-galactopyranosyl)-D-glucopyranose, lactose laurate] (**4b**) [27]. Yield: 44% (0.058 g). ^{1}H NMR (400 MHz, DMSO) δ: 0.86 (t, 3H, J = 6.6 Hz, CH_3), 1.19–1.30 [m, 16H, $(CH_2)_n$], 1.48–1.57 (m, 2H, CH_2CH_2COOR), 2.31 (t, 2H, J = 7.3 Hz, CH_2COOR), 3.17 (ddd, 1H, $J_{2\text{–}1}$ = 4.0 Hz, $J_{2\text{–OH2}}$ = 7.0 Hz, $J_{2\text{–}3}$ = 9.5 Hz, H^2), 3.27 (dd, 1H, $J_{4\text{–}3} \cong J_{4\text{–}5}$ = 9.5 Hz, H^4), 3.33–3.38 (m, 2H, H^8, H^9), 3.56 (dd, 1H, $J_{3\text{–}2} \cong J_{3\text{–}4}$ = 9.5 Hz, H^3), 3.60–3.67 (m, 3H, H^{6a}, H^{6b}, H^{10}), 3.68–3.76 (m, 2H, H^5, H^{11}), 4.09 (dd, 1H, $J_{12b\text{–}11}$ = 4.5 Hz, $J_{12b\text{–}12a}$ = 11.5 Hz, H^{6a}), 4.17 (dd, 1H, $J_{12a\text{–}11}$ = 8.5 Hz, $J_{12a\text{–}12b}$ = 11.5 Hz, H^{6b}), 4.20–4.24 (m, 2H, H^7, OH^3), 4.43 (dd, 1H, $J_{OH6\text{–}6a} \cong J_{OH6\text{–}6b}$ = 6.0 Hz, OH^6), 4.56 (d, 1H, $J_{OH2\text{–}2}$ = 7.0 Hz, OH^2), 4.79 (d, 1H, $J_{OH10\text{–}10}$ = 5.0 Hz, OH^{10}), 4.86 (d, 1H, J = 5.0 Hz, OH), 4.90 (dd, 1H, $J_{1\text{–OH1}} \cong J_{1\text{–}2}$ = 4.0 Hz, H^1), 5.16 (d, 1H, J = 4.0 Hz, OH), 6.34 (d, 1H, $J_{OH1\text{–}1}$ = 4.0 Hz, OH^1) ppm. ^{13}C NMR (100 MHz, DMSO) δ: 14.4, 22.6, 24.8, 28.9, 29.2, 29.4, 29.46, 29.48, 31.8, 33.8, 60.9, 63.8, 68.7, 70.2, 70.7, 71.7, 72.7, 72.9, 73.3, 81.6, 92.5, 104.0, 173.4 ppm.

[6′-O-Tetradecanoyl-4-O-(β-D-galactopyranosyl)-D-glucopyranose, lactose myristate] (**4c**) [27]. Yield: 65% (0.090 g). ^{1}H NMR (400 MHz, DMSO) δ: 0.86 (t, 3H, J = 6.6 Hz, CH_3), 1.17–1.32 [m, 20H, $(CH_2)_n$], 1.48–1.57 (m, 2H, CH_2CH_2COOR), 2.30 (t, 2H, J = 7.4 Hz, CH_2COOR), 3.16 (ddd, 1H, $J_{2\text{–}1}$ = 4.0 Hz, $J_{2\text{–OH2}}$ = 7.0 Hz, $J_{2\text{–}3}$ = 9.5 Hz, H^2), 3.27 (dd, 1H, $J_{4\text{–}3} \cong J_{4\text{–}5}$ = 9.5 Hz, H^4), 3.31–3.37 (m, 2H, H^8, H^9), 3.56 (dd, 1H, $J_{3\text{–}2} \cong J_{3\text{–}4}$ = 9.5 Hz, H^3), 3.60–3.66 (m, 3H, H^{6a}, H^{6b}, H^{10}), 3.67–3.76 (m, 2H, H^5, H^{11}), 4.08 (dd, 1H, $J_{12b\text{–}11}$ = 4.5 Hz, $J_{12b\text{–}12a}$ = 11.5 Hz, H^{12b}), 4.16 (dd, 1H, $J_{12a\text{–}11}$ = 8.5 Hz, $J_{12a\text{–}12b}$ = 11.5 Hz, H^{12a}), 4.20–4.25 (m, 2H, H^7, OH^3), 4.47 (dd, 1H, $J_{OH6\text{–}6a} \cong J_{OH6\text{–}6b}$ = 6.0 Hz, OH^6), 4.60 (d, 1H, $J_{OH2\text{–}2}$ = 7.0 Hz, OH^2), 4.82 (d, 1H, $J_{OH10\text{–}10}$ = 5.0 Hz, OH^{10}), 4.89 (d, 1H, J = 4.0 Hz, OH), 4.90 (dd, 1H, $J_{1\text{–OH1}} \cong J_{1\text{–}2}$ = 4.0 Hz, H^1), 5.19 (d, 1H, J = 4.0 Hz, OH), 6.37 (d, 1H, $J_{OH1\text{–}1}$ = 4.0 Hz, OH^1) ppm. ^{13}C NMR (100 MHz, DMSO) δ: 14.4, 22.6, 24.8, 29.0, 29.18, 29.19, 29.4, 29.48, 29.51, 29.53, 31.8, 33.8, 60.9, 63.8, 68.7, 70.2, 70.7, 71.7, 72.7, 72.9, 73.3, 81.6, 92.5, 104.0, 173.4 ppm.

[6′-O-Esadecanoyl-4-O-(β-D-galactopyranosyl)-D-glucopyranose, lactose palmitate] (**4d**) [27]. Yield: 80% (0.116 g). ^{1}H NMR (400 MHz, DMSO) δ: 0.86 (t, 3H, J = 6.6 Hz, CH_3), 1.18–1.32 [m, 24H, $(CH_2)_n$], 1.47–1.58 (m, 2H, CH_2CH_2COOR), 2.31 (t, 2H, J = 7.4 Hz, CH_2COOR), 3.18 (ddd, 1H, $J_{2\text{–}1}$ = 4.0 Hz, $J_{2\text{–OH2}}$ = 7.0 Hz, $J_{2\text{–}3}$ = 9.5 Hz, H^2), 3.27 (dd, 1H, $J_{4\text{–}3} \cong J_{4\text{–}5}$ = 9.5 Hz, H^4), 3.32–3.38 (m, 2H, H^8, H^9), 3.57 (dd, 1H, $J_{3\text{–}2} \cong J_{3\text{–}4}$ = 9.5 Hz, H^3), 3.61–3.67 (m, 3H, H^{6a}, H^{6b}, H^{10}), 3.68–3.76 (m, 2H, H^5, H^{11}), 4.09 (dd, 1H, $J_{12b\text{–}11}$ = 4.5 Hz, $J_{12b\text{–}12a}$ = 11.5 Hz, H^{12b}), 4.17 (dd, 1H, $J_{12a\text{–}11}$ = 8.5 Hz, $J_{12a\text{–}12b}$ = 11.5 Hz, H^{12a}), 4.20–4.28 (m, 2H, H^7, OH^3), 4.39 (dd, 1H, $J_{OH6\text{–}6a} \cong J_{OH6\text{–}6b}$ = 6.0 Hz, OH^6), 4.51 (d, 1H, $J_{OH2\text{–}2}$ = 7.0 Hz, OH^2), 4.75 (d, 1H, $J_{OH10\text{–}10}$ = 5.0 Hz, OH^{10}), 4.82 (br s, 1H, OH), 4.90 (dd, 1H, $J_{1\text{-OH1}} \cong J_{1\text{–}2}$ = 4.0 Hz, H^1), 5.12 (br s, 1H, OH), 6.31 (d, 1H, $J_{OH1\text{–}1}$ = 4.0 Hz, OH^1) ppm. ^{13}C NMR (100 MHz, DMSO) δ: 14.4,

22.5, 24.8, 29.0, 29.1, 29.2, 29.4, 29.46, 29.50, 31.7, 33.8, 61.0, 63.7, 68.7, 70.2, 70.8, 71.7, 72.7, 72.9, 73.3, 81.6, 92.5, 104.0, 173.4 ppm.

2.4. Surface Tension Measurements

Surface tension of different concentrations of surfactant solutions in water was measured using a platinum cylindrical rod probe with wetted length of 1.6 mm (K100-Krüss force tensiometer, Hamburg, Germany) at room temperature. Approximately 1 mL of each surfactant solution was placed onto a Teflon plate and the surface of the liquid was aspirated to remove any remaining impurities. Then, the rod probe was immersed 2 mm into the liquid. Data are expressed as the mean of three repeated measurements performed at room temperature. The critical micelle concentration and the surface tension at the CMC (γCMC) were calculated through the straight-line interception method, while the Gibbs surface excess (Γ_{max}) was calculated from the following equation:

$$\boldsymbol{\Gamma}_{max} = \frac{\mathbf{1}}{\mathbf{2.303} \times \text{n} \times \text{R} \times \text{T}} \left(\frac{\delta_\gamma}{\delta \boldsymbol{logC}} \right) \quad (1)$$

where T is the absolute temperature, R is the gas constant (8.314 J/mol K), C is the surfactant concentration, n = 1 for a non-ionic candidate. $\delta_\gamma / \delta \boldsymbol{logC}$ was calculated from the maximum slope of the plot surface tension vs. surfactant concentration in the linear region before CMC.

The minimum area per surfactant molecule at the air-water interface (A_{min}) was determined as follow:

$$\boldsymbol{A}_{min} = \frac{\mathbf{10^{18}}}{\boldsymbol{N} \times \boldsymbol{\Gamma}_{max}} \quad (2)$$

where N is the Avogadro number.

2.5. MTT Cell Viability Assays

Caco-2 and Calu-3 cells were seeded in sterile 96-well culture plates at a density of 3×10^4 cells per well. The cells were incubated to attain at least 80% confluence before the experiment. Stock solutions of surfactants were prepared in phosphate buffered saline (PBS). They were diluted at various concentrations (from 0.0078 to 1 mg/mL) in cell culture medium before added to the cells. Complete culture media were used as control. The cytotoxic effect of each surfactant was evaluated using the MTT cell viability assay. After 24 h of incubation, surfactant solution was discarded and replaced by MTT solution (0.8 mg/mL). The cells were subjected to MTT treatment for 2 h. Formazan crystals formed were then dissolved in absolute isopropanol and incubated with gentle shaking at room temperature for 15 min. Absorbance was measured at 570 nm using a microplate reader (Multiskan™ GO Microplate Spectrophotometer Thermo Scientific, Waltham, MA, USA). Percentage of viable cells was calculated using untreated cells as control with 100% cell viability. The percentage of viable cells was plotted against log concentration of the surfactants. IC_{50} (mg/mL), the concentration of surfactant that caused a 50% reduction in cell viability was calculated by fitting the experimental data with dose–response model (Prism 6, Version 6.0b, GraphPad Software).

2.6. Lactate Dehydrogenase (LDH) Release Assay

LDH assay was used to evaluate the membrane disruption effect exhibited by the surfactants. Caco-2 and Calu-3 cells were seeded in sterile 96-well culture plates at a density of 3×10^4 cells per well. Surfactant solutions (at the same concentration as in MTT assay described above) were added to the cells and incubated at 37 °C for 24 h. Triton X-100 at 1% v/v was used as positive control. LDH release assay was conducted according to the manufacturer's protocol. The percentage of released LDH was calculated relative to the controls by taking samples treated with Triton X-100 as complete LDH release and untreated cells as nil LDH release.

The concentration of surfactant that caused a 50% release of LDH (IC_{50}, mM), was calculated by fitting the experimental data with dose–response model (Prism 6, Version 6.0b, GraphPad Software).

2.7. Mitochondrial Membrane Potential (JC-1 Assay)

Caco-2 and Calu-3 cells were seeded in sterile 96 well plates at a density of 1×10^4 cells per well and cultured for 24 h. As above, surfactant solutions were applied in Hank's balanced salt solution (HBSS) for 24 h. One millimolar FCCP was employed as the positive, mitochondrial depolarizing control. Following exposure, treatments were removed and cells were washed twice with PBS prior to the addition of 50 μL (5 μg/mL) JC-1 dye diluted in complete DMEM (without antibiotics) per well for 15 min at 37 °C. Dye solution was then removed and wells washed with PBS followed by addition of 50 μL/well PBS prior to measuring fluorescence at 550/600 nm ($\lambda_{ex}/\lambda_{em}$) for detection of JC-1 J-aggregates and 485/535 nm ($\lambda_{ex}/\lambda_{em}$) for detection of JC-1 monomers. A ratio between JC-1 aggregates and JC-1 monomer signals was then taken, and data normalized by setting the untreated control as a value of 1.0 and the positive control (1.0 mM FCCP) as a value of 0.0.

2.8. Caspase 3/7 Activation (CellEvent™ Assay)

Caco-2 and Calu-3 cells were seeded in sterile 96 well plates at a density of 1×10^4 cells per well and cultured for 24 h. Following 24 h exposure on cells, surfactant solutions were removed, and cells washed twice with PBS followed by the addition of 100 μL 1.0% CellEvent™ Caspase-3/7 detection reagent diluted in HBSS buffer per well for 60 min. Fluorescence was then analyzed at 490/540 nm ($\lambda_{ex}/\lambda_{em}$), and data presented normalized to the untreated control set as a value of 1.0.

2.9. Nuclear Membrane Permeability (CellTox™ Green Cytotoxicity Assay)

Caco-2 and Calu-3 cells were seeded at a density of 1×10^4 cells per well in sterile 96 well plates for 24 h prior to assaying. Cells were exposed to treatments for 24 h, followed by the addition of 100 μL (2×) CellTox™ Green reagent (1:500 dilution of CellTox™ Green Dye in Assay Buffer) per well. The resulting solution was incubated at room temperature for 15 min and fluorescence then measured at 495/519 nm ($\lambda_{ex}/\lambda_{em}$). CellTox™ green signals were normalized by setting the untreated control as 0% and the positive control (1% Triton X-100) as 100% permeabilization of cell nuclei.

2.10. Measurement of Trans-Epithelial Electrical Resistance (TEER)

Caco-2 and Calu-3 cells were seeded at a density of 2×10^5 cells per well on filter inserts (Transwell® Permeable Support 12 mm Insert, Corning Life Sciences, Tewksbury, MA, USA) and cultured to confluence under air-liquid interface conditions. Culture media on the baso-lateral sides of the cells were changed every 24 h. For TEER measurements, culture medium was discarded from the cell layer and replaced with Kreb's Balanced Saline Solutions (KBSS) on both the apical and baso-lateral sides of the monolayers. Cell layers were allowed equilibrating in KBSS at 37 °C, 5% CO_2 for 45 min prior to sample application. Baseline TEER was measured before the treatment with surfactants. For each surfactant, concentrations that caused 50% cell viability, and the highest concentration that maintained 100% cell viability (according to the MTT assay) were added to the apical sides of the cell layers and incubated for 2 h. TEER was then measured at 5, 30, 60, 90 and 120 min after surfactant addition. Between TEER measurements, cells were incubated at normal cell culture conditions. After 120 min, surfactant was removed, and culture media were added to both sides of the filter inserts. TEER measurement was conducted again after 24 h to evaluate the recovery of cell monolayers. A volt-ohmmeter (Millcell® ERS-2 Voltohmmeter, Millipore, Burlington, MA, USA) equipped with a pair of electrodes was used for TEER measurement. Baseline TEER measured from cell layers incubated in KBSS was used as control and the change in TEER was presented as a percentage relative to baseline value. Three independent experiments were performed in duplicate.

3. Results and Discussion

3.1. *Surface Tension and CMC Determination*

Figure 1 shows the variation of surface tension over concentrations for each lactose fatty acid monoester. From the plotted curves, it is possible to observe the relevant influence of the carbon chain length on the surface properties of the amphiphiles.

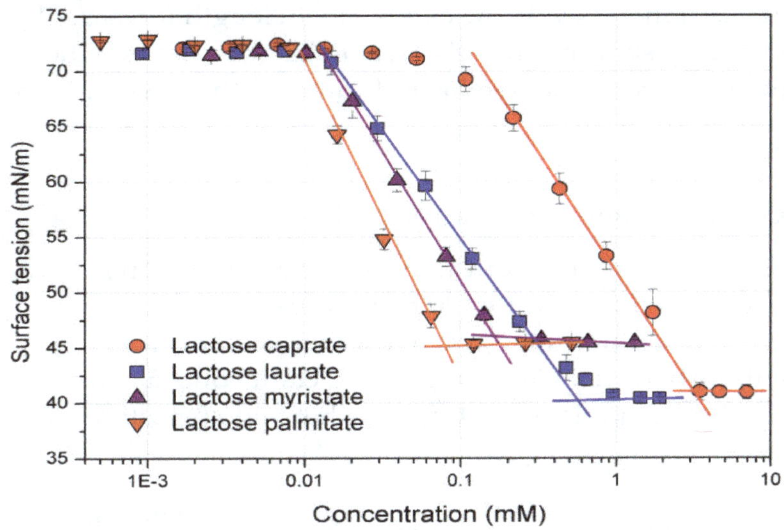

Figure 1. Surface tension (mN/m) vs. concentration (mM) plot for the lactose fatty acid monoester surfactants. Surface tension data are the mean of three repeated measurements (n = 3) performed at room temperature. The CMC (critical micelle concentration) is calculated from the straight-line interception method [28].

A clear relationship between the calculated CMC values (Table 1) and the carbon chain length can be established.

Table 1. Air-water surface parameters (critical micelle concentration (CMC), surface tension at CMC (γCMC), maximum surface excess (Γ_{max}) and minimum area per surfactant molecule (A_{min})) of the synthetized lactose fatty acid monoesters determined by tensiometry.

Entry	CMC (mM)	γCMC (mN/m)	$\Gamma_{max} \times 10^{-6}$ (mol/m^2)	A_{min} (Å^2)
Lactose caprate	2.58 ± 0.32	40.6 ± 0.04	9.52 ± 0.11	17.46 ± 0.25
Lactose laurate	0.55 ± 0.02	40.4 ± 0.02	9.52 ± 0.05	17.45 ± 0.09
Lactose myristate	0.14 ± 0.05	45.6 ± 0.19	8.37 ± 0.46	19.86 ± 0.80
Lactose palmitate	0.08 ± 0.03	45.1 ± 0.33	6.46 ± 0.11	25.69 ± 0.43

Indeed, lactose esters with longer carbon chains show a lower CMC because of the higher hydrophobicity. This translates in a lower water solubility and micellization reasonably occurs at lower concentrations. These results agree with those previously reported by Becerra et al. and Garofalakis et al. [24,29].

The surface tension at the CMC (γCMC) was calculated to be around 40 mN/m for lactose caprate and lactose laurate, while it was around 45 mN/m for derivatives with a longer hydrocarbon chain (C14 and C16), demonstrating the potential application of these compounds as surface-active agents (Table 1).

The absorption of the surfactants at the interface is described by the maximum surface excess concentration (Γ_{max}), according to the Gibbs isotherm.

The packing ability of surfactants at the interface is influenced by both the hydrocarbon chain length and polar head group. Surfactants with the bulkiest organization are generally characterized by a higher area per surfactants (A_{min}). In fact, as previously reported, A_{min} depends not only on the hydrophilic head group dimensions (number of hydroxyl group), but also on packing and stereochemistry of the whole structure [29].

According to Becerra et al., the surface excess is inversely dependent on the hydrocarbon chain length, therefore as the carbon chain length increase, the Γ_{max} decreases. Conversely, the area occupied by each molecule of surfactant increases as the carbon chain length increases [24]. Lactose caprate and lactose laurate, characterized by short hydrocarbon chain lengths, showed the highest Γ_{max}, suggesting the organization in a more packed monolayer as indicated by the lower area per molecule.

3.2. Biocompatibility Studies

3.2.1. MTT and LDH Assays on Calu-3 and Caco-2 Cells

MTT and LDH assays were carried out to assess the cytotoxicity of various concentration of lactose esters on Calu-3 and Caco-2 cells after 24 h exposure.

Results from the MTT assay (Figure 2) clearly suggest that cell viability of Calu-3 and Caco-2 cells is influenced by both carbon chain length and surfactant concentration. It is interesting to notice how, by increasing the carbon chain length of the synthetized surfactants, cell viability decreases at lower concentrations.

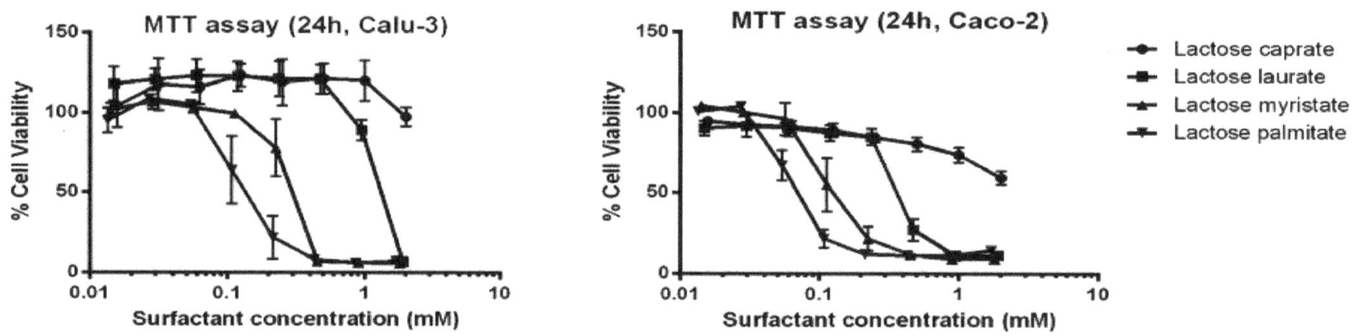

Figure 2. MTT assay of the lactose ester surfactants on Calu-3 and Caco-2 cell lines. The graph plots cell viability (%) as a function of different surfactant concentrations. Data are expressed as mean ± SD (n = 3).

A similar toxicological profile of lactose surfactants was observed when tested on both Caco-2 and Calu-3 cell lines.

Besides the MTT assay, another commonly employed in vitro cytotoxicity assay (LDH assay) was performed. The LDH assay highlights the effect of lactose esters on the cell membrane integrity, confirming the influence of the carbon chain length on the surfactant cytotoxicity on both cell lines (Figure 3).

A comparison on the cytotoxicity of lactose surfactants can be performed by calculation IC_{50} values, which is the concentration of surfactant that causes 50% maximum effect, in terms of 50% reduction of viable cells (MTT assay) or 50% release of LDH (LDH assay) (Table 2).

IC_{50} values decrease from lactose caprate to lactose palmitate independently from the cytotoxicity tests (MTT or LDH assay) or cell lines (Calu-3 and Caco-2). Indeed, for lactose caprate surfactant an IC_{50} value cannot be calculated since it is higher than the tested concentration range, confirming it has the lowest cytotoxicity. For the other lactose surfactants, it is noted that comparable IC_{50} values were calculated from the LDH assay between the two cell lines, while slightly higher IC_{50} values were found in Calu-3 with respect to Caco-2 from the MTT assay.

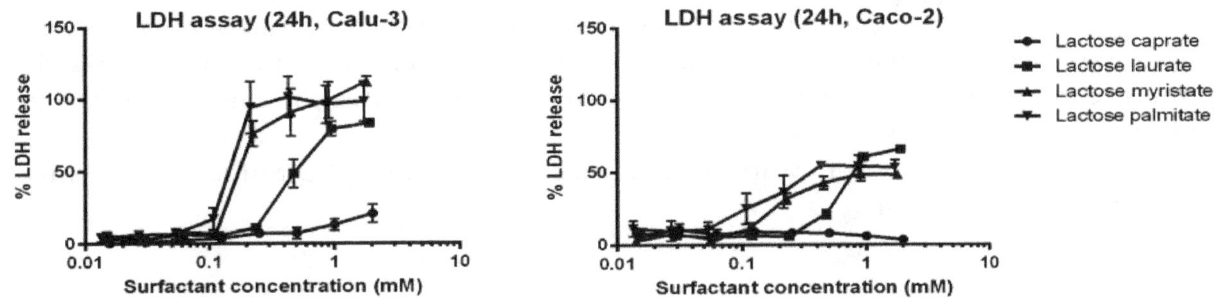

Figure 3. LDH assay of the series of lactose surfactants. The graph plots LDH release (%) from Calu-3 and Caco-2 cell lines as a function of different surfactant concentrations. Data are expressed as mean ± SD (n = 3).

Table 2. MTT and LDH cytotoxicity studies of the lactose ester surfactants on Calu-3 and Caco-2 cells. IC_{50} is the concentration of surfactant that causes 50% maximum effect, thus 50% reduction of viable cells (MTT assay) or 50% release of LDH (LDH assay).

Entry	MTT Assay IC_{50} (mM)		LDH Assay IC_{50} (mM)	
	Calu-3	Caco-2	Calu-3	Caco-2
Lactose caprate	>2	>2	>2	>2
Lactose laurate	1.069	0.376	0.452	0.597
Lactose myristate	0.261	0.112	0.189	0.194
Lactose palmitate	0.122	0.060	0.142	0.163

Interestingly, previous studies demonstrate the relationship between the hydrocarbon chain length and the cytotoxicity of sugar-based surfactants. The cytotoxic effect results from the interplay of different factors such as the ability of the hydrocarbon chain to insert into the lipid bilayer and to perturb membrane as well as the availability of free surfactant molecules, as indicated by CMC value [30,31]. Perinelli et al. recently investigated the correlation between the CMC and the cytotoxicity of *N*-decanoyl amino acid-based surfactants with different polar head groups. The authors demonstrated that toxicity is affected by both the polar head and the hydrocarbon chain length, with the latter parameter causing the main effect [32,33].

Lactose palmitate, which is characterized by the lowest CMC (0.08 mM), demonstrated the highest cytotoxicity in both cell lines. The calculated IC_{50} values for lactose palmitate, were 0.122 mM (Calu-3) and 0.060 mM (Caco-2) for the MTT assay and 0.142 mM (Calu-3) and 0.194 mM (Caco-2) for the LDH assay, respectively.

Moreover, IC_{50} values were compared to the CMC values, since it has already been demonstrated that surfactants with high cytotoxicity, show IC_{50} values lower than the CMC [33,34]. All the surfactants demonstrated IC_{50} values higher or comparable to the CMC in both cell lines (MTT and LDH assays), showing a low toxicity potential of the investigated lactose ester series on the two selected cell lines under defined conditions. This result obtained on cell-based methods in vitro is a preliminary evaluation of the toxicological profile of these surfactants, which should be confirmed by in vivo studies to assess the safety of these amphiphiles for pharmaceutical applications.

3.2.2. JC-1 Assay to Monitor Mitochondrial Health on Caco-2 and Calu-3

To examine the effect of lactose surfactants on the variation of mitochondrial membrane potential ($\Delta\Psi_m$), the ratiometric dye JC-1 assay was employed. The JC-1 dye readily permeates across the cell plasma membrane where it specifically accumulates in active mitochondria, in a potential dependent way. When present in the mitochondria, the dye forms J-aggregates, emitting fluorescence at red 595 nm wavelength, distinct from the dye presents in the cytoplasm which remains in monomeric form emitting fluorescence at green 530 nm wavelength [34]. Mitochondrial depolarization, due to the dissipation of negative charges across the mitochondrial membrane because of mitochondrial disruption, is consequently indicated by a decrease in the J-aggegrate:monomer intensity ratio, thus representing an arbitrary value for $\Delta\Psi_m$.

The effect of different concentration of lactose surfactants on the mitochondrial membrane potential is reported in Figure 4.

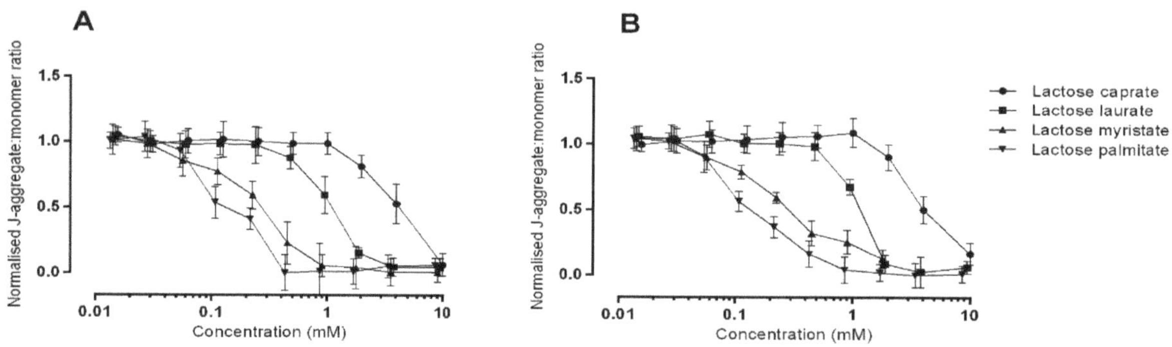

Figure 4. Mitochondrial membrane potential as measured by JC-1 assay in (**A**) Caco-2 and (**B**) Calu-3 cells. Responses are relative to those induced by untreated (HBSS buffer) which were set to a value of 1.0 and to 1.0 mM FCCP (carbonyl cyanide 4-(trifluoromethoxy) phenylhydrazone), known to induce total depolarization of mitochondrial membrane which were set to a value of 0.0. Data represents mean ± SD of triplicates from three independent experiments except for data for Caco-2 dosing of lactose myristate 3.6 mM and 9.0 mM, which comes from one repeat.

Loss of mitochondrial membrane potential is influenced by both concentration and hydrocarbon chain length of the tested surfactants, thus reflecting the results obtained from the MTT and LDH assays. In general, all the surfactants exert a similar toxicological profile in the two cell lines. When applied at the same concentrations, the highest cytotoxic effect is observed with lactose palmitate, as indicated by the lower J-aggretates:J-monomers ratio.

It is likely that the decline in metabolic activity measured by the MTT assay, observed above (Figure 2), is related to the interruption of mitochondrial respiration that would occur because of mitochondrial membrane potential disruption.

A common cause of mitochondrial depolarization is the induction of apoptosis. Both intrinsic and extrinsic apoptosis cause depolarization, which induces the release of key pro-apoptotic proteins/messengers from the mitochondria.

Depolarization of the mitochondrial membrane potential is commonly caused by the formation of pores or channels across the inner mitochondrial membrane, such as the permeability transition pore that is activated by the pro-apoptotic Bcl-2 family members [35]. Various accounts demonstrate that the dissipation of mitochondrial membrane potential occurs shortly after the permeabilization of the outer mitochondrial membrane [36]. Once the outer membrane is permeabilized, the soluble proteins present in the inner mitochondrial space are released [37,38], many of which play crucial roles in the induction of apoptosis. Therefore, the results gathered suggest the potentially involvement of apoptosis in surfactant toxicity and is explored further in the next section.

3.2.3. Caspase 3/7 Detection

Detection of activated effector caspases 3/7 is a well-recognized marker of programmed cell death. CellEvent™ Caspase-3/7 detection reagent is a four-amino acid peptide (DEVD) conjugated to a specific dye, thus inhibiting its ability to bind to DNA. The conjugated dye is non-fluorescent until the DEVD peptide sequence is recognized and cleaved by activated caspase-3/7, which in turn enables the dye to bind to DNA.

Figure 5 shows the detection of activated caspase 3/7 induced by the tested lactose surfactants as a function of the applied concentration, in Caco-2 and Calu-3 cells. Based on these results, it is reasonable to assume that the compounds induce caspase 3/7 activation, indicating that apoptosis is occurring. Furthermore, the induction of activated caspases occurs in a compound-dependent manner; therefore, as carbon chain length is increased, the potency to elicit apoptosis increases also since caspase 3/7 activation occurs at lower concentrations. Nevertheless, starting from a certain concentration, the normalized level of caspase 3/7 activation decreases, returning to the baseline values (or lower as is the case for lactose palmitate).

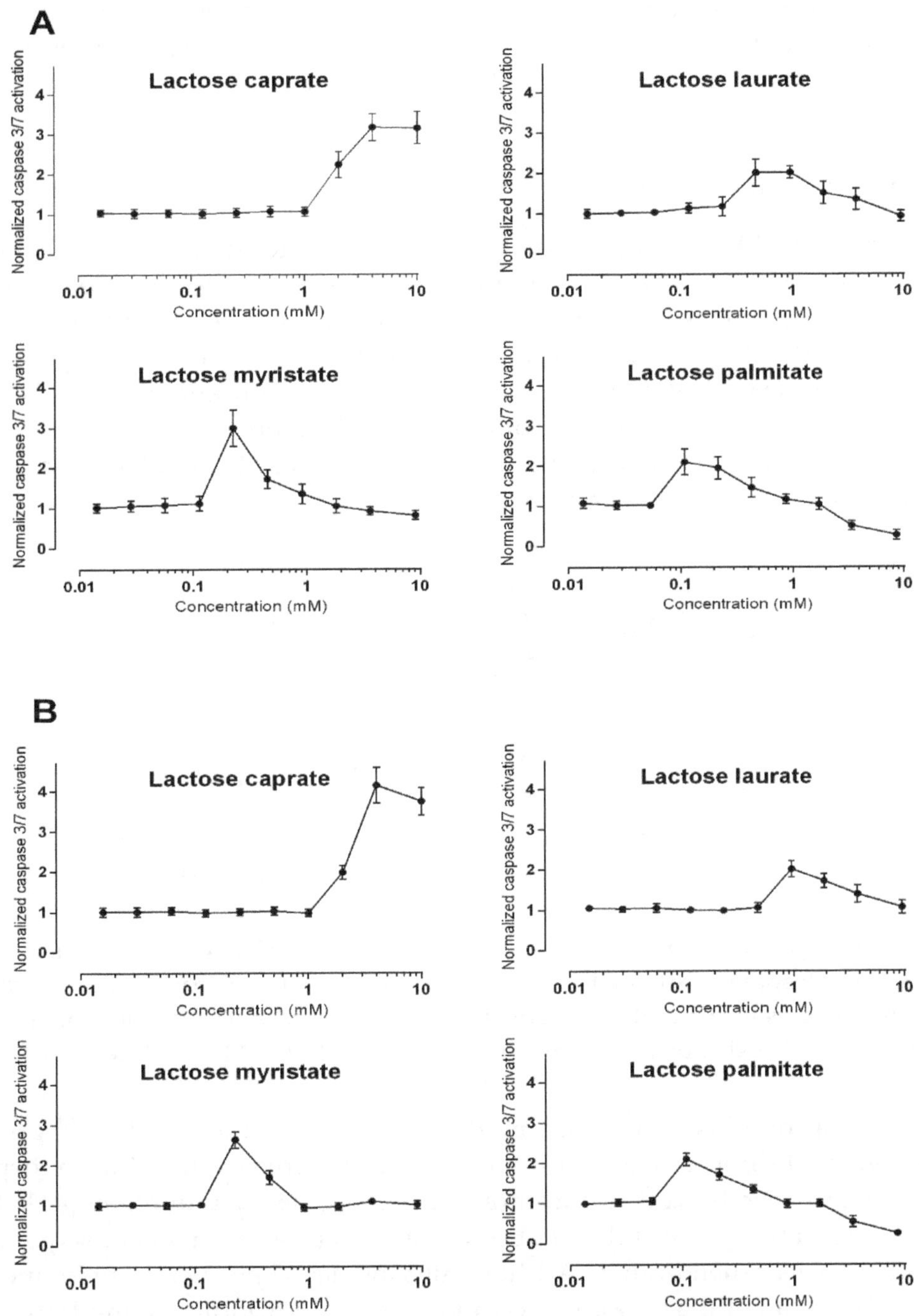

Figure 5. Detection of activated caspase 3/7 in (**A**) Caco-2 and (**B**) Calu-3 cells. Responses are displayed normalized to those induced by vehicle control (HBSS buffer). Data is presented as mean ± SD and represents triplicates from three experiments except for data for dosing of lactose myristate 3.6 mM and 9.0 mM in both Caco-2 and Calu-3 cells, which comes from one repeat.

These unusual profiles (Figure 5) observable for all the lactose surfactants may be explained by the dynamic and transient nature of caspase expression. Once cellular death has occurred, indicated by total loss of metabolic activity, the apoptotic process is likely over, therefore cellular expression of effector caspases is no longer necessary. When a cell population undergoes apoptosis, however, caspase levels significantly increase, and the breakdown of the cellular components occurs.

An alternative interpretation to the obtained results that should not be overlooked, is the induction of necrosis at higher concentrations rather than apoptosis, as was observed with quaternary ammonium surfactants [39]. This data set could therefore benefit from the inclusion of an intermediate exposure point (6 or 12 h) which could test the theory based on dynamic caspase expression discussed above. Additional approaches, such as the detection of apoptotic DNA fragmentation, would also aid in deciphering if apoptosis is occurring at higher surfactant concentrations or indeed if necrosis was prevalent.

3.2.4. CellTox™ Green Cytotoxicity Assay

CellTox™ green is a DNA binding dye that measures changes in membrane integrity that occurs because of cell death [40]. Signal generation occurs when the cell-impermeable dye binds DNA, and this can occur when DNA is released from cells. Thus, this assay detects for both loss of cellular and nuclear membrane integrity. Alternatively, compounds that enhance membrane permeability can also facilitate dye entry via permeabilization of the cell and nuclear membrane, thus binding to intracellular DNA. Figure 6 shows the results obtained from CellTox™ green assay in Caco-2 and Calu-3 cells treated with different concentration of lactose surfactants. It is possible to observe a concentration and compound dependent increase in nuclear permeability.

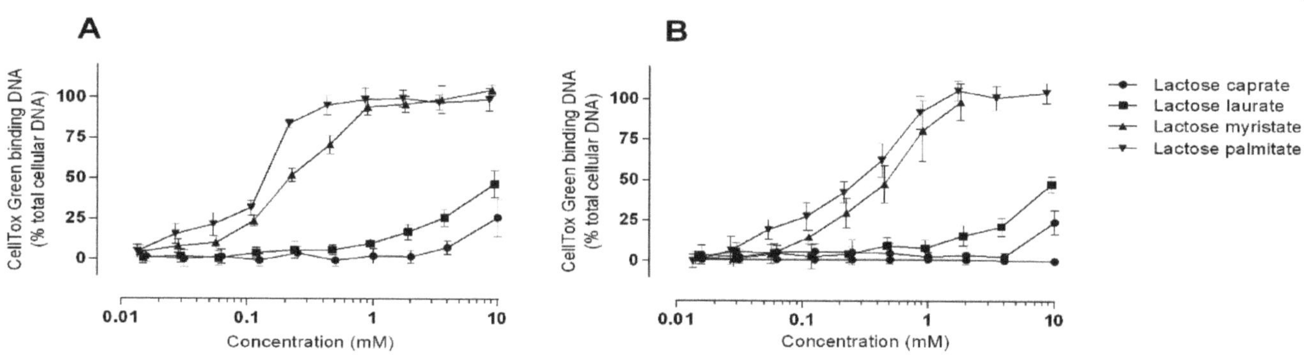

Figure 6. Nuclear membrane permeability as measured using the CellTox™ green assay in (**A**) Caco-2 and (**B**) Calu-3 cells. Responses are relative to those caused by 1.0% Triton X-100, which were set to 100%. Data is presented as mean ± SD and represents triplicates from three independent experiments except for data for Caco-2 dosing of lactose myristate 3.6 mM and 9.0 mM, which comes from one repeat.

Permeabilization of the plasma membrane that may enable the CellTox™ green dye to enter the cell is likely an effect of direct surfactant interaction and incorporation into phospholipid bilayer resulting in altered membrane fluidity, a commonly observed surfactant effect [41]. The increases in nuclear membrane permeability could then subsequently occur as a direct consequence of surfactant incorporation into the nuclear membranes. Additionally, increased permeability in nuclear membranes may be induced because of cellular apoptosis—a late event in apoptosis, mediating the formation of apoptotic bodies. Thus, taken together with the activation of caspase-3/7, increased nuclear membrane permeability at low surfactant concentrations may be occurring in an apoptotic manner. However, at higher concentrations the presence of LDH release alongside increased nuclear membrane permeabilization is likely indicative of surfactant-mediated perturbation of cellular membranes.

3.3. *Trans-Epithelial Electrical Resistance (TEER) Studies in Calu-3 and Caco-2 Cells*

TEER studies were performed in Calu-3 and Caco-2 cells to evaluate the ability of lactose surfactants to act as absorption enhancers, through transmucosal perturbation possibly by transiently opening tight junctions (Figure 7). Results obtained from TEER measurements should be interpreted carefully with the toxicological profile of the tested compounds to ensure that the changes in TEER was not due to the permeant damage of the membrane integrity. In fact, a transient modulation of tight junction opening commonly translates in a reversible effect on the TEER, while a permanent perturbation of the membrane integrity, on the other hand, is evidenced by a non-reversible effect on the TEER. However, it should also be noted that reversible effect on TEER could be a consequence of mechanisms other than tight junction opening.

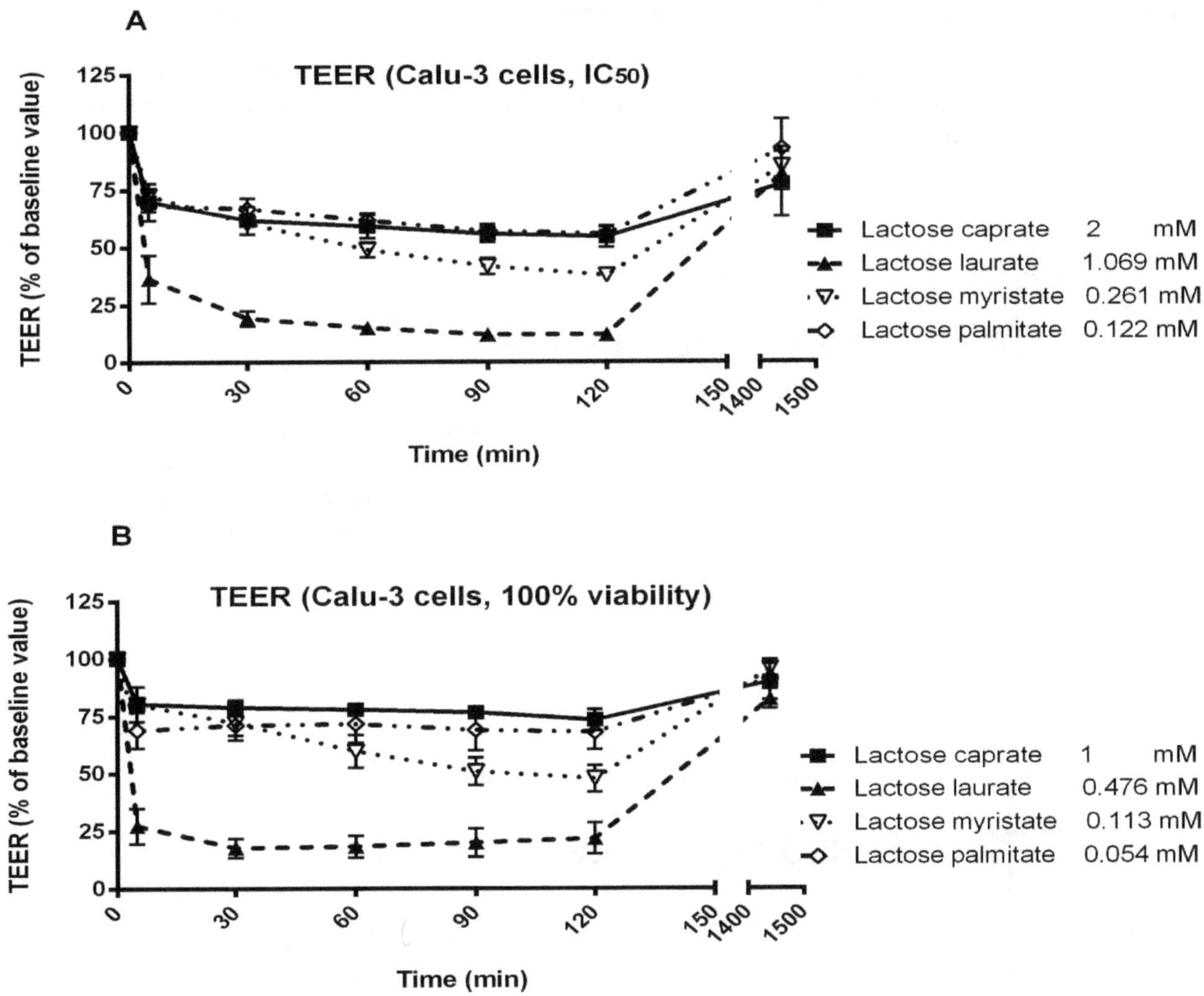

Figure 7. Effect of two different concentrations of lactose surfactants on Calu-3 cell monolayer TEER. (**A**) IC_{50} calculated from MTT assay and (**B**) the highest concentration that shows 100% viability from MTT assay. Data are presented as the mean of three independent experiments.

In the present study, two concentrations of each lactose surfactant were selected for TEER studies, specifically the IC_{50} calculated from MTT assay and the highest concentration that shows 100% viability in MTT assay, to evaluate the potential application of lactose surfactants within this range of concentrations. Hence, the effect observed on TEER for each surfactant must be correlated with the specific applied concentration, in addition to the structure of the compound (hydrocarbon chain length).

Regarding Calu-3 cells, lactose laurate was found to be the most effective surfactant in decreasing the TEER at both tested concentrations, while all the other surfactants showed only a moderate decrease in the TEER. Lactose laurate was effective in decreasing the TEER at the lowest applied concentration (0.476 mM; 0.025% *w*/*v*), with an effect comparable to the highest applied concentration (1.069 mM; 0.056% *w*/*v*). On the other hand, lactose caprate, applied at a similar concentration (1 mM), only slightly affected the TEER. It is noted that the surfactants were tested at different concentrations according to their toxicity profile. The ability of lactose laurate to lower the TEER significantly at the tested concentrations indicated that this surfactant exhibits a good balance between safety and efficacy.

Interestingly, TEER reversed to the initial value after 25 h with all the tested surfactants and concentrations, suggesting a transient effect on the membrane permeability, possibly by tight junction opening. To elucidate the mechanism and to confirm whether the surfactants could be serve as permeation enhancers, a macromolecule permeability assay could be performed in future study.

Regarding Caco-2 cells, different concentrations of surfactants were selected for TEER experiments, based on the IC_{50} calculated from the MTT assay (Figure 8). Due to the higher cytotoxicity displayed on Caco-2 cells, surfactants were tested at lower concentrations.

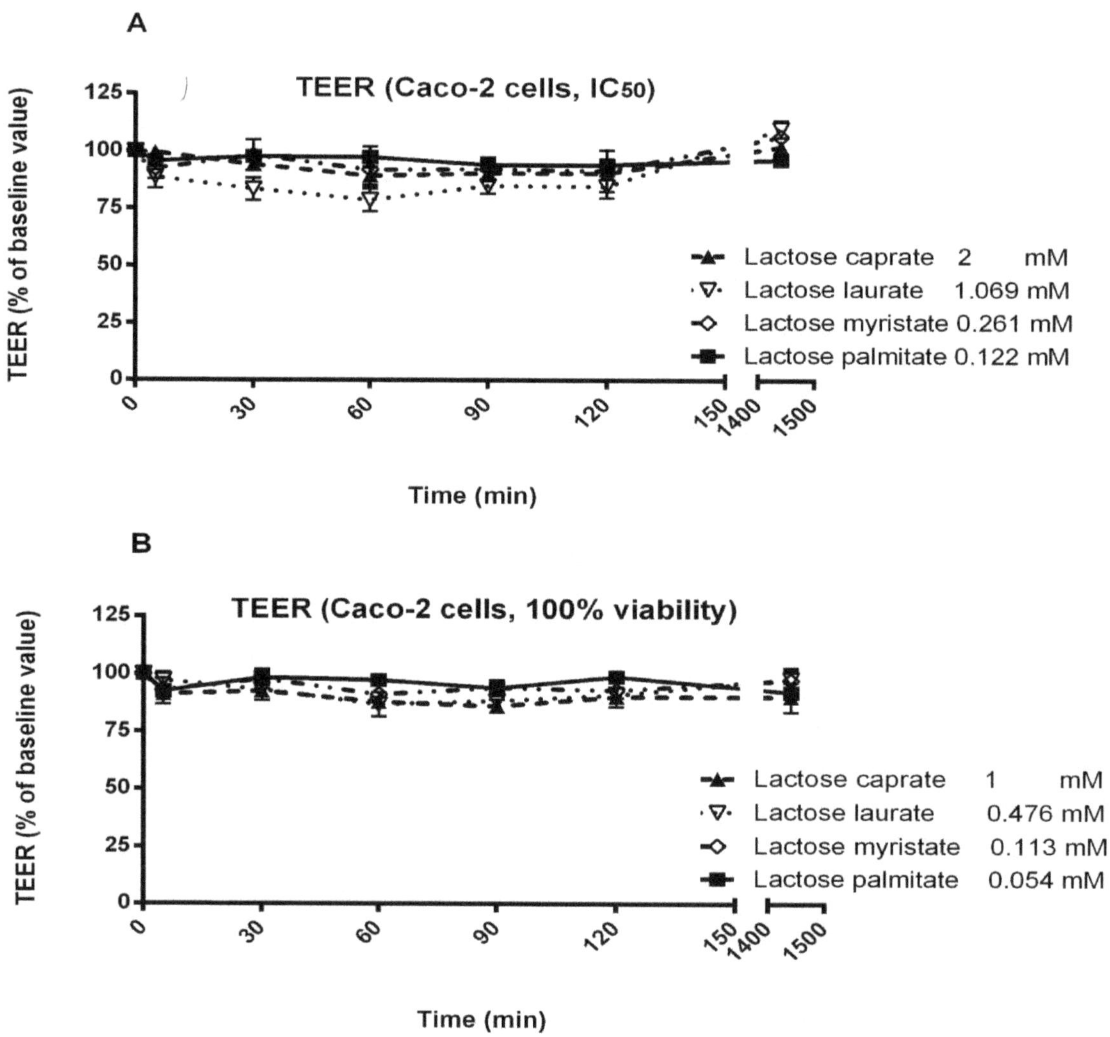

Figure 8. Effect of two different concentrations of lactose surfactants on Caco-2 cell monolayer TEER. (**A**) IC_{50} calculated from MTT assay and (**B**) the highest concentration that shows 100% viability from MTT assay. Data are presented as the mean of three independent experiments.

Caco-2 cells were significantly less sensitive than Calu-3 cells. This was mainly because Caco-2 cells were more prone to the cytotoxic effect of the surfactants, hence a much lower concentrations were used in the TEER study than on Calu-3 cells, rendering the rather poor response on this cell line. Lactose caprate tested at 2 mM, induced a more significant decrease in TEER in Calu-3 cells compared to Caco-2 cells. All the surfactants, tested at their IC_{50} concentration, only poorly affected the TEER, suggesting a reduced efficacy in tight junction opening or other membrane perturbation mechanisms. Nevertheless, lactose laurate showed a more significant effect, with a moderate reduction of TEER. On the other hand, all the surfactants tested at the lowest concentration (100% cell viability from MTT assay) did not induced a significant decrease of TEER.

4. Conclusions

This work reports an extensive and comprehensive study of the cytotoxicity profile of selected lactose-based surfactants, as function of their structure (different hydrocarbon chain length) and concentration. Cytotoxicity of the tested surfactants was found to be closely related to their hydrocarbon tail for this specific homologues series in cell cultures tested, thus increasing the hydrocarbon chain length also increased the cytotoxicity. Hence, higher IC_{50} values were observed in presence of more hydrophilic compounds (shorter hydrocarbon chain length). Moreover, comparing CMC and IC_{50} values reveals that the CMCs of the surfactants are lower or similar, thus showing a low toxicity potential on the selected cell lines. Furthermore, the compounds tested showed a comparable cytotoxicity in Caco-2 colonic epithelium and Calu-3 airway epithelium according to both MTT and LDH assay. When applied for 24 h the compounds induced, in a dose-dependent manner, depolarization of the mitochondrial membrane potential and permeabilization of plasma and nuclear membranes, as shown by JC-1 assay and CellTox^{TM} green assay, respectively. The activation of caspase-3/7 suggests apoptosis may play a role in surfactant-induced cell death, particularly at lower surfactant concentrations; however, at higher concentrations, surfactant-mediated membrane perturbation may possibly result in necrotic-like cell death. The initiating factor behind induction of apoptosis remains unknown but is likely associated to alterations in membrane fluidity and the subsequent effect on ion gradient homeostasis and intracellular redox environment. Interestingly, lactose laurate showed a good ability to decrease the TEER at a concentration close to IC_{50} value, while all the other surfactants showed only a moderate effect on membrane perturbation across cell monolayer.

Overall, results from cytotoxicity assays suggest a possible "mild behavior" of lactose monoester surfactants in term of toxicological profile, providing a preliminary evidence regarding one of the possible advantages of using these amphiphiles in different fields.

Author Contributions: Conceptualization, L.C., S.L., A.D., J.W.K.L. and S.S.; Methodology, S.L., R.C., M.C. and D.R.P.; Formal Analysis, S.L., M.C., R.C., D.R.P. and W.L.; Investigation, L.F., R.C., W.L. and D.R.P.; Resources, L.C., A.D., J.W.K.L. and S.S.; Writing-Original Draft Preparation, L.F. R.C., D.R.P., S.L. and L.C.; Writing-Review and Editing, L.C., A.D., S.L., D.R.P. and R.C.; Supervision, L.C., A.D., S.S. and J.W.K.L.

Acknowledgments: The authors wish to thank Fabio De Belvis for the design and realization of the graphical abstract.

References

1. Plou, F.J.; Cruces, M.A.; Ferrer, M.; Fuentes, G.; Pastor, E.; Bernabé, M.; Christensen, M.; Comelles, F.; Parra, J.L.; Ballesteros, A. Enzymatic acylation of di- and trisaccharides with fatty acids: Choosing the appropriate enzyme, support and solvent. *J. Biotechnol.* **2002**, *96*, 55–66. [CrossRef]
2. Hill, K.; Rhode, O. Sugar-based surfactants for consumer products and technical applications. *Lipid* **1999**, *101*, 25–33. [CrossRef]

3. Neta, N.S.; Teixeira, J.A.; Rodrigues, L.R. Sugar Ester Surfactants: Enzymatic Synthesis and Applications in Food Industry. *Crit. Rev. Food Sci. Nutr.* **2015**, *55*, 595–610. [CrossRef] [PubMed]
4. Plat, T.; Linhardt, R.J. Syntheses and applications of sucrose-based esters. *J. Surfactants Deterg.* **2001**, *4*, 415–421. [CrossRef]
5. Szuts, A.; Szabó-Révész, P. Sucrose esters as natural surfactants in drug delivery systems—A mini-review. *Int. J. Pharm.* **2012**, *433*, 1–9. [CrossRef] [PubMed]
6. De, S.; Malik, S.; Ghosh, A.; Saha, R.; Saha, B. A review on natural surfactants. *RSC Adv.* **2015**, *5*, 65757–65767. [CrossRef]
7. Zhang, X.; Wei, W.; Cao, X.; Feng, F. Characterization of enzymatically prepared sugar medium-chain fatty acid monoesters. *J. Sci. Food Agric.* **2015**, *95*, 1631–1637. [CrossRef] [PubMed]
8. Zhao, K.-H.; Cai, Y.-Z.; Lin, X.-S.; Xiong, J.; Halling, P.; Yang, Z. Enzymatic Synthesis of Glucose-Based Fatty Acid Esters in Bisolvent Systems Containing Ionic Liquids or Deep Eutectic Solvents. *Molecules* **2016**, *21*, 1294. [CrossRef] [PubMed]
9. Cruces, M.A.; Plou, F.J.; Ferrer, M.; Bernabé, M.; Ballesteros, A. Improved synthesis of sucrose fatty acid monoesters. *J. Am. Oil Chem. Soc.* **2001**, *78*, 541–546. [CrossRef]
10. Zhang, X.; Song, F.; Taxipalati, M.; Wei, W.; Feng, F. Comparative Study of Surface-Active Properties and Antimicrobial Activities of Disaccharide Monoesters. *PLoS ONE* **2014**, *9*, e114845. [CrossRef] [PubMed]
11. Ferrer, M.; Comelles, F.; Plou, F.J.; Cruces, M.A.; Fuentes, G.; Parra, J.L.; Ballesteros, A. Comparative Surface Activities of Di- and Trisaccharide Fatty Acid Esters. *Langmuir* **2002**, *18*, 667–673. [CrossRef]
12. Lucarini, S.; Fagioli, L.; Campana, R.; Cole, H.; Duranti, A.; Baffone, W.; Vllasaliu, D.; Casettari, L. Unsaturated fatty acids lactose esters: Cytotoxicity, permeability enhancement and antimicrobial activity. *Eur. J. Pharm. Biopharm.* **2016**, *107*, 88–96. [CrossRef] [PubMed]
13. Perinelli, D.R.; Lucarini, S.; Fagioli, L.; Campana, R.; Vllasaliu, D.; Duranti, A.; Casettari, L. Lactose oleate as new biocompatible surfactant for pharmaceutical applications. *Eur. J. Pharm. Biopharm.* **2018**, *124*, 55–62. [CrossRef] [PubMed]
14. Kiss, L.; Hellinger, É.; Pilbat, A.-M.; Kittel, Á.; Török, Z.; Füredi, A.; Szakács, G.; Veszelka, S.; Sipos, P.; Ózsvári, B.; et al. Sucrose esters increase drug penetration, but do not inhibit p-glycoprotein in caco-2 intestinal epithelial cells. *J. Pharm. Sci.* **2014**, *103*, 3107–3119. [CrossRef] [PubMed]
15. Maher, S.; Heade, J.; McCartney, F.; Waters, S.; Bleiel, S.B.; Brayden, D.J. Effects of surfactant-based permeation enhancers on mannitol permeability, histology, and electrogenic ion transport responses in excised rat colonic mucosae. *Int. J. Pharm.* **2018**, *539*, 11–22. [CrossRef] [PubMed]
16. Aguirre, T.A.S.; Rosa, M.; Guterres, S.S.; Pohlmann, A.R.; Coulter, I.; Brayden, D.J. Investigation of coco-glucoside as a novel intestinal permeation enhancer in rat models. *Eur. J. Pharm. Biopharm.* **2014**, *88*, 856–865. [CrossRef] [PubMed]
17. Maher, S.; Mrsny, R.J.; Brayden, D.J. Intestinal permeation enhancers for oral peptide delivery. *Adv. Drug Deliv. Rev.* **2016**, *106*, 277–319. [CrossRef] [PubMed]
18. McCartney, F.; Gleeson, J.P.; Brayden, D.J. Safety concerns over the use of intestinal permeation enhancers: A mini-review. *Tissue Barriers* **2016**, *4*, e1176822. [CrossRef] [PubMed]
19. Touitou, E. Enhancement of intestinal peptide absorption. *J. Control. Release* **1992**, *21*, 139–144. [CrossRef]
20. Ghadiri, M.; Canney, F.; Pacciana, C.; Colombo, G.; Young, P.M.; Traini, D. The use of fatty acids as absorption enhancer for pulmonary drug delivery. *Int. J. Pharm.* **2018**, *541*, 93–100. [CrossRef] [PubMed]
21. Scholnick, F.; Sucharski, M.K.; Linfield, W.M. Lactose-derived surfactants (I) fatty esters of lactose. *J. Am. Oil Chem. Soc.* **1974**, *51*, 8–11. [CrossRef]
22. Staroń, J.; Dąbrowski, J.M.; Cichoń, E.; Guzik, M. Lactose esters: Synthesis and biotechnological applications. *Crit. Rev. Biotechnol.* **2018**, *38*, 245–258. [CrossRef] [PubMed]
23. Drummond, C.J.; Wells, D. Nonionic lactose and lactitol based surfactants: Comparison of some physico-chemical properties. *Colloids Surf. A Physicochem. Eng. Asp.* **1998**, *141*, 131–142. [CrossRef]
24. Becerra, N.; Toro, C.; Zanocco, A.L.; Lemp, E.; Günther, G. Characterization of micelles formed by sucrose 6-O-monoesters. *Colloids Surf. A Physicochem. Eng. Asp.* **2008**, *327*, 134–139. [CrossRef]
25. Neta, N.D.A.S.; dos Santos, J.C.S.; de Oliveira Sancho, S.; Rodrigues, S.; Gonçalves, L.R.B.; Rodrigues, L.R.; Teixeira, J.A. Enzymatic synthesis of sugar esters and their potential as surface-active stabilizers of coconut milk emulsions. *Food Hydrocoll.* **2012**, *27*, 324–331. [CrossRef]

26. Thelwall, L.A.W.; Hough, L.; Richardson, A.C. Sugar Acetals, Their Preparation and Use. U.S. Patent 4,284,763, 2 April 1980.
27. Sarney, D.B.; Kapeller, H.; Fregapane, G.; Vulfson, E.N. Chemo-enzymatic synthesis of disaccharide fatty acid esters. *J. Am. Oil Chem. Soc.* **1994**, *71*, 711–714. [CrossRef]
28. Mukherjee, I.; Moulik, S.P.; Rakshit, A.K. Tensiometric determination of Gibbs surface excess and micelle point: A critical revisit. *J. Colloid Interface Sci.* **2013**, *394*, 329–336. [CrossRef] [PubMed]
29. Garofalakis, G.; Murray, B.S.; Sarney, D.B. Surface Activity and Critical Aggregation Concentration of Pure Sugar Esters with Different Sugar Headgroups. *J. Colloid Interface Sci.* **2000**, *229*, 391–398. [CrossRef] [PubMed]
30. Lu, B.; Vayssade, M.; Miao, Y.; Chagnault, V.; Grand, E.; Wadouachi, A.; Postel, D.; Drelich, A.; Egles, C.; Pezron, I. Physico-chemical properties and cytotoxic effects of sugar-based surfactants: Impact of structural variations. *Colloids Surf. B. Biointerfaces* **2016**, *145*, 79–86. [CrossRef] [PubMed]
31. Li, X.; Turánek, J.; Knötigová, P.; Kudláčková, H.; Mašek, J.; Parkin, S.; Rankin, S.E.; Knutson, B.L.; Lehmler, H.-J. Hydrophobic tail length, degree of fluorination and headgroup stereochemistry are determinants of the biocompatibility of (fluorinated) carbohydrate surfactants. *Colloids Surf. B Biointerfaces* **2009**, *73*, 65–74. [CrossRef] [PubMed]
32. Perinelli, D.R.; Casettari, L.; Cespi, M.; Fini, F.; Man, D.K.W.; Giorgioni, G.; Canala, S.; Lam, J.K.W.; Bonacucina, G.; Palmieri, G.F. Chemical–physical properties and cytotoxicity of *N*-decanoyl amino acid-based surfactants: Effect of polar heads. *Colloids Surf. A Physicochem. Eng. Asp.* **2016**, *492*, 38–46. [CrossRef]
33. Perinelli, D.R.; Cespi, M.; Casettari, L.; Vllasaliu, D.; Cangiotti, M.; Ottaviani, M.F.; Giorgioni, G.; Bonacucina, G.; Palmieri, G.F. Correlation among chemical structure, surface properties and cytotoxicity of *N*-acyl alanine and serine surfactants. *Eur. J. Pharm. Biopharm.* **2016**, *109*, 93–102. [CrossRef] [PubMed]
34. Sakamuru, S.; Li, X.; Attene-Ramos, M.S.; Huang, R.; Lu, J.; Shou, L.; Shen, M.; Tice, R.R.; Austin, C.P.; Xia, M. Application of a homogenous membrane potential assay to assess mitochondrial function. *Physiol. Genom.* **2012**, *44*, 495–503. [CrossRef] [PubMed]
35. Marzo, I.; Brenner, C.; Zamzami, N.; Jürgensmeier, J.M.; Susin, S.A.; Vieira, H.L.; Prévost, M.C.; Xie, Z.; Matsuyama, S.; et al. Bax and adenine nucleotide translocator cooperate in the mitochondrial control of apoptosis. *Science* **1998**, *281*, 2027–2031. [CrossRef] [PubMed]
36. Kroemer, G.; Galluzzi, L.; Brenner, C. Mitochondrial Membrane Permeabilization in Cell Death. *Physiol. Rev.* **2007**, *87*, 99–163. [CrossRef] [PubMed]
37. Patterson, S.D.; Spahr, C.S.; Daugas, E.; Susin, S.A.; Irinopoulou, T.; Koehler, C.; Kroemer, G. Mass spectrometric identification of proteins released from mitochondria undergoing permeability transition. *Cell Death Differ.* **2000**, *7*, 137–144. [CrossRef] [PubMed]
38. Van Loo, G.; Demol, H.; van Gurp, M.; Hoorelbeke, B.; Schotte, P.; Beyaert, R.; Zhivotovsky, B.; Gevaert, K.; Declercq, W.; Vandekerckhove, J.; et al. A matrix-assisted laser desorption ionization post-source decay (MALDI-PSD) analysis of proteins released from isolated liver mitochondria treated with recombinant truncated Bid. *Cell Death Differ.* **2002**, *9*, 301–308. [CrossRef] [PubMed]
39. Inácio, Â.S.; Costa, G.N.; Domingues, N.S.; Santos, M.S.; Moreno, A.J.M.; Vaz, W.L.C.; Vieira, O.V. Mitochondrial dysfunction is the focus of quaternary ammonium surfactant toxicity to mammalian epithelial cells. *Antimicrob. Agents Chemother.* **2013**, *57*, 2631–2639. [CrossRef] [PubMed]
40. McDougall, M.; Dwight, S. Nucleic Acid Binding Dyes and Uses Therefor. U.S. Patent 8,598,198 B2, 3 December 2013.
41. Heerklotz, H. Interactions of surfactants with lipid membranes. *Q. Rev. Biophys.* **2008**, *41*, 205–264. [CrossRef] [PubMed]

3

Homogenization of Amorphous Solid Dispersions Prepared by Electrospinning in Low-Dose Tablet Formulation

Gergő Fülöp [1,2], Attila Balogh [2], Balazs Farkas [2], Attila Farkas [2], Bence Szabó [2], Balázs Démuth [2], Enikő Borbás [2], Zsombor Kristóf Nagy [2,*] and György Marosi [2]

1 Gedeon Richter Plc., Formulation R&D, Gyömrői Street 19-21, H-1103 Budapest, Hungary; fulop.gergo89@gmail.com

2 Department of Organic Chemistry and Technology, Budapest University of Technology and Economics, Budafoki út 8. 3, H-1103 Budapest, Hungary; baloghattila5@gmail.com (A.B.); farkasbalazs09@gmail.com (B.F.); farkas.attila88@gmail.com (A.F.); szabob@oct.bme.hu (B.S.); demuth@oct.bme.hu (B.D.); eniko.borbas@gmail.com (E.B.); gmarosi@mail.bme.hu (G.M.)

* Correspondence: zsknagy@oct.bme.hu

Abstract: Low-dose tablet formulations were produced with excellent homogeneity based on drug-loaded electrospun fibers prepared by single-needle as well as scaled-up electrospinning (SNES and HSES). Carvedilol (CAR), a BCS II class compound, served as the model drug while poly (vinylpyrrolidone-*co*-vinyl acetate) (PVPVA64) was adopted as the fiber-forming polymer. Scanning electron microscopy (SEM) imaging was used to study the morphology of HSES and SNES samples. Different homogenization techniques were compared to maximize homogeneity: mixing in plastic bags and in a high-shear granulator resulting in low-shear mixing (LSM) and high-shear mixing (HSM). Drug content and homogeneity of the tablets were measured by UV-Vis spectrometry, the results revealed acceptably low-dose fluctuations especially with formulations homogenized with HSM. Sieve analysis was used on the final LSM and HSM powder mixtures in order to elucidate the observed differences between tablet homogeneity. Tablets containing drug-loaded electrospun fibers were also studied by Raman mapping demonstrating evenly distributed CAR within the corpus.

Keywords: carvedilol; poly (vinylpyrrolidone-*co*-vinyl acetate); high-speed electrospinning; high-shear mixing; homogenization; Raman mapping; sieve analysis

1. Introduction

Tablets are generally regarded as the most popular and accepted dosage forms in pharmaceutical technology. Their ease of manufacturing and high patient compliance make them an ideal choice for both the industry and therapeutics [1]. Tablets are available with doses ranging from very low (micrograms) to very high (1–2 g). In such extreme cases, manufacturing becomes more challenging which is especially true for microgram dosed formulations. Handling low quantities of active pharmaceutical ingredients (APIs) can often lead to decreased drug content and high relative standard deviation (RSD) values in the final batches [2]. Proper content uniformity (CU) among others is one of the basic requirements of tablets by Pharmacopeias across the world [3] ensuring high quality and patient safety.

In terms of formulation development, amorphous solid dispersions (ASD) are getting more recognition since enhanced dissolution and bioavailability can be achieved this way [4]. Techniques capable of manufacturing ASDs on the industrial scale, such as spray drying (SD) [5] and hot-melt extrusion (HME) [6] have already produced FDA approved formulations such as Raplixa [7] and NuvaRing [8]. However, SD generally requires high capital investment for the equipment and its maintenance, while it has a low thermal efficiency due to the large volume of hot air circulating in the drying chamber [9]. HME usually operates at even higher temperatures that should be avoided in case of thermosensitive components and it is not applicable for ASD formation in case of APIs of very high melting points [10].

On the other hand, both SD and HME are continuous technologies, which are heavily encouraged by the leading regulatory agencies [11]. Continuous manufacturing has multiple advantages over traditional batch methods, such as huge improvement in productivity, time-efficiency, less energy requirement and a reduced amount of actual waste [12]. As of today, three products have been produced and approved this way in the following chronological order: Orkambi (lumacaftor/ivacaftor) manufactured by Vertex [13], Prezista (darunavir) produced by Janssen [14] and Symdeko (tezacaftor/ivacaftor and ivacaftor) also developed by Vertex [15].

Electrospinning (ES) is a unique method enabling the production of ASDs from a polymer solution or melt [16,17]. Applying ES polymer fibers are formed in the micro and nanometer scale by the creation and elongation of an electrified fluid jet [18]. In comparison with the aforementioned ASD producing technologies, ES operates at ambient conditions resulting in a gentle drying process at minimal costs [19]. The electrospun fibers have an enormous surface area where the API is often molecularly dispersed in a polymer matrix, producing a nano-amorphous solid dispersion (NASD) [20–23]. ES is also being investigated for various biomedical purposes for its advantages in controlled delivery [24–27], tissue engineering [28,29], wound dressing, enzyme immobilization and biodrug delivery [30].

Regarding scaled-up nanofiber production, the high-speed electrospinning (HSES) technology has the capability to produce approximately half kg of product per hour [31] in accordance with industrial guidelines, while the traditional single-needle electrospinning (SNES) technique can only produce a few grams per hour at best [32,33]. HSES achieves this increased output by combining electrostatic and high-speed rotational jet generation [34,35]. There are also other alternate methods such as pressurized gyration [36], infusion gyration [37] and pressure-coupled infusion gyration [38], that have shown the capability of increased nanofiber output. The latest results and their possible future implications are assembled in a most recent review article [39].

The tableting of electrospun nanofibrous materials is a rather new concept so only a few studies have been reported that tackle this field [40–42]. However, there is no publication dealing with the homogeneity challenges in tablet formulation. Based on our previous experiences, this can be mainly attributed to the flowability concerns during downstream processing of the ES material. Moreover, ensuring homogeneity, and thus, appropriate CU can be a tall order when very low doses are needed especially in the case of tablets based on electrospun fibers [43].

To produce ES-based tablets on the industrial scale at any dose, the homogenization characteristics need to be better comprehended and implemented. This work aimed at developing a suitable technology to provide low-dose tablets with proper homogeneity containing electrospun substance prepared by an industrial HSES process. For this purpose, a direct compression (DC) technology was intended to be applied along with industrial tableting by a tablet rotary press. A model system was selected containing carvedilol (CAR, Figure 1), an antihypertensive drug, and PVPVA64, a copolymer as the matrix forming agent (the model drug was selected for analytical reasons, not for any biological relevance at such a low concentration).

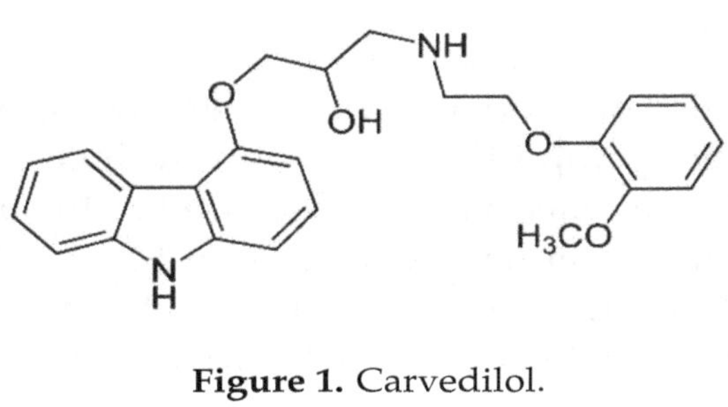

Figure 1. Carvedilol.

2. Materials and Methods

2.1. Materials

Carvedilol (CAR) was provided by Sigma-Aldrich (Budapest, Hungary) with purity ≥ 98% and a melting point of 117 °C. Kollidon VA 64 (Copovidone, PVPVA64) was supplied by BASF (Ludwigshafen, Germany), is a vinylpyrrolidone/vinylacetate amorphous copolymer (6:4) with a molecular weight in the range of 45–70 kDa. Lactose monohydrate (Flowlac 100 mesh) was provided by Meggle Pharma (Wasserburg, Germany), while microcrystalline cellulose (Vivapur 112), Croscarmellose sodium (Vivasol) and sodium stearyl fumarate (Pruv) were supplied by JRS Pharma (Rosenberg, Germany).

2.2. Single-Needle Electrospinning (SNES)

The single-needle electrospinning experiments were carried out using a spinneret equipped with an NT-35 high voltage DC supply (Unitronik Ltd., Nagykanizsa, Hungary). An electric potential of 25 kV was applied to the spinneret electrode. Sample collection was obtained using a grounded aluminum plate completely covered by aluminum foil. The distance of the spinneret from the collector was set at 15 cm, and the experiments were executed at ambient temperature (25 °C). The electrospinnable solution (Table 1) was dosed utilizing a SEP-10S Plus type syringe pump (Aitecs, Vilnius, Lithuania). The feed rate was 6 mL/h.

Table 1. Tablet composition.

Applied Tableting Ingredients	Amount (mg)/Tablet	Amount (%)/Tablet	Total Amount of Materials (Batch Size 5000 Tablets)
Electrospun/Crys. Carvedilol	0.05	0.05	0.25 g
poly (vinylpyrrolidone-*co*-vinyl acetate) (PVPVA64)	4.95	4.95	24.75 g
Flowlac 100 mesh (amorphous lactose)	65.00	65.00	325 g
Microcrystalline cellulose (MCC) 112	25.50	25.50	127.5 g
Croscarmellose sodium (CCS)	3.00	3.00	15.0 g
Sodium stearyl fumarate (Pruv)	1.5	1.50	7.5 g
Σ	100.0	100.0	500.00 g

2.3. High-Speed Electrospinning (HSES)

The scaled-up electrospinning productions were achieved by adopting a high-speed electrostatic spinning setup made up of a stainless steel spinneret with sharp edges and spherical cap geometry controlled by a high-speed motor. The electrospinnable solution was dosed by means of a SEP-10S Plus syringe pump. The flow rate was set at 750 mL/h. A rotational speed of 35,000 rpm was applied to the spinneret, while the voltage was 35 kV through the experiments (NT-65 high voltage DC supply Unitronik Ltd., Nagykanizsa, Hungary). The grounded collector completely covered by aluminum foil was positioned 35 cm from the spinneret in each case. The manufacture of fibers was carried out at ambient temperature (25 °C). More details about HSES can be found in the literature [44].

2.4. Low-Shear and High-Shear Homogenization

Homogenizations were carried out in plastic bags (low-shear mixing, LSM) or in a Diosna P-06 high-shear mixer (HSM). The tablet composition is detailed in Table 1.

A 100-mesh amorphous lactose called Flowlac was used as the filler, microcrystalline cellulose type 112 was applied as the binder, croscarmellose sodium (CCS) was adopted as the superdisintegrant and sodium stearyl fumarate (SSF) was implemented as the lubricant.

In the HSM setup, the chopper blades are set horizontally, which is standard for Diosna high-shear mixers.

In practice, all ingredients except the API and SSF were placed into plastic bags (LSM) or into the HSM, where they were pre-homogenized in 2 min (200 rpm impeller, 600 rpm chopper for HSM). Then the electrospun product or the crystalline CAR was added to the mixture, where it was homogenized in 7 min (200 rpm impeller, 850 rpm chopper for HSM). Upon completion, the mixtures were sieved applying a 500 μm sieve. Finally, SSF was added and blended with the other components in 30 s (200 rpm impeller, 0 rpm chopper for HSM).

2.5. Tableting and in Process Control (IPC) Tests

The average tablet weight was set to 100 mg, with the dose of CAR at 50 μg. Tableting was performed on a Riva Piccola tablet rotary press machine using 8 tablet dies with 6 mm diameter and no markings. Table speed was 40 rpm, Fill-O-Matic was 7 rpm and compression force was between 1–1.5 kN. A reference batch was also produced containing crystalline carvedilol as the API. Each batch consisted of 5000 tablets.

The compressed tablets were evaluated by IPC tests, such as tablet weight, thickness, hardness, friability measurement and time of disintegration. The first 3 were determined by an Erweka MultiCheck apparatus, while friability tests were conducted in a Pharmatest PTFR-A analyzer and disintegration time was measured in a Pharmatest PTZ-Auto disintegration tester. All in all 10 tablets were examined by the MultiCheck, 6 tablets were studied by the PTZ-Auto and tablets with the sum weight of 6.5 g were evaluated by the PTFR-A. Friability tests were made according to the Pharmacopeias with 100 turns in 4 min [45].

2.6. Scanning Electron Microscopy (SEM) and Fiber Diameter Analysis

Sample morphology was studied by applying a JEOL 6380LVa (JEOL, Tokyo, Japan) type scanning electron microscope. Initially, the samples were secured by virtue of a conductive double-sided carbon adhesive tape, then were coated with an alloy consisting of gold-palladium prior to investigation. The applied accelerating voltage was between 15 and 25 kV, while the working distance was in the range of 12–16 mm. A randomized fiber diameter determination method developed in-house was implemented as described in our previous work [46], $n = 100$ measurements were made on each sample.

2.7. Differential Scanning Calorimetry (DSC)

The differential scanning calorimetry (DSC) experiments were made with a DSC 92 Setaram device (Caluire, France). The average sample weight of ~10–15 mg was placed in a closed aluminum pan. A nitrogen purge gas flow of 50 mL/min was used in all experiments. The temperature program started with a preliminary isothermal period that lasted for 1 min at 25 °C. Upon completion, a subsequent linear heating phase ensued from 25 °C to 200 °C at a rate of 10 °C/min. Purified indium standard was applied for calibration.

2.8. Raman Mapping

Raman mapping was performed using Horiba Jobin-Yvon LabRAM-type microspectrometer with external 785 nm diode laser source and Olympus BX-40 optical microscope. The laser beam was focused by an objective of 20 × (NA = 0.4) to the tablet surface. The confocal hole of 1000 μm was used in the confocal system. 950 groove/mm grating monochromator dispersed the backscattered light. The spectral range of 460–1680 cm^{-1} was detected as the relevant range with 5 cm^{-1} resolution. Spectral data were collected from 41 × 41 points with 25 μm step size. The acquisition time was 40 s and two spectra were averaged per point. The classical least squares (CLS) method was applied to calculate the concentration of the different materials. All reference spectra (excipients and ES samples) were recorded and the combination of these was used to approximate the spectra of the maps. The so-obtained coefficients were depicted in the maps.

2.9. Content Uniformity Analysis

Content uniformity (CU) was measured by UV-Vis spectrometry. Ten random tablets were individually put into 10 mL volumetric flasks where they were disintegrated in an acidic buffer (pH 1) within an ultrasonic bath in 15 min. Upon completion they were filtered by a 0.45 µm polytetrafluoroethylene (PTFE) syringe filter and the concentration of CAR in the acidic buffer (pH 1) was determined by a Hewlett-Packard HP 8453G UV-Vis spectrophotometer (Palo Alto, CA, USA) at a wavelength of 241 nm based on a former calibration.

2.10. Sieve Analysis

Sieve analyses were made on the pure ES material and the final powder mixtures by a Fritsch Analysette 3 Pro Vibratory Sieve Shaker (Idar-Oberstein, Germany). A total weight of 25 g was investigated in each case. The pure ES material and the final powder mixtures were sieved for 10 min with the amplitude set at 0.5. Upon completion, the sieved fractions were weighed and evaluated.

3. Results and Discussion

As briefly mentioned at the beginning of this paper, the goal was to achieve highly homogenous NASD containing tablets with low doses of API. By doing so, we could develop a standard method for producing high-quality electrospun products, which meet the requirements of the Pharmacopeias. Fiber morphology of the HSES fibers was studied and compared with SNES samples by SEM. CU was evaluated by UV-Vis spectrometry, while API distribution in the tablets was also studied with Raman mapping and final powder mixture homogeneity was evaluated by sieve analysis.

3.1. Electrospinning

The preparation of the ES samples is detailed in Table 2.

Table 2. Comparison of the details of manufacturing using SNES and HSES.

Sample	Preparation Method	Applied Solvent	Dissolved PVPVA64 and CAR (99:1) in 10 mL of Solvent (g)	Flow Rate (mL/h)	Productivity for Dried Material (g/h)
PVPVA64 +1% CAR SNES	Single-needle electrospinning	96% EtOH	4.00	6	1.8
PVPVA64 +1% CAR HSES	High-speed electrospinning	96% EtOH	4.00	750	225

Single-needle electrospinning (SNES) is the basic method for preparing NASD; however, its production rate (few grams of product an hour) is way too limited for industrial purposes and applications. Our results fell in line with these assessments since our fiber production with SNES was only 1.8 g per hour. On the other hand, HSES offered a much higher output rate resulting in 225 g of fiber production per hour. In both cases, 96% ethanol was adopted as the solvent since it is accepted by the Pharmacopeia. Using this new technology, it was possible to increase our productivity 125-fold in regard to the dried product. It is encouraging that the output could have been further increased, but in this case, it was only a secondary objective.

3.2. Fiber Morphology

Once the ES materials were obtained their morphology were investigated with SEM. The images are shown in Figure 2. Upon inspecting them the average diameter was 1.02 ± 1.00 µm and 0.80 ± 0.31 µm for the HSES and SNES samples, respectively. However, the HSES sample contained more beads indicating that further research is required to reach optimal morphology. This outcome is likely the result of the fiber-forming technology. No crystalline objects were visible in either case, suggesting their amorphous states.

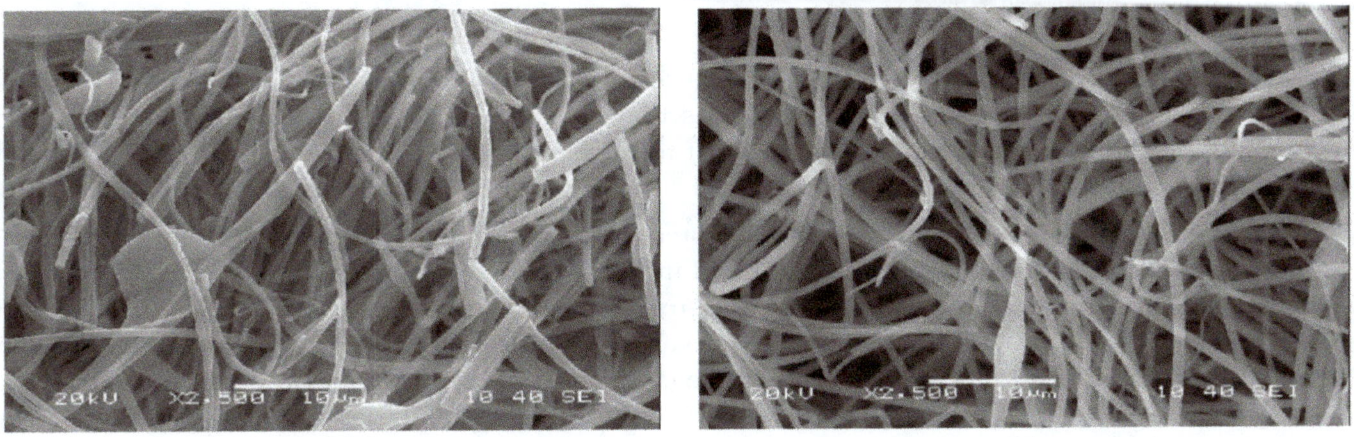

(a) (b)

Figure 2. Scanning electron microscopic images of PVPVA64 + 1% CAR fibers prepared by high-speed electrospinning (**a**) and single-needle electrospinning (**b**).

3.3. Differential Scanning Calorimetry

To examine the physical state of carvedilol in the electrospun samples, differential scanning calorimetry measurements were carried out. Physical mixture and pure polymer were used as reference.

The DSC curves are detailed in Figure 3.

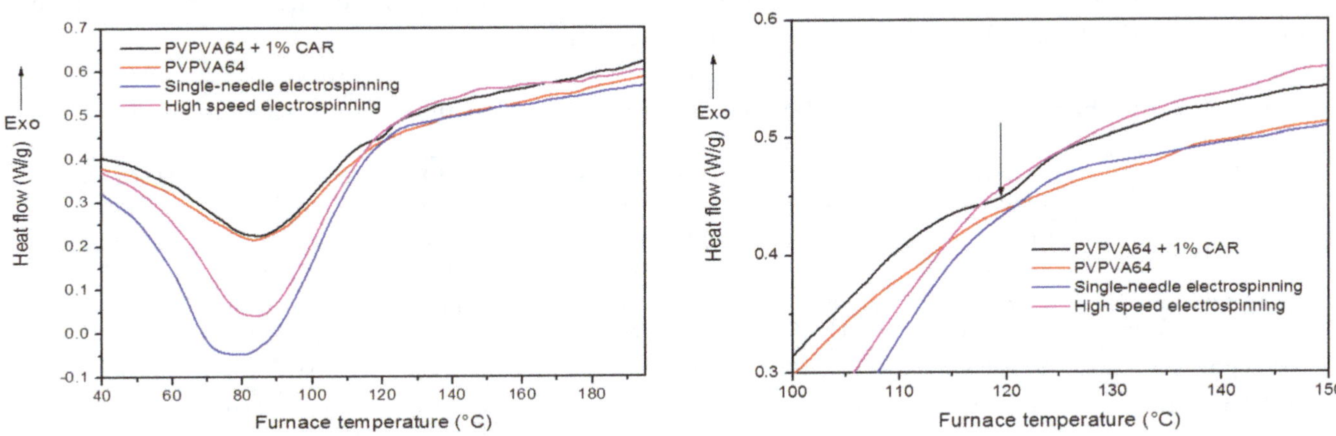

(a) (b)

Figure 3. (**a**,**b**) Differential scanning calorimetry (DSC) thermograms of PVPVA64, PVPVA64 + 1% CAR physical mixture and fibers prepared by single-needle and high-speed electrospinning.

According to the thermograms, no endotherm melting peaks of API origin were observable in the electrospun fibers and only a very slight curvature was detected at 120 degrees Celsius in the physical mixture (3.b). Based on these results, we can assume that this faint signal comes from the minimal amount of crystalline carvedilol melting in the aforementioned sample.

These data further indicate that total amorphization was achieved in both the scaled up (HSES) and regular (SNES) ES samples. The wide endotherm peaks at lower temperatures are related to water evaporation.

3.4. Tableting

Once the ES products proved to be amorphous, a direct compression (DC) technology was developed to compress them. DC technology is the safest, easiest and most economical way to produce tablets since it takes the least amount of toll on the ingredients through simple and short homogenization steps [47].

However, in order to successfully apply the technology, proper tableting materials are needed. For our purposes, as they are briefly summarized in Table 1, an amorphous lactose with exceptional flowability called Flowlac was co-processed with microcrystalline cellulose (with low water content < 1.5%). The application of this MCC subtype was preferable since ES products are hygroscopic. The adoption of both materials was desirable since (as it was described in our previous work [48]) the electrospun samples can adhere to their surfaces. Ultimately, this phenomenon sets the foundation to achieve proper homogenization.

Croscarmellose sodium, specifically developed for manufacturing tablets was used as the superdisintegrant. These agents provide superior disintegration properties compared to regular disintegrants while maintaining a low-dose (1–4%) in the formulation [49]. Lastly, Sodium stearyl fumarate (Pruv), was adopted to lubricate the tablets. It is a hydrophilic agent, that has advantages compared to magnesium stearate such as less sensitivity to over-lubrication [50].

For the DC technology only plastic bags, a high-shear mixer, and a tablet rotary press were required. Only the HSES samples were compressed into tablets since the production of sufficient amounts of ingredients by SNES would have taken days to fabricate. Overall, 6 batches were produced 4 of which contained ES product. Two were manually homogenized in plastic bags emulating industrial container homogenization and the other two were homogenized in an HSM. The final two batches contained crystalline carvedilol serving as reference. One was homogenized in LSM conditions and the other by HSM. The batch characteristics are detailed in Table 3.

Table 3. Batch characteristics and their IPC results (A and B are repetitions of the same technology).

Characteristics	LSM Reference	HSM Reference	LSM HSES Batch A	LSM HSES Batch B	HSM HSES Batch A	HSM HSES Batch B
API type	Crystalline CAR	Crystalline CAR	Electrospun CAR	Electrospun CAR	Electrospun CAR	Electrospun CAR
Method of homogenization	Manual (LSM)	High-shear (HSM)	Manual (LSM)	Manual (LSM)	High-shear (HSM)	High-shear (HSM)
Weight (mg)	99.9 ± 0.5	99.2 ± 0.7	99.2 ± 0.8	100.2 ± 0.7	100.9 ± 1.0	99.8 ± 1.1
Thickness (mm)	3.08 ± 0.44	3.02 ± 0.54	3.06 ± 0.69	3.04 ± 0.57	3.05 ± 0.60	3.03 ± 0.52
Hardness (N)	64.3 ± 7.62	69.2 ± 6.22	60.6 ± 5.67	63.8 ± 7.51	68.6 ± 5.11	62.7 ± 6.71
Diameter (mm)	5.97 ± 0.19	5.95 ± 0.22	5.97 ± 0.27	5.98 ± 0.17	5.99 ± 0.29	5.97 ± 0.21
Friability (%)	0.21	0.31	0.39	0.25	0.20	0.27
Disintegration (s)	84	95	103	119	138	125

The HSM suitable for executing multiple technological steps, such as homogenization, granulation, and drying, was expected to work well with the ES product [51]. Once the homogenizations were completed, the mixtures were compressed into tablets using a tablet rotary press without any problems. IPC tests were carried out to evaluate the oral dosage forms. The summary of the results is detailed in Table 3.

According to the IPC results, all batches had roughly the same properties without any unacceptable data. Friability was well below the 1% limit, while disintegration [52] was easily achieved within 30 min both criteria set by the Pharmacopeias.

3.5. Content Uniformity

The measured average API contents and their homogeneity are detailed in Table 4. The batches containing crystalline carvedilol yielded expected results with acceptable API content and high RSD values. These results can be linked to the low quantity of API (250 mg) applied and to the fact that the average particle size of crystalline carvedilol is quite large, that makes its proper homogenization quite difficult in such a small dose. This phenomenon could not be solved even in the HSM since SD and RSD values were still too high, 4.65 and 5.13 respectively. Out of the ES samples, the batches homogenized in HSM proved to be much better than the LSM tablets homogenized in plastic bags under low-shear conditions. To differentiate between the samples, additional measurements were carried out.

Table 4. UV-Vis results.

Sample Number	Carvedilol %					
	LSM Reference	HSM Reference	LSM ES A	LSM ES B	HSM ES A	HSM ES B
Average	98.76	97.68	94.19	93.21	97.63	96.71
SD (%)	7.43	4.65	9.50	6.80	2.04	2.49
RSD	7.52	5.13	10.08	7.30	2.09	2.58

3.6. Raman Mapping Results

To evaluate the homogeneity differences between LSM and HSM ES tablets, Raman maps were taken of the aforementioned solid dosage forms. Raman mapping is a non-destructive analytical method enabling API homogeneity measurements in pharmaceuticals [53]. Analyses were conducted on individual tablet surfaces, one from each batch.

Since directly searching for the API at such a low-dose (50 μg) with Raman spectrometry is a very challenging task, an indirect method was applied. Given the fact, that the API is molecularly dispersed in the PVPVA64 polymer matrix [54], we can assume that the homogeneity of the API is related to the homogeneity of the polymer. Consequently, the maps were taken accordingly. These results are shown in Figure 4.

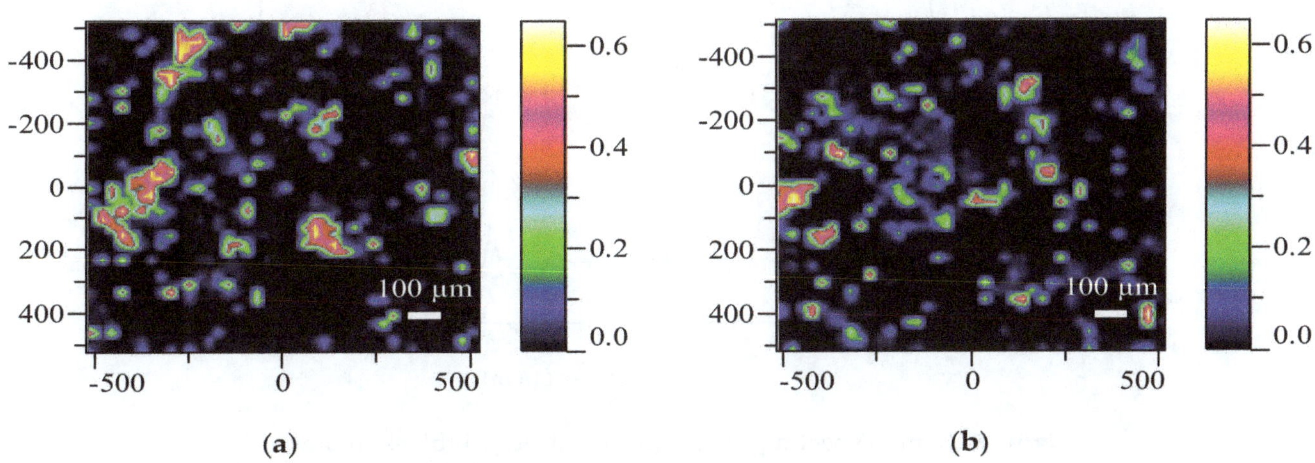

Figure 4. Raman maps of LSM (**a**) and HSM (**b**) ES tablets (colorful images show the distribution of the PVPVA64 polymer).

Upon inspecting the maps, the distribution of API could be indirectly investigated, but only slight differences were detected within the standalone tablets. This result indicates, that the API containing polymer is evenly distributed in the single solid dosage forms. However, this still does not explain the large inhomogeneity deviations discovered by the CU measurement, which is a result of evaluating multiple tablets at once.

3.7. *Sieve Analysis*

Since the analysis of single tablets did not clarify the deviations between the LSM and HSM, sieve analysis was chosen as an alternative method. A total weight of 25 g (the equivalent of 250 tablets) of LSM and HSM final powder mixtures along with the pure fibers were analyzed, whose results are detailed in Table 5. Both LSM and HSM tablets are mainly (more than 90%) made up of lactose and microcrystalline cellulose tableting materials, whose average particle sizes are 150 and 130 μm respectively.

Table 5. Sieve analysis results (the mixtures contain 5% ES material).

Sieve Size (μm)	Pure ES Material (g)	LSM Final Powder Mixture (g)	HSM Final Powder Mixture (g)
355	13.80	0.22	0.02
180	1.61	5.02	5.41
90	1.03	9.22	9.35
sub 90	8.56	10.54	10.22

According to the weighed sieve fractions, HSM homogenization was able to decrease the 355 μm portion by more than ten times compared to LSM mixing. This is crucial since the bulk of the pure electrospun materials was recovered on this sieve and, more importantly for complete homogenization, particle sizes should be as close to each other as possible to avoid segregation [55]. Based on these results, the high-performance impeller and chopper blades present in the HSM can further reduce the average particle sizes (due to high shear forces) of the fibrous materials, thus superior mixing of materials can be realized. These aforementioned fractions were also evaluated by Raman spectroscopy to look for traces of electrospun material. The spectra are shown in Figure 5.

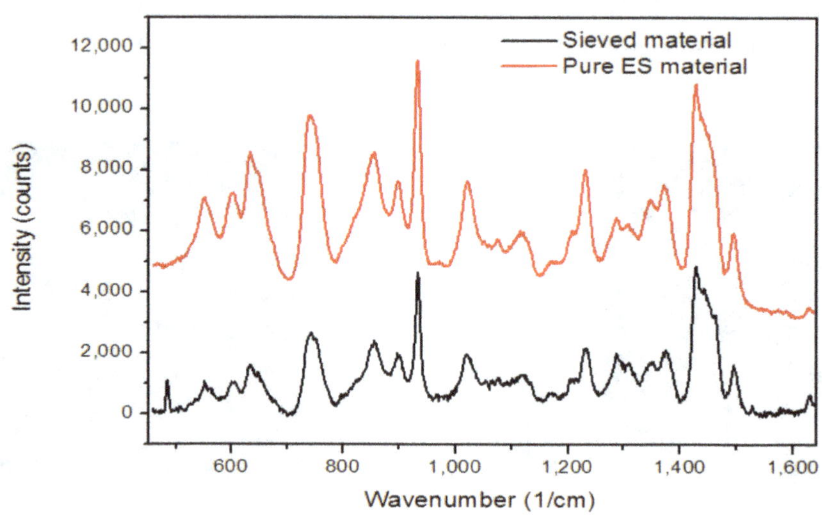

Figure 5. Raman spectra pure ES (red) and sieved (black) material.

It is clear that the spectrum of the sieved material is almost identical to the spectrum of the starting ES material ultimately proving that the API containing polymer was detected in the sieved mixture. In the end, this resulted in higher inhomogeneity among LSM tablets compared to HSM tablets. This outcome can be linked to Table 4 where the high SD and RSD values of the LSM tablets validate these findings.

Based on these results it is clear that a greater sample size was needed to be evaluated in order to identify the causes of homogeneity differences observed between the mixing methods. By implementing sieve analysis, the equivalent of 250 tablets could be screened, which enables broader examination compared to single tablet Raman mapping.

This outcome proves that the high-shear mixer coupled with the direct compression technology should be the first method of choice when proper homogenization of electrospun samples is required.

4. Conclusions

A low-dose, highly homogenous tablet formulation made from drug-loaded electrospun fibers was demonstrated by applying HSM homogenization. Carvedilol, an antihypertensive drug was used as the model API, while PVPVA64 was adopted as the matrix forming polymer. Electrospinning was carried out by HSES with increased productivity, while the SNES technology was applied as the reference. Homogenizations were made in plastic bags (LSM) and in an HSM, while tableting was performed by a tablet rotary press. Tablet batches containing crystalline carvedilol served as reference. Sieve analysis was used to study the particle size distribution in the final LSM and HSM powder mixtures. API content and homogeneity were measured by UV-Vis spectrometry, while the latter was also studied by Raman mapping.

HSM homogenization seems to be the preferred method of choice for preparing highly homogenous tablets containing electrospun NASDs. Their RSD values were much lower than their LSM counterparts. It is encouraging that this was achievable, despite setting a low API dose (50 μg) for the tablets. The technology can be scaled up easily, which could be truly beneficial for both academic researchers at universities and pharmaceutical technologists in the industry.

Author Contributions: G.F. designed and accomplished the experiments, like electrospinning and homogenization. A.F. performed and evaluated the Raman mapping measurements. A.B. carried out the SEM analysis, while B.F. performed and evaluated the fiber diameter measurements. E.B., B.D., and B.S. evaluated the results. Z.K.N. and G.M. finalized the manuscript.

Acknowledgments: This project was supported by the New Széchenyi Plan (project ID: TÁMOP-4.2.1/B-09/1/KMR-2010-0002), OTKA grant KH 124541, PD 116122, PD-121051, GINOP-2.1.1-15-2015-00541, ÚNKP-17-4-I and ÚNKP-17-4-II New National Excellence Program of the Ministry of Human Capacities, BME-KKP and the János Bolyai Research Scholarship of the Hungarian Academy of Sciences. This work was supported by the National Research, Development and Innovation in the frame of FIEK_16-1-2016-0007 (Higher Education and Industrial Cooperation Center) project.

References

1. Lieberman, H.A.; Lachman, L. *Pharmaceutical Dosage Forms: Tablets*; M. Dekker: New York, NY, USA, 1981.
2. Muselik, J.; Franc, A.; Dolezel, P.; Gonec, R.; Krondlova, A.; Lukasova, I. Influence of process parameters on content uniformity of a low dose active pharmaceutical ingredient in a tablet formulation according to GMP. *Acta Pharm.* **2014**, *64*, 355–367. [CrossRef] [PubMed]
3. US Pharmacopeia. Uniformity of Dosage Units/Content Uniformity. Available online: http://www.drugfuture.com/Pharmacopoeia/usp35/PDF/0420-0423%20[905]%20UNIFORMITY%20OF%20DOSAGE%20UNITS.pdf (accessed on 8 February 2017).
4. Baghel, S.; Cathcart, H.; O'Reilly, N.J. Polymeric amorphous solid dispersions: A review of amorphization, crystallization, stabilization, solid-state characterization, and aqueous solubilization of biopharmaceutical classification system class II drugs. *J. Pharm. Sci.* **2016**, *105*, 2527–2544. [CrossRef] [PubMed]
5. Paudel, A.; Worku, Z.A.; Meeus, J.; Guns, S.; Van den Mooter, G. Manufacturing of solid dispersions of poorly water soluble drugs by spray drying: Formulation and process considerations. *Int. J. Pharm.* **2013**, *453*, 253–284. [CrossRef] [PubMed]
6. Patil, H.; Tiwari, R.V.; Repka, M.A. Hot-melt extrusion: From theory to application in pharmaceutical formulation. *AAPS Pharm. Sci. Technol.* **2016**, *17*, 20–42. [CrossRef] [PubMed]

7. BioPharm. FDA Approves First Spray-Dried Biologic. Available online: http://www.biopharminternational.com/fda-approves-first-spray-dried-biologic (accessed on 7 May 2017).
8. Review, A.P. Recent Innovations in Pharmaceutical Hot Melt Extrusion. Available online: https://www.americanpharmaceuticalreview.com/Featured-Articles/179317-Recent-Innovations-in-Pharmaceutical-Hot-Melt-Extrusion/ (accessed on 4 June 2017).
9. Sosnik, A.; Seremeta, K.P. Advantages and challenges of the spray-drying technology for the production of pure drug particles and drug-loaded polymeric carriers. *Adv. Colloid Interface Sci.* **2015**, *223*, 40–54. [CrossRef] [PubMed]
10. Crowley, M.M.; Zhang, F.; Repka, M.A.; Thumma, S.; Upadhye, S.B.; Kumar Battu, S.; McGinity, J.W.; Martin, C. Pharmaceutical applications of hot-melt extrusion: Part I. *Drug Dev. Ind. Pharm.* **2007**, *33*, 909–926. [CrossRef] [PubMed]
11. Lee, S.L.; O'Connor, T.F.; Yang, X.; Cruz, C.N.; Chatterjee, S.; Madurawe, R.D.; Moore, C.M.V.; Yu, L.X.; Woodcock, J. Modernizing pharmaceutical manufacturing: From batch to continuous production. *J. Pharm. Innov.* **2015**, *10*, 191–199. [CrossRef]
12. Poechlauer, P.; Manley, J.; Broxterman, R.; Gregertsen, B.; Ridemark, M. Continuous processing in the manufacture of active pharmaceutical ingredients and finished dosage forms: An industry perspective. *Org. Process Res. Dev.* **2012**, *16*, 1586–1590. [CrossRef]
13. Vertex. FDA Approves Orkambi™ (Lumacaftor/Ivacaftor)—The First Medicine to Treat the Underlying Cause of Cystic Fibrosis for People Ages 12 and Older with Two Copies of the F508del Mutation. Available online: http://investors.vrtx.com/releasedetail.cfm?releaseid=920512 (accessed on 8 June 2017).
14. Pharmtech. EMA Approves Janssen Drug Made via Continuous Manufacturing. Available online: http://www.pharmtech.com/ema-approves-janssen-drug-made-continuous-manufacturing (accessed on 7 July 2017).
15. Pharmtech. Vertex Receives FDA Approval for Continuously Manufactured Drug Product. Available online: http://www.pharmtech.com/vertex-receives-fda-approval-continuously-manufactured-drug-product (accessed on 4 July 2017).
16. Lukáš, D.; Sarkar, A.; Martinová, L.; Vodsed' álková, K.; Lubasová, D.; Chaloupek, J.; Pokorný, P.; Mikeš, P.; Chvojka, J.; Komárek, M. Physical principles of electrospinning (electrospinning as a nano-scale technology of the twenty-first century). *Text. Prog.* **2009**, *41*, 59–140. [CrossRef]
17. Hutmacher, D.W.; Dalton, P.D. Melt electrospinning. *Chem. Asian J.* **2011**, *6*, 44–56. [CrossRef] [PubMed]
18. Reneker, D.H.; Yarin, A.L. Electrospinning jets and polymer nanofibers. *Polymer* **2008**, *49*, 2387–2425. [CrossRef]
19. Hu, X.; Liu, S.; Zhou, G.; Huang, Y.; Xie, Z.; Jing, X. Electrospinning of polymeric nanofibers for drug delivery applications. *J. Control. Release* **2014**, *185*, 12–21. [CrossRef] [PubMed]
20. Wang, Q.; Yu, D.-G.; Zhang, L.-L.; Liu, X.-K.; Deng, Y.-C.; Zhao, M. Electrospun hypromellose-based hydrophilic composites for rapid dissolution of poorly water-soluble drug. *Carbohydr. Polym.* **2017**, *174*, 617–625. [CrossRef] [PubMed]
21. Vuddanda, P.R.; Mathew, A.P.; Velaga, S. Electrospun nanofiber mats for ultrafast release of ondansetron. *React. Funct. Polym.* **2016**, *99*, 65–72. [CrossRef]
22. Illangakoon, U.E.; Gill, H.; Shearman, G.C.; Parhizkar, M.; Mahalingam, S.; Chatterton, N.P.; Williams, G.R. Fast dissolving paracetamol/caffeine nanofibers prepared by electrospinning. *Int. J. Pharm.* **2014**, *477*, 369–379. [CrossRef] [PubMed]
23. Lopez, F.L.; Shearman, G.C.; Gaisford, S.; Williams, G.R. Amorphous formulations of indomethacin and griseofulvin prepared by electrospinning. *Mol. Pharm.* **2014**, *11*, 4327–4338. [CrossRef] [PubMed]
24. Balogh, A.; Farkas, B.; Domokos, A.; Farkas, A.; Démuth, B.; Borbás, E.; Nagy, B.; Marosi, G.; Nagy, Z.K. Controlled-release solid dispersions of eudragit® FS 100 and poorly soluble spironolactone prepared by electrospinning and melt extrusion. *Eur. Polym. J.* **2017**, *95*, 406–417. [CrossRef]
25. Hamori, M.; Yoshimatsu, S.; Hukuchi, Y.; Shimizu, Y.; Fukushima, K.; Sugioka, N.; Nishimura, A.; Shibata, N. Preparation and pharmaceutical evaluation of nano-fiber matrix supported drug delivery system using the solvent-based electrospinning method. *Int. J. Pharm.* **2014**, *464*, 243–251. [CrossRef] [PubMed]
26. Shen, X.; Yu, D.; Zhu, L.; Branford-White, C.; White, K.; Chatterton, N.P. Electrospun diclofenac sodium loaded eudragit® l 100-55 nanofibers for colon-targeted drug delivery. *Int. J. Pharm.* **2011**, *408*, 200–207. [CrossRef] [PubMed]

27. Karthikeyan, K.; Guhathakarta, S.; Rajaram, R.; Korrapati, P.S. Electrospun zein/eudragit nanofibers based dual drug delivery system for the simultaneous delivery of aceclofenac and pantoprazole. *Int. J. Pharm.* **2012**, *438*, 117–122. [CrossRef] [PubMed]
28. Sill, T.J.; von Recum, H.A. Electrospinning: Applications in drug delivery and tissue engineering. *Biomaterials* **2008**, *29*, 1989–2006. [CrossRef] [PubMed]
29. Xue, J.; Xie, J.; Liu, W.; Xia, Y. Electrospun nanofibers: New concepts, materials, and applications. *Acc. Chem. Res.* **2017**, *50*, 1976–1987. [CrossRef] [PubMed]
30. Agarwal, S.; Wendorff, J.H.; Greiner, A. Use of electrospinning technique for biomedical applications. *Polymer* **2008**, *49*, 5603–5621. [CrossRef]
31. Nagy, Z.K.; Balogh, A.; Demuth, B.; Pataki, H.; Vigh, T.; Szabo, B.; Molnar, K.; Schmidt, B.T.; Horak, P.; Marosi, G.; et al. High speed electrospinning for scaled-up production of amorphous solid dispersion of itraconazole. *Int. J. Pharm.* **2015**, *480*, 137–142. [CrossRef] [PubMed]
32. Williams, G.R.; Chatterton, N.P.; Nazir, T.; Yu, D.G.; Zhu, L.M.; Branford-White, C.J. Electrospun nanofibers in drug delivery: Recent developments and perspectives. *Ther. Deliv.* **2012**, *3*, 515–533. [CrossRef] [PubMed]
33. Ignatious, F.; Sun, L.; Lee, C.P.; Baldoni, J. Electrospun nanofibers in oral drug delivery. *Pharm. Res.* **2010**, *27*, 576–588. [CrossRef] [PubMed]
34. Lukas, D.; Sarkar, A.; Pokorny, P. Self-organization of jets in electrospinning from free liquid surface: A generalized approach. *J. Appl. Phys.* **2008**, *103*, 084309. [CrossRef]
35. Sebe, I.; Szabó, B.; Nagy, Z.K.; Szabó, D.; Zsidai, L.; Kocsis, B.; Zelkó, R. Polymer structure and antimicrobial activity of polyvinylpyrrolidone-based iodine nanofibers prepared with high-speed rotary spinning technique. *Int. J. Pharm.* **2013**, *458*, 99–103. [CrossRef] [PubMed]
36. Raimi-Abraham, B.T.; Mahalingam, S.; Davies, P.J.; Edirisinghe, M.; Craig, D.Q.M. Development and characterization of amorphous nanofiber drug dispersions prepared using pressurized gyration. *Mol. Pharm.* **2015**, *12*, 3851–3861. [CrossRef] [PubMed]
37. Zhang, S.; Karaca, B.; Vanoosten, S.; Yuca, E.; Mahalingam, S.; Edirisinghe, M.; Tamerler, C. Coupling infusion and gyration for the nanoscale assembly of functional polymer nanofibers integrated with genetically engineered proteins. *Macromol. Rapid Commun.* **1322**, *36*, 1322–1328. [CrossRef] [PubMed]
38. Hong, X.; Mahalingam, S.; Edirisinghe, M. Simultaneous application of pressure-infusion-gyration to generate polymeric nanofibers. *Macromol. Mater. Eng.* **2017**, *302*, 1600564. [CrossRef]
39. Heseltine Phoebe, L.; Ahmed, J.; Edirisinghe, M. Developments in pressurized gyration for the mass production of polymeric fibers. *Macromol. Mater. Eng.* **2018**, 1800218. [CrossRef]
40. Hamori, M.; Nagano, K.; Kakimoto, S.; Naruhashi, K.; Kiriyama, A.; Nishimura, A.; Shibata, N. Preparation and pharmaceutical evaluation of acetaminophen nano-fiber tablets: Application of a solvent-based electrospinning method for tableting. *Biomed. Pharmacother.* **2016**, *78*, 14–22. [CrossRef] [PubMed]
41. Demuth, B.; Farkas, A.; Balogh, A.; Bartosiewicz, K.; Kallai-Szabo, B.; Bertels, J.; Vigh, T.; Mensch, J.; Verreck, G.; Van Assche, I.; et al. Lubricant-induced crystallization of itraconazole from tablets made of electrospun amorphous solid dispersion. *J. Pharm. Sci.* **2016**, *105*, 2982–2988. [CrossRef] [PubMed]
42. Poller, B.; Strachan, C.; Broadbent, R.; Walker, G.F. A minitablet formulation made from electrospun nanofibers. *Eur. J. Pharm. Biopharm.* **2017**, *114*, 213–220. [CrossRef] [PubMed]
43. Demuth, B.; Nagy, Z.K.; Balogh, A.; Vigh, T.; Marosi, G.; Verreck, G.; Van Assche, I.; Brewster, M.E. Downstream processing of polymer-based amorphous solid dispersions to generate tablet formulations. *Int. J. Pharm.* **2015**, *486*, 268–286. [CrossRef] [PubMed]
44. Vigh, T.; Démuth, B.; Balogh, A.; Galata, D.L.; Van Assche, I.; Mackie, C.; Vialpando, M.; Van Hove, B.; Psathas, P.; Borbás, E.; et al. Oral bioavailability enhancement of flubendazole by developing nanofibrous solid dosage forms. *Drug Dev. Ind. Pharm.* **2017**, *43*, 1126–1133. [CrossRef] [PubMed]
45. US Pharmacopeia. Tablet Friability. Available online: https://www.usp.org/sites/default/files/usp/document/harmonization/gen-chapter/g06_pf_ira_32_2_2006.pdf (accessed on 7 August 2017).
46. Balogh, A.; Farkas, B.; Farago, K.; Farkas, A.; Wagner, I.; Van Assche, I.; Verreck, G.; Nagy, Z.K.; Marosi, G. Melt-blown and electrospun drug-loaded polymer fiber mats for dissolution enhancement: A comparative study. *J. Pharm. Sci.* **2015**, *104*, 1767–1776. [CrossRef] [PubMed]
47. Pharmtech. Direct Compression Versus Granulation. Available online: http://www.pharmtech.com/direct-compression-versus-granulation (accessed on 7 September 2017).

48. Démuth, B.; Farkas, A.; Szabó, B.; Balogh, A.; Nagy, B.; Vágó, E.; Vigh, T.; Tinke, A.P.; Kazsu, Z.; Demeter, Á.; et al. Development and tableting of directly compressible powder from electrospun nanofibrous amorphous solid dispersion. *Adv. Powder Technol.* **2017**, *28*, 1554–1563. [CrossRef]
49. Battu, S.K.; Repka, M.A.; Majumdar, S.; Rao, Y.M. Formulation and evaluation of rapidly disintegrating fenoverine tablets: Effect of superdisintegrants. *Drug Dev. Ind. Pharm.* **2007**, *33*, 1225–1232. [CrossRef] [PubMed]
50. Shah, N.H.; Stiel, D.; Weiss, M.; Infeld, M.H.; Malick, A.W. Evaluation of two new tablet lubricants-sodium stearyl fumarate and glyceryl behenate. Measurement of physical parameters (compaction, ejection and residual forces) in the tableting process and the effect on the dissolution rate. *Drug Dev. Ind. Pharm.* **1986**, *12*, 1329–1346. [CrossRef]
51. Pharmaapproach. High-Shear Granulator. Available online: http://pharmapproach.com/high-shear-granulator/ (accessed on 1 August 2017).
52. EMA. Ich Topic q4b Annex 5 Disintegration Test General Chapter. Available online: http://www.ema.europa.eu/docs/en_GB/document_library/Scientific_guideline/2009/09/WC500003292.pdf (accessed on 2 September 2017).
53. Gordon, K.C.; McGoverin, C.M. Raman mapping of pharmaceuticals. *Int. J. Pharm.* **2011**, *417*, 151–162. [CrossRef] [PubMed]
54. Vo, C.L.-N.; Park, C.; Lee, B.-J. Current trends and future perspectives of solid dispersions containing poorly water-soluble drugs. *Eur. J. Pharm. Biopharm.* **2013**, *85*, 799–813. [CrossRef] [PubMed]
55. Williams, J.C. The segregation of particulate materials. A review. *Powder Technol.* **1976**, *15*, 245–251. [CrossRef]

4

Strategies for Hyaluronic Acid-Based Hydrogel Design in Drug Delivery

Sonia Trombino †, Camilla Servidio †, Federica Curcio and Roberta Cassano *

Department of Pharmacy, Health and Nutritional Science, University of Calabria, Arcavacata, 87036 Rende, Italy
* Correspondence: roberta.cassano@unical.it
† These authors contributed equally to this work.

Abstract: Hyaluronic acid (HA) is a natural, linear, endogenous polysaccharide that plays important physiological and biological roles in the human body. Nowadays, among biopolymers, HA is emerging as an appealing starting material for hydrogels design due to its biocompatibility, native biofunctionality, biodegradability, non-immunogenicity, and versatility. Since HA is not able to form gels alone, chemical modifications, covalent crosslinking, and gelling agents are always needed in order to obtain HA-based hydrogels. Therefore, in the last decade, different strategies for the design of physical and chemical HA hydrogels have been developed, such as click chemistry reactions, enzymatic and disulfide crosslinking, supramolecular assembly via inclusion complexation, and so on. HA-based hydrogels turn out to be versatile platforms, ranging from static to smart and stimuli-responsive systems, and for these reasons, they are widely investigated for biomedical applications like drug delivery, tissue engineering, regenerative medicine, cell therapy, and diagnostics. Furthermore, the overexpression of HA receptors on various tumor cells makes these platforms promising drug delivery systems for targeted cancer therapy. The aim of the present review is to highlight and discuss recent advances made in the last years on the design of chemical and physical HA-based hydrogels and their application for biomedical purposes, in particular, drug delivery. Notable attention is given to HA hydrogel-based drug delivery systems for targeted therapy of cancer and osteoarthritis.

Keywords: hyaluronic acid; hydrogel; cancer; drug delivery; click chemistry; biomaterial

---

1. Introduction

Hydrogels are three-dimensional, hydrated polymeric networks, formed by crosslinked hydrophilic polymers with a high affinity for water and biological fluids, capable of absorbing from 10% up to thousands of times their dry weight in water [1].

In recent years, thanks to their unique properties such as biocompatibility, biodegradability, flexibility, softness, etc., hydrogels have been widely investigated for biomedical applications like cell therapy, tissue engineering, drug delivery, and diagnostics [2]. For example, hydrogels made of pectin, carboxymethylcellulose and propylene glycol or polyethylene glycol (PEG) and propylene glycol are used as wound dressings [3,4], keratin- or polyvinyl alcohol-based hydrogels as scaffolds for cell growth [5,6], PEG-based hydrogel (DEXTENZA®), recently approved by the Food and Drug Administration, as ophthalmic inserts, etc. [7].

Among biopolymers, hyaluronic acid (HA) represents one of the most used in the design of hydrogels for biomedical applications due to its biocompatibility, native biofunctionality, biodegradability, non-immunogenicity, and versatility.

HA is a natural linear polysaccharide that consists of alternating units of D-glucuronic acid and *N*-acetyl-D-glucosamine, connected by β-1,3- and β-1,4-glycosidic bonds.

HA is a non-sulfated glycosaminoglycan that is widely found in the epithelial and connective tissues of vertebrates and it is the major component of the extracellular matrix (ECM) [8]. It is synthesized by hyaluronan synthase at the plasma membrane and it is then extruded to the extracellular matrix [9]. HA is found in a wide range of molecular weights from 20,000 up to several million Daltons, depending on the enzyme that catalyzes its synthesis.

Around 30% of HA present in the body is rapidly degraded by hyaluronidases and oxidative species, while the remaining 70% is catabolized by liver and lymphatic vessels endothelial cells, with tissue half-lives going from minutes in the bloodstream to weeks in cartilage [10]. Upon physiological conditions, HA is a polyanion associated with extracellular cations (Na^+, Ca^{2+}, Mg^{2+}, K^+) known as hyaluronan [11].

HA plays important physiological and biological roles in the human body. In the extracellular matrix of most tissues it contributes to maintain the tissue's mechanical integrity, homeostasis, viscoelasticity and lubrication thanks to its high molecular weight and its capacity to absorb a high quantity of water [12]. Furthermore, it also plays an important role in intracellular functions; in fact, it is able to regulate, due to its binding to cell surface specific receptors (such as CD44 or RHAMM), cell adhesion, migration, proliferation, and differentiation and, consequently, processes like inflammation, wound healing, tissue development, morphogenesis, tumor progression, and metastasis [13].

For these reasons, in recent years, hydrogels built from HA have been developed and investigated for biomedical applications like tissue regeneration, tissue engineering, drug delivery, gene therapy, diagnostics, etc.

Nowadays several HA-based hydrogels are already used in medicine as dermal fillers, viscosupplements, wound dressings, etc., and the market is continuously increasing worldwide. They are now progressing in their design to be responsive to several triggers, to have various features like stability, complex structures, and biochemical cues. The aim of the present review is to highlight and discuss recent advances made in the last years on the design of chemical and physical HA-based hydrogels and their application for biomedical purposes, in particular, drug delivery.

2. Physical and Chemical Hydrogels

Hydrogels can be classified into "physical" and "chemical" gels, depending on the type of bond that is formed between the polymer chains from which they derive.

Hydrogels are called "reversible" or "physical" if the networks are formed as a result of weak physical interactions between the macromolecular chains such as ionic, H-bonding, Van der Waals interactions, hydrophobic forces, or molecular entanglements [14].

Physical hydrogels can be synthesized by warming or cooling polymer solution, mixing solution of polyanion and polycation, combining polyelectrolyte with multivalent ions of opposite charge, etc. [1].

Physical hydrogels are often heterogeneous, unstable, and reversible; in fact, they are not able to maintain their structural integrity and dissolve easily by changing environmental factors like temperature, pH, etc.

Instead, hydrogels are called "permanent" or "chemical" if the polymeric chains are connected by covalent bonds [15]. For this reason, these materials, after swelling, retain their structural integrity, even if it is possible a degradation when particular bonds, sensitive to chemical or enzymatic hydrolysis, are present in the structure.

Chemical hydrogels can be generated by crosslinking polymers with radiations, chemical crosslinkers, polyfunctional compounds, free radical generating compounds, etc. [1]. Consequently, these systems have a better chemical, mechanical, and thermal stability compared to physical hydrogels.

Even though HA, due to its conformation and molecular weight, can form molecular networks in solution, it is not able to form physical gel alone. For this reason, chemical modifications, covalent crosslinking, and gelling agents are needed in order to obtain HA hydrogels.

HA turns out to be a functional and suitable polymer for chemical modification with reactive species due to its chemical structure; in particular, the chemical modifications concern three functional groups: the carboxylic acid group, the hydroxyl group, and the amino group (after deacetylation) [16].

This section reviews the different modified HA macromers and chemical techniques described in the literature in the last years used for the design of physical and chemical HA-based hydrogels.

2.1. Chemical Hydrogels

Chemical crosslinking turns out to be a versatile method to obtain hydrogels with excellent chemical, mechanical and thermal stability. However, this approach presents some limitations like the use of metal catalysts, photoinitiators, low reaction yield, etc. [17]. With regard to the chemical approach, HA-based hydrogels can be obtained via condensation reactions, enzymatic crosslinking, disulfide crosslinking, click chemistry, polymerization, etc. HA can be directly crosslinked by divinyl sulfone [18], glutaraldehyde [19], carbodiimide [20], bisepoxide [21], etc.; however, direct crosslinking cannot be considered suitable for hydrogels design since it requires harsh reaction condition, toxic by-products can be formed and the crosslinking agents used are cytotoxic. Nowadays, one of the most promising strategies for hydrogels preparation turns out to be click chemistry due to its high specificity, high yield, bioorthogonality, and mild reaction conditions [22].

2.1.1. Diels Alder Reaction (Click Chemistry)

In recent years, a particular interest has been addressed to the Diels–Alder reaction between furan and maleimide moieties for hydrogels design due to its selectivity, efficiency, and thermoreversibility [23].

In this regard, Fisher et al. recently developed a HA-based hydrogel with tunable properties to use as a platform to investigate breast cancer cells invasion. The hydrogel was obtained via a Diels–Alder click reaction between furan modified HA and bismaleimide functional peptides with the aim of mimicking ECM [24]. A similar approach was reported by Yu et al. in order to obtain a 3D patterned hydrogel. In this work Diels–Alder click chemistry has been used in order to get a HA-based hydrogel that can be subsequently subjected to thiol-ene photocoupling allowing its spatiotemporal patterning [25].

2.1.2. Azide-Alkyn Huisgen Cycloaddition (Click Chemistry)

The Huisgen reaction is a cycloaddition between an azide and an alkyne to produce triazoles which requires the presence of a catalyst (Cu^+) as reported by Rostovtsev et al. [26]. In recent years it has become one of the most used strategies for hydrogels preparation thanks to its high yield, efficiency, excellent bioorthogonality, fast reaction rate, etc. [27,28]. For example, Manzi et al. fabricated nanohydrogels based on derivatives of HA and riboflavin obtained by Cu^+ catalyzed Huisgen cycloaddition [29].

Despite the various advantages offered by this reaction, the use of copper as a catalyst can be problematic since it is a cytotoxic element. However, recently, it has been observed that cyclooctyne functionalized molecules are able to react rapidly with azide without the presence of copper [30]. This alternative reaction, called strain-promoted azide-alkyne cycloaddition, is currently more used for hydrogels design since it presents biosafety as well as the advantages of the previous reaction. On this matter, Fu et al. fabricated an injectable HA-PEG based hydrogel [31]. In particular, cyclooctyne modified HA was synthesized by reacting HA with 2-(aminoethoxy)cyclooctyne (Figure 1); subsequently, it was reacted with azide functionalized PEG in order to obtain the hydrogel. Interestingly, the resulting hydrogel showed fast gelation time, excellent mechanical properties, and high stability.

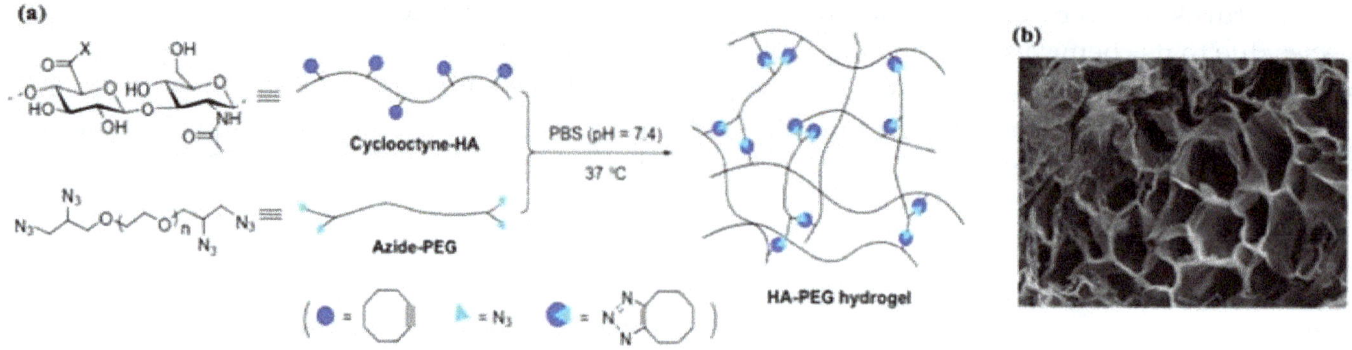

Figure 1. Preparation of the HA-PEG hydrogel (**a**), SEM image of the hydrogel (**b**) [31]. Reproduced with permission from Elsevier, 2017.

2.1.3. Thiol-ene Photocoupling (Click Chemistry)

The thiol-ene reaction consists of a radical addition (induced by light) between a thiol and enes which has a high yield, efficiency, specificity and a fast reaction rate [32]. This method is particularly attractive for hydrogels preparation because it is solvent free and allows the hydrogels spatiotemporal control; for this reason, it is particularly investigated for the design of hydrogels to use as scaffolds for tissue engineering and cell culture or as drug delivery systems [33,34]. Different vinyl groups are employed for thiol-ene click chemistry like norbornene [35], vinyl sulfone [36], maleimide, etc. The thiol-norbornene reaction is characterized by greater specificity compared to the use of other functional groups. For example, Gramlich et al. employed this method for the synthesis of a photopatterned HA-based hydrogel by reacting norbornene modified HA (NorHA) with dithiothreitol (Figure 2) [37]. Hydrogels with an elastic modulus ranging from 1000 Pa to 70,000 Pa were obtained by varying the quantity of crosslinker. Furthermore, they reported that a secondary thiol-norbornene reaction can be performed to the hydrogel by reducing the initial amount of crosslinker.

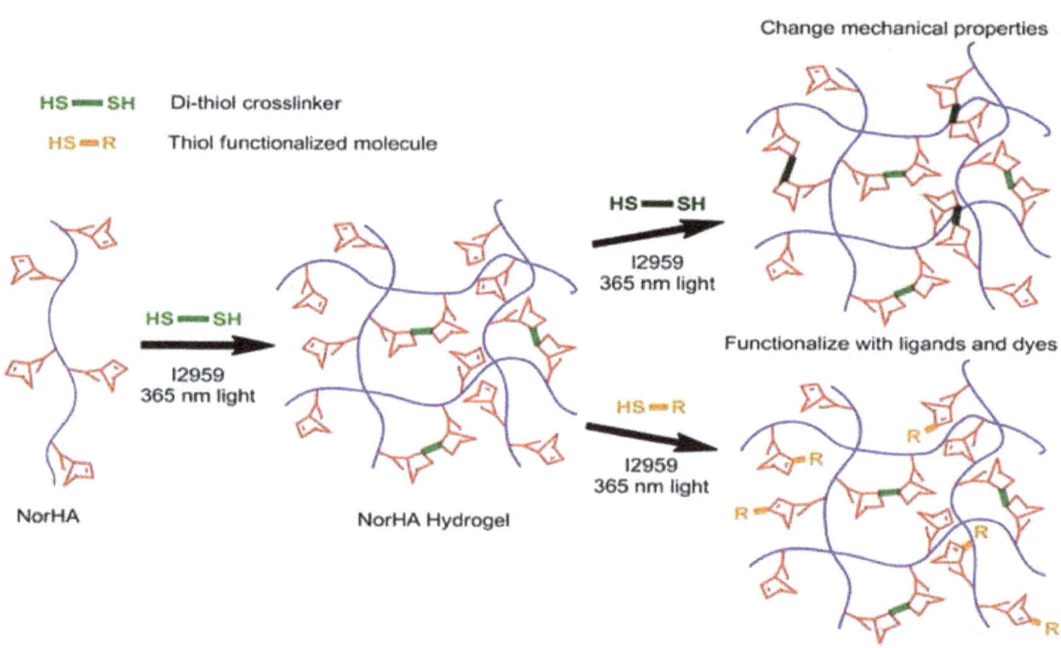

Figure 2. Synthesis scheme of hydrogel [37]. Reproduced with permission from Elsevier, 2013.

In this context, we also find the thiol-Michael addition which, however, is characterized by lower orthogonality. In this regard, Khetan et al. designed and prepared a 3D hydrogel via a two step crosslinking process: firstly, via a thiol-Michael addition between methacrylate-maleimide functionalized HA and thiols of peptides and, subsequently, via methacrylates photopolymerization [38].

2.1.4. Aldehyde-Hydrazide Coupling (Click Chemistry)

The aldehyde-hydrazide reaction has currently attracted interest in hydrogels design due to its high efficiency, cytocompatibility, simplicity, reversibility, and mild reaction conditions [39–41]. In particular, covalent hydrazone crosslinked hydrogels seem to be a promising approach for tissue engineering. In this regard, Chen et al. recently developed an injectable HA-pectin based hydrogel, by reacting HA adipic dihydrazide with biofunctionalized pectin-dialdehyde, and investigated its use as a scaffold for cartilage tissue engineering (Figure 3) [42]. Interestingly, the resulting hydrogel exhibited a fast gelation rate, good mechanical properties, biocompatibility, and cytocompatibility that make it a potential platform suitable for tissue regeneration. To further improve the structural integrity of hydrazone crosslinked hydrogels, Wang et al. recently reported the design and the preparation of an elastin-like protein/HA-based hydrogel by combining two different crosslinking processes (covalent and thermal) [43]. Firstly, the hydrogel was obtained via an aldehyde-hydrazide coupling between hydrazine modified elastin-like protein and aldehyde modified HA; the use of a thermoresponsive protein allowed a secondary thermal crosslinking that improved its structural integrity and stability. The resulting hydrogel showed shear-thinning and self-healing properties, easy injectability and protection of cells from the mechanical stress of injection and for these reasons can be considered a promising candidate for stem cells delivery.

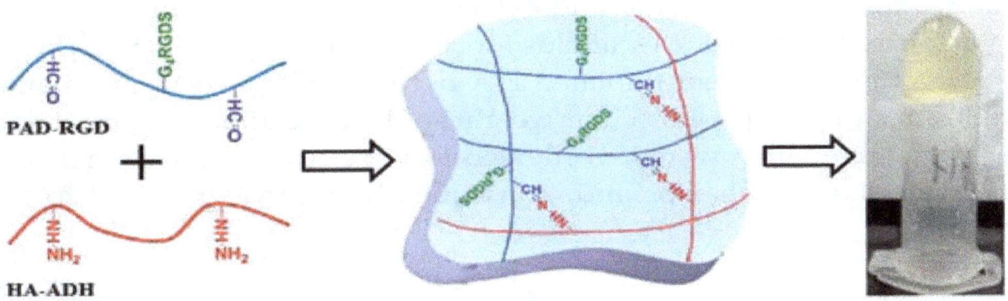

Figure 3. Hydrogels synthetic scheme [42]. Reproduced with permission from Elsevier, 2017.

2.1.5. Enzymatic Crosslinking

Enzymatic crosslinking represents an interesting approach for HA-based hydrogels preparation because it is characterized by mild reaction condition, fast gelation rate and leads to obtaining hydrogels with excellent mechanical properties [44,45]. Among different enzymes, horseradish peroxidase (HRP) turns out to be one of the most employed; it is usually employed in combination with hydrogen peroxide and the reaction can be summarized as follows: $2Ph + H_2O_2 \rightarrow 2Ph\cdot + H_2O$ [46]. In literature are reported various tyramine modified HA-based hydrogels which are formed as a result of an enzymatic crosslinking process that occurs through oxidation of tyramine which causes the formation of di-tyramine bonds [47]. In this regard, Xu et al. designed and fabricated HA-tyramine hydrogels by crosslinking tyramine moieties of HA in the presence of HRP and hydrogen peroxide (Figure 4) [48]. By varying the amounts of the enzyme and hydrogen peroxide, hydrogels with different mechanical strength were formed and were investigated in order to obtain a stable scaffold for stem cells culture. Interestingly, it was observed that the hydrogel with an elastic modulus of 350 Pa supported the proliferation of stem cells. A similar approach was reported by Raia et al. that enzymatically crosslinked tyramine functionalized HA and silk fibroin in order to increase the mechanical strength and the stability of tyramine-HA-based hydrogels [49]. By changing polymers concentration, hydrogels with tunable properties were obtained, resulting in versatile platforms that can be employed for various applications in tissue engineering.

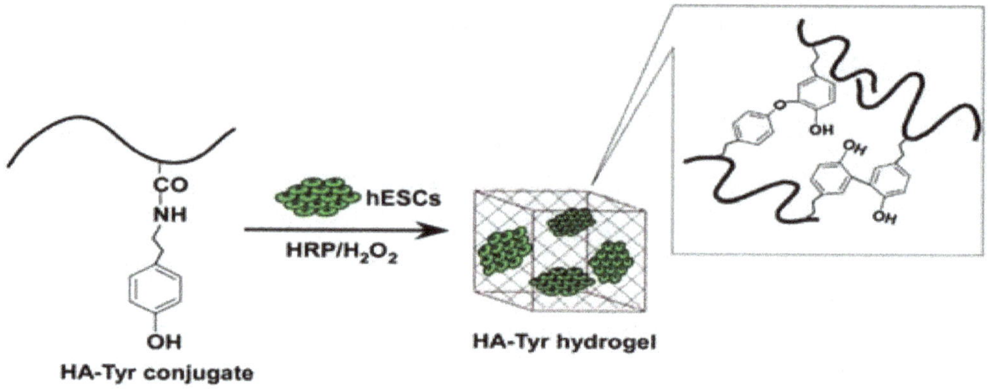

Figure 4. Schematic representation of hydrogels preparation and of encapsulation of human embryonic stem cells (hESCs) [48]. Reproduced with permission from Elsevier, 2015.

2.1.6. Disulfide Crosslinking

In the last years, disulfide crosslinked hydrogels have attracted growing attention because this crosslinking method presents various advantages such as biosafety, ease of execution, reversibility and permits to obtain hydrogels with *in-situ* gelation properties and responsiveness to reductant stimuli. Generally, disulfide bonds are formed via oxidation of thiols induced by air or oxidating agents like Cu(II)SO_4 [50]. Disulfide crosslinked HA hydrogels are currently investigated for tissue regeneration thanks to their degradability since they can be cleaved enzymatically by hyaluronidase and by physiological reductants like glutathione and cysteine [51]. For example, Bian et al. proposed self-crosslinking HA-based hydrogels as scaffolds for cell culture (Figure 5) [52]. They were prepared through exposition to air of different thiolated HA derivatives which were obtained by varying the degree of thiol substitution and molecular weights of HA. Gelation rate, mechanical properties, swelling degree, and degradation were investigated and the resulting hydrogel showed excellent biocompatibility, degradation behavior and, consequently, a great potential for applications in tissue engineering.

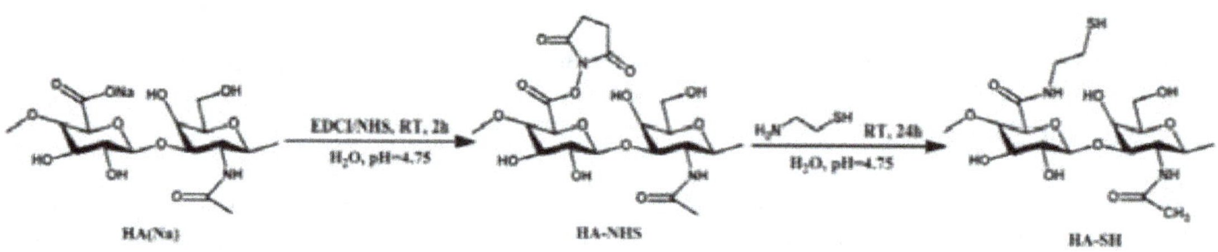

Figure 5. Synthesis scheme of thiol modified HA [52]. Reproduced with permission from Elsevier, 2016.

However, disulfide crosslinking presents some disadvantages like long reaction times, the presence of strong oxidants, etc. To overcome these limitations, an interesting strategy for disulfide crosslinked HA hydrogels preparation has been recently proposed by Velasco et al. [53]. Herein, the authors investigated the effects of the presence of various electron-withdrawing groups at the β position of thiol modified HA (cysteine, *N*-acetyl-L-cysteine). Interestingly, HA functionalized with cysteine or *N*-acetyl-L-cysteine showed fast gelation rate at physiological pH, while HA-thiol did not form any gel in the same conditions. Furthermore, the resulting hydrogels showed excellent mechanical properties and hydrolytic stability.

2.1.7. Crosslinking by Radical Polymerization

Hydrogels can be formed via radical polymerization of monomers in the presence of crosslinking agents and an initiator like a redox pair or a photoinitiator [54]. Methacrylates represent the most common groups used for HA-based hydrogels preparation and they can be introduced to HA by reacting it with glycidyl methacrylate or methacrylic anhydride [55,56]. An advantage of methacrylated HA-based hydrogels is that it is possible to tune their properties by varying HA molecular weight, the concentration of the functional monomer, the degree of substitution, etc. [57]. In this regard, Tavsanli et al. developed silk/HA-based hydrogels and investigated their mechanical properties [58]. The hydrogels were prepared by reacting methacrylated HA (MeHA) and silk fibroin (SF) in aqueous solution in the presence of *N,N,N′,N′*-tetramethylethylenediamine (TEMED), ammonium persulfate (APS), and *N,N*-dimetylacrylamide (DMMA) which has the function of connecting methacrylated HA macromers via their vinyl groups (Figure 6). Interestingly, the resulting hydrogels showed bicompatibility, excellent mechanical properties and stability thanks to the presence of SF since its β-sheet domains act as physical crosslinks.

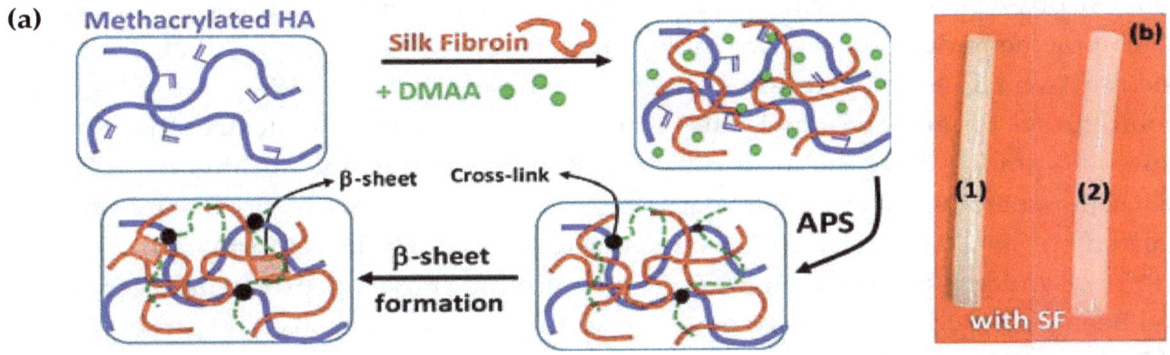

Figure 6. Schematic formation of HA-SF based hydrogel (**a**) and photographs of hydrogels with SF (**b**) [58]. Adapted with permission from Elsevier, 2019.

2.1.8. Crosslinking by Condensation Reactions

Condensation reactions are often applied for hydrogels synthesis. Considering the chemical structure of HA, among the different condensation reactions, esterification turns out to be one of the most commonly employed for hydrogels design. In this regard, Larrañeta et al. recently developed an attractive eco-friendly strategy for the synthesis of HA-based hydrogels [59]. For this purpose, Gantrex S97 was used as crosslinking agent and the hydrogels were obtained via esterification between the hydroxyl groups of HA and the carboxylic groups of Gantrex S97 (Figure 7). Since the reaction takes place in solid phase inside a microwave or an oven, the process can be considered green because it does not need organic solvents or toxic substances. Furthermore, the release capabilities and the antimicrobial properties were investigated. Interestingly, the resulting hydrogel showed a sustained release and anti-infective properties resulting in a promising candidate for the design of drug delivery systems and wound dressings.

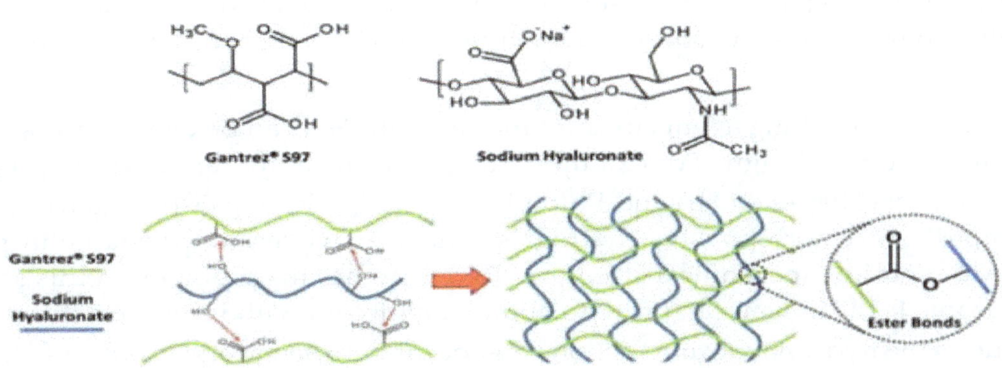

Figure 7. Schematic crosslinking mechanism between sodium hyaluronate and Gantrez® S97 [59]. Reproduced with permission from Elsevier, 2018.

2.2. Physical Hydrogels

In recent years, non-covalent bonds and supramolecular interactions have been widely investigated for hydrogels design thanks to their singular features. First of all, since these interactions are reversible, the non-covalent assembly allows to obtain hydrogels with tunable properties and responsivity to various cues like light, pH, temperature, etc. [60,61]. In contrast to covalent crosslinking, physical crosslinking leads to the formation of less mechanically and chemically stable hydrogels. However, this aspect can be considered an advantageous feature since it can be exploited in order to obtain hydrogels with shear-thinning and self-healing properties [17].

In this context, inclusion complexation represents one of the most used strategies for the preparation of physical gels. It can be considered the result of supramolecular interactions and structural complementarity between two molecules called "host" and "guest" [62]. Cyclodextrins are one of the most widely employed hosts which have hydrophobic cavities with a high affinity for hydrophobic guests. Several guest molecules employed in pair with cyclodextrins have been reported in literature and among these the most representative is adamantane. In this regard, Rodell et al. designed a self-assembling HA hydrogel based on supramolecular interactions between adamantane functionalized HA and β-cyclodextrin functionalized HA [63]. Hydrogel formation occurred rapidly by mixing host and guest molecules in aqueous solution. Physical properties were investigated and it has been observed that were dependent on the crosslink density and structure that can be modified by varying host and guest concentrations, molar ratio, etc. The obtained hydrogel displayed shear-thinning properties resulting in a promising injectable system. Another investigated pair for inclusion complexation broadly reported in literature is represented by α- or β-cyclodextrin and azobenzenes since *trans*-azobenzene has a high binding affinity for α- or β-cyclodextrin, while *cis*-azobenzene has a low binding affinity for them. On this subject, Rosales et al. recently developed a supramolecular HA-based hydrogel using HA functionalized with β-cyclodextrin and azobenzene [64]. It has been shown that it is possible to modulate hydrogel properties with light; in fact, upon irradiation ($\lambda = 365$ nm), isomerization of azobenzene occurs changing the binding affinity between host/guest molecules and, consequently, the network connectivity and the elastic modulus of the hydrogel. Furthermore, the release capabilities were investigated, highlighting the possibility to tune drugs release profile with light exposure. A similar approach was reported by Rowland et al. using cucurbit [8] uril and cysteine-phenylalanine as host/guest pair in order to obtain a supramolecular HA-based hydrogel [65]. Another interesting non-covalent approach for HA-based hydrogels design is represented by functionalization of HA with hydrophobic molecules in order to render it amphiphilic and consequently determine the macromers self assembly in nanogels. In this regard, Montanari et al. designed HA-based hydrogels via self-assembly of macromers in water after the functionalization of HA with cholesterol [66]. In particular, the self-assembly of macromers occurs due to the hydrophobic interactions between the cholesterol cores and the hydrophilic interactions between the shells formed by HA.

Moreover, the use of gelling agents in combination with HA can be considered a valid strategy for HA physical hydrogels design. For example, Jung et al. recently reported the preparation of a thermosensitive hydrogel based on HA and Pluronic F-127 [67]. Pluronic F-127 is a triblock copolymer able to form rapidly thermoresponsive hydrogels which, however, are unstable in physiological conditions due to their low mechanical strength. To overcome this problem, in this study HA was mixed with Pluronic F-127 in water in order to obtain a hydrogel with improved structural integrity and stability due to the hydrophobic interactions that occur between acetyl groups of HA and methyl groups of Pluronic F-127. Interestingly, the resulting hydrogel not only showed an increased mechanical strength but also a sustained drug release, reducing the typical burst release observed in Pluronic F-127-based hydrogels.

3. HA-Based Hydrogels for Biomedical Applications

Currently, HA-based hydrogels are widely investigated for biomedical purposes like drug delivery, tissue engineering, regenerative medicine thanks to their biocompatibility, biodegradability, non–immunogenicity, responsivity to various cues, and tunable properties [68–70]. This section reviews the main biomedical applications of HA-based hydrogels reported in literature in the last few years, focusing in particular on drug delivery.

3.1. *Drug Delivery*

HA-based hydrogels are particularly interesting for drug delivery since, in addition to above cited features, allow to have a controlled and targeted drug release in response to different triggers that turns out to be attractive when aiming for targeted therapy [71,72].

3.1.1. Stimuli-Responsive Hydrogels

Various smart hydrogels responsive to different environmental factors such as pH, temperature, light, biochemical molecules have been developed as drug delivery systems. With regard to stimuli-responsive platforms, physical crosslinking is preferred since supramolecular interactions are reversible and consequently results easier to tune hydrogels properties.

In this context, Highley et al. recently proposed an interesting strategy for the design of a near infrared light (NIR)/temperature responsive platform [73]. In this study, the platform was prepared in a microfluidic mixing device by combining gold nanorods with a HA supramolecular hydrogel obtained via the inclusion complexation of β-cyclodextrin and adamantane. The presence of nanorods caused heating in response to NIR irradiation causing consequently the breakage of supramolecular interactions and the networks disruption. The release capability of the resulting platform in response to different NIR exposures was evaluated, and interestingly it has been observed that the drug release can be modulated by varying two parameters: irradiation time, and light intensity; specifically, the quantity of the molecule released from the platform increased with increasing power and irradiation time.

Inclusion complexation employing azobenzene/cyclodextrin as host/guest pair has been broadly investigated for photoresponsive hydrogels design since the supramolecular host/guest interactions can be disrupted upon *trans-cis* photoisomerization of azobenzene induced by ultraviolet (UV) light [74]. An interesting example of a photoresponsive drug delivery platform has been described by Rosales et al. [64]. Thus, HA was functionalized with azobenzene and β-cyclodextrin in order to obtain self-assembled hydrogels. The resulting hydrogels showed reversible changes in crosslink density and, consequently, in mesh size, upon UV exposures. These changes were exploited to modulate drug release profiles and, therefore, the release capability upon different UV irradiations was evaluated. In particular, a fluorescently labeled protein was loaded as a model drug and it has been observed that upon irradiation hydrogels released a double amount of protein compared to the non irradiated ones.

Even if physical crosslinking is preferred for smart hydrogels preparation, also the chemical approach has been recently investigated. In this regard, Kwon et al. reported the preparation of pH-sensitive hydrogels based on hydroxyethyl cellulose and hyaluronic acid and investigated their potential use as transdermal delivery systems for the treatment of skin lesions [75]. In this study, the hydrogels were synthesized via Michael addition between HA and hydroxyethyl cellulose by using divinyl sulfone as crosslinking agent and their physicochemical properties were investigated. Hydrogels were then loaded with isoliquiritigenin, which has antimicrobial activity, and its release efficiency has been investigated by in vitro measurements at different values of pH. Experimental data showed that the quantity of isoliquiritigenin released increased with increasing pH beyond 7 due to electrostatic repulsions between the carboxylate groups of HA that cause consequently an increase of mesh size.

3.1.2. HA-Based Hydrogels for Targeted Cancer Treatment

As already reported, HA regulates different cellular functions such as cell adhesion, differentiation, migration, proliferation, etc., which arise as a result of HA binding to specific membrane surface receptors, called hyaldherins, like CD44, LYVE-1, and RHAMM [76]. In particular, CD44 is the main receptor involved in cellular proliferation, differentiation, and migration pathways and consequently in tumor progression and metastasis; moreover, it is overexpressed in various types of tumors like melanoma, chondrosarcoma, breast, gastrointestinal, prostate, bladder, lung, and pancreatic cancers, and different studies have reported a relationship between CD44 expression and poor prognosis [77]. For these reasons, HA has recently emerged as a promising molecule for the design of anticancer drug delivery systems for active targeting of malignant tumors [78]. Comprehensive reviews by Huang et al. and Choi et al. supply an interesting description of HA-based drug delivery systems developed for targeted cancer treatment [79,80].

In the last years, several HA-based hydrogels have been studied for the delivery of different antitumor drugs such as doxorubicin, paclitaxel, cisplatin, etc., in order to improve their antitumor activity and reduce their systemic side effects [81,82]; some of the most interesting and recent examples will now be presented.

Aiming at preparing a suitable drug delivery platform for the targeted release of doxorubicin, Yang et al. prepared various HA-based nanogels via copolymerization of methacrylated HA with di(ethylene glycol) diacrylate [83]. Nanogels with a diameter of about 70 nm and a spherical shape were obtained, which were then loaded with doxorubicin by an incubation method. In vitro studies showed a CD44-dependent cellular uptake and consequently a greater internalization of nanogels in tumor cell lines that overexpress CD44 receptor (Figure 8).

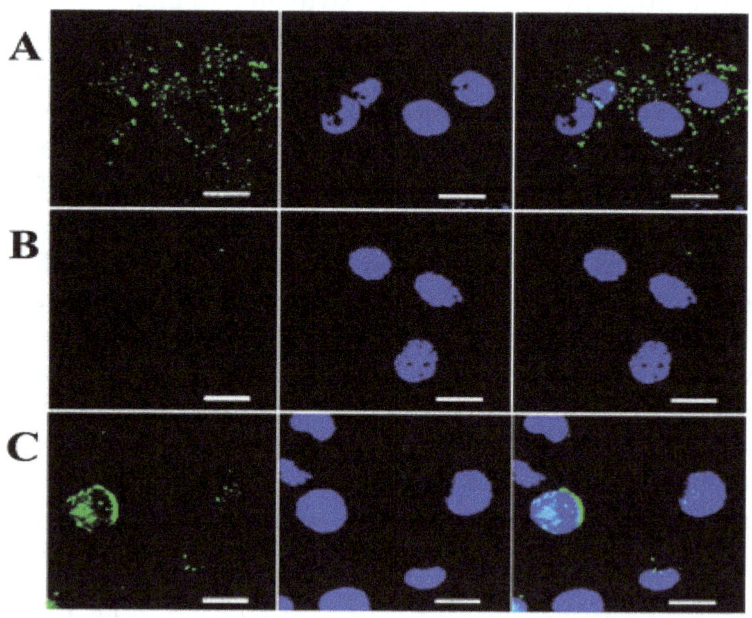

Figure 8. Confocal laser scanning microscopy of (**a**) A549, (**b**) NIHT3T, and (**c**) H22 cells incubated with FITC-labeled HA nanogels [83], The scale bar =10μm. Reproduced with permission from Elsevier, 2015.

Furthermore, the nanogels showed higher accumulation in the tumor site and a superior antitumor activity compared with the free doxorubicin, resulting in a promising drug delivery system for cancer therapy.

A noteworthy further example of doxorubicin delivery platform has been reported by Jhan et al. [84]. In this study, injectable thermosensitive hydrogels based on Pluronic F-127 and HA-doxorubicin nanocomplexes were prepared via physical mixing and their physiochemical properties were investigated. The doxorubicin release profile was studied in vitro, while nanogels antitumor activity both in vivo and in vitro. Experimental data showed a pH sensitive and sustained release of doxorubicin from hydrogels with a faster release rate at tumoral pH. Moreover, hydrogels showed an excellent cytotoxic activity against tumor cell lines that overexpress CD44 receptor and a high affinity targeting to the lymphonodes, resulting in promising injectable formulations for the treatment of local and metastatic tumors.

Furthermore, in this context, an efficient approach for metastatic breast cancer treatment has been recently described by Chen et al. [85]. In particular, the authors prepared saporin loaded epidermal growth factor receptor (EGFR) and CD44 dual targeted HA nanogels by combining inverse nanoprecipitation and tetrazole-alkene photocoupling. Nanogels with a diameter of about 160 nm and a spherical shape were obtained and evaluated for the treatment of metastatic breast cancer. In vitro studies showed an excellent internalization of nanogels in 4T1 breast cancer cell line that overexpresses both EGFR and CD44. Furthermore, in vivo studies in metastatic 4T1-luc breast tumor bearing mice displayed that the nanogels enhanced the therapeutic efficacy of saporin, showing an excellent inhibition of tumor growth and lung metastasis.

Currently intraperitoneal (IP) chemotherapy is emerging as an efficient strategy for the treatment of solid tumors present in the peritoneal cavity [86]. However, the delivery systems suitable for the IP chemotherapy should have some requirements like biocompatibility, biodegradability, non-immunogenicity and the capacity to control the drug release. Since HA hydrogels have these features, they are now also studied for the design of drug delivery platforms for IP chemotherapy. In this regard, Cho et al. recently reported the design of in situ crosslinkable HA-based gels and evaluated their potential use as IP carriers of platinum for the treatment of ovarian cancer [87]. Firstly, they prepared platinum loaded nanoparticles that were incorporated in HA-based hydrogels obtained via the aldehyde-hydrazide coupling. The obtained platforms showed sustained platinum release, good anti-tumor activity and a long permanence in the peritoneal cavity resulting attractive for IP chemotherapy of ovarian cancer.

Unfortunately, one problem that can occur sometimes when using hydrogels as drug delivery systems is the burst release [88]; with the attempt to reduce the burst release of drugs from hydrogels, Zhang et al. proposed an innovative strategy for HA-based hydrogels design [89]. In this regard, they prepared multilayer hydrogel capsules based on chitosan, HA and doxorubicin via the ionotropic crosslinking method. Release studies concerning these hydrogels showed a pH-sensitive, controlled release of doxorobucin with a notable reduction of the burst release due to their particular structure; in fact, the multilayer structure reduced the drug concentration gradient between the capsules external layer and the surrounding environment limiting the release of doxorubicin adsorbed on the surface of the hydrogels.

3.1.3. HA-Based Hydrogels for Osteoarthritis Treatment

Osteoarthritis is an inflammatory, chronic joint disorder characterized by progressive cartilage erosion. Currently, osteoarthritis treatment is limited to anti-inflammatory drugs administration, viscosupplementation and, if necessary, prosthesis graft at the last stage [90].

As already reported, HA performs multiple biological functions: at the articular level, thanks to its viscoelasticity, it acts as a lubricant, increasing the viscosity of the synovial fluid, and as a cushioning, allowing the separation of the articular surfaces under load.

HA presents also chondroprotective and anti-inflammatory effects [91]. Furthermore, some studies reported the overexpression of CD44 receptor on human articular chondrocytes [92]. For these reasons, HA-based hydrogels are widely investigated and used as viscosupplements and delivery platforms for osteoarthritis treatment.

In this regard, Jung et al. recently reported the preparation of an injectable thermosensitive hydrogel via physical mixing of HA and Pluronic F-127 [67]. As previously reported, Pluronic F-127 is a gelling agent able to rapidly form thermoresponsive hydrogels that however are instable in physiological conditions due to their low mechanical strength. To overcome this problem, in this study,

HA was physically mixed with Pluronic F-127 in order to obtain a hydrogel with improved structural integrity and stability due to the hydrophobic interactions that occur between HA and Pluronic. The hydrogel was then loaded with piroxicam and evaluated for the treatment of osteoarthritis. In Vitro release studies showed a 10 days sustained and slow release of piroxicam from HA-Pluronic F-127 hydrogel, while Pluronic F-127 based hydrogels displayed a faster release behavior (Figure 9). Furthermore, in vivo pharmacokinetic studies reported an increase of drug bioavailability and half-life in comparison to a commercial Paclitaxel formulation.

(a) (b)

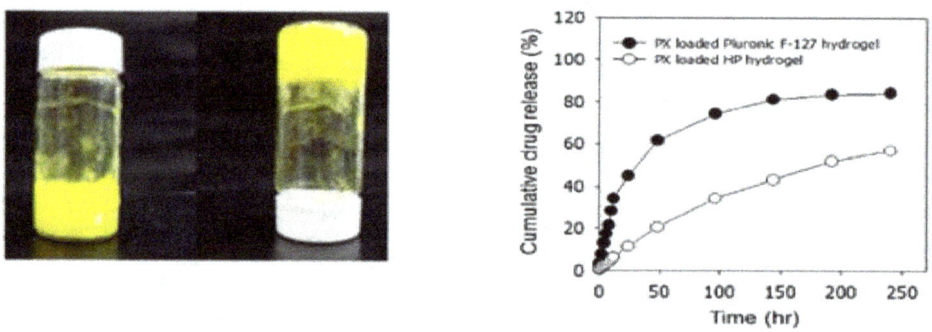

Figure 9. Photographs of the hydrogel (**a**) and in vitro Paclitaxel release from Pluronic F-127 and Pluronic F-127/HA-based hydrogels (**b**) [67]. Reproduced with permission from Elsevier, 2016.

In addition to the classical therapeutic approaches, nowadays gene silencing of signal molecules, proteins, enzymes, that play an important role in osteoarthritis degenerative events, is emerging as a promising strategy for osteoarthritis treatment.

In this regard, Cai et al. recently developed a HA-based hydrogel loaded with gapmer antisense oligonucleotides that was studied for silencing target gene expression in osteoarthritis [93]. In particular, the hydrogel was prepared via Schiff reaction between aldehyde modified HA and chitosan, and subsequently, it was loaded with a gapmer oligonucleotide, obtaining a high encapsulation efficiency (~97%), in order to reduce COX-2 expression. In vitro studies showed a sustained release of COX-2 gapmer up to five days with a low burst release and, furthermore, a 10–14 days long COX-2 gene silencing activity in osteoarthritis chondrocytes. A similar approach was recently reported by Garcia et al. in order to obtain a HA-based hydrogel for the delivery of chondrocytes and antisense oligonucleotides [94]. In this case hydrogels made of HA and fibrin were loaded with an antisense oligonucleotide in order to modulate the expression of genes that codify for ADAMTS (A Disintegrin and Metallo Proteinase with Thrombospondin Motifs) enzymes which showed to play a key role in causing proteoglycans loss in osteoarthritis [95]; chondrocytes were also incorporated in the scaffolds in order to have both regenerative and therapeutic effects. In Vitro studies showed 14-day long sustained release and an efficient and long genes inhibition in both incorporated and resident chondrocytes. These features make this platform a potential formulation for osteoarthritis treatment.

4. Conclusions

In recent decades, HA has emerged as an attractive molecule for hydrogels design thanks to its biocompatibility, native biofunctionality, biodegradability, non-immunogenicity, and versatility. Nowadays, several HA-based hydrogels are already used in medicine as dermal fillers, viscosupplements, wound dressings, etc., and the market is continuously increasing worldwide.

Since HA is not able to form gels alone, new crosslinking methods, like click chemistry reactions, disulfide crosslinking, enzymatic crosslinking, or supramolecular assembly methods like inclusion complexation, functionalization with lipophilic molecules, etc., have been widely investigated resulting in efficient strategies for chemical and physical hydrogels design. However, these current synthetic strategies present several advantages as well as some limitations. For example, various chemical crosslinking techniques often require organic solvents, metal catalysts, reaction by-product can be formed, etc. Thus, in this respect, research is aimed at developing new advantageous synthetic strategies.

HA-based hydrogels turn out to be versatile platforms ranging from passive and static matrices to smart, stimuli-responsive platforms with tunable properties and consequently they showed to have great potential as drug delivery systems, scaffolds for tissue engineering and regenerative medicine, and so on. In particular, their tunability is exploited for the design of platforms for controlled and targeted drug delivery; in this regard, a notable attention is given to inclusion complexation employing cyclodextrin and azobenzene as a host/guest pair, which allows obtaining phototoresponsive drug delivery systems. Furthermore, since HA receptors were found to be overexpressed on various tumor cells and on chondrocytes, different HA-based hydrogels have been broadly developed for these purposes, showing promising results for targeted cancer and osteoarthritis therapies.

Nowadays, one of the main goals is the design of intelligent hydrogels with various features like stability, complex structures, biochemical cues and responsive to several triggers that, surely, will find a place into clinical practice.

References

1. Hoffman, A.S. Hydrogels for biomedical applications. *Adv. Drug Deliv. Rev.* **2012**, *64*, 18–23. [CrossRef]
2. Seliktar, D. Designing cell-compatible hydrogels for biomedical applications. *Science* **2012**, *336*, 1124–1128. [CrossRef] [PubMed]
3. ConvaTec Website. Available online: https://www.convatec.it/ (accessed on 12 June 2019).
4. Covidien Website. Available online: https://www.covidien.com/ (accessed on 12 June 2019).
5. Blanchard, C.R.; Timmons, S.F.; Smith, R.A. Keratin-Based Hydrogel for Biomedical Applications and Method of Production. U.S. Patent 6,379,690 B2, 30 April 2002.
6. Kumar, A. Hydrogel scaffolds for tissue engineering. U.S. Patent 2013/0236971 A1, 12 September 2013.
7. Ocular Therapeutix Website. Available online: https://www.ocutx.com/products/dextenza/ (accessed on 12 June 2019).
8. Fraser, J.R.E.; Laurent, T.C.; Laurent, U. Hyaluronan: Its nature, distribution, functions and turnover. *J. Intern. Med.* **1997**, *242*, 27–33. [CrossRef] [PubMed]
9. Prehm, P. Hyaluronate is synthesized at plasma membranes. *Biochem. J.* **1984**, *220*, 597–600. [CrossRef] [PubMed]
10. Fallacara, A.; Baldini, E.; Manfredini, S.; Vertuani, S. Hyaluronic acid in the third millennium. *Polymers* **2018**, *10*, 701. [CrossRef]
11. Laurent, T.C.; Fraser, J. Hyaluronan. *FASEB J.* **1992**, *6*, 2397–2404. [CrossRef]
12. Dicker, K.T.; Gurski, L.A.; Pradhan-Bhatt, S.; Witt, R.L.; Farach-Carson, M.C.; Jia, X. Hyaluronan: A simple polysaccharide with diverse biological functions. *Acta Biomater.* **2014**, *10*, 1558–1570. [CrossRef]
13. Toole, B.P. Hyaluronan: From extracellular glue to pericellular cue. *Nat. Rev. Cancer* **2004**, *4*, 528. [CrossRef]
14. Ahmed, E.M. Hydrogel: Preparation, characterization, and applications: A review. *J. Adv. Res.* **2015**, *6*, 105–121. [CrossRef]
15. Caló, E.; Khutoryanskiy, V.V. Biomedical applications of hydrogels: A review of patents and commercial products. *Eur. Polym. J.* **2015**, *65*, 252–267. [CrossRef]
16. Schanté, C.E.; Zuber, G.; Herlin, C.; Vandamme, T.F. Chemical modifications of hyaluronic acid for the synthesis of derivatives for a broad range of biomedical applications. *Carbohydr. Polym.* **2011**, *85*, 469–489. [CrossRef]
17. Appel, E.A.; del Barrio, J.; Loh, X.J.; Scherman, O.A. Supramolecular polymeric hydrogels. *Chem. Soc. Rev.* **2012**, *41*, 6195–6214. [CrossRef] [PubMed]
18. Ibrahim, S.; Kang, Q.K.; Ramamurthi, A. The impact of hyaluronic acid oligomer content on physical, mechanical, and biologic properties of divinyl sulfone-crosslinked hyaluronic acid hydrogels. *J. Biomed. Mater. Res. Part A* **2010**, *94*, 355–370. [CrossRef] [PubMed]
19. Crescenzi, V.; Francescangeli, A.; Taglienti, A. New gelatin-based hydrogels via enzymatic networking. *Biomacromolecules* **2002**, *3*, 1384–1391. [CrossRef] [PubMed]

20. Kuo, J.W.; Swann, D.A.; Prestwich, G.D. Chemical modification of hyaluronic acid by carbodiimides. *Bioconj. Chem.* **1991**, *2*, 232–241. [CrossRef]
21. Segura, T.; Anderson, B.C.; Chung, P.H.; Webber, R.E.; Shull, K.R.; Shea, L.D. Crosslinked hyaluronic acid hydrogels: A strategy to functionalize and pattern. *Biomaterials* **2005**, *26*, 359–371. [CrossRef]
22. Jiang, Y.; Chen, J.; Deng, C.; Suuronen, E.J.; Zhong, Z. Click hydrogels, microgels and nanogels: Emerging platforms for drug delivery and tissue engineering. *Biomaterials* **2014**, *35*, 4969–4985. [CrossRef]
23. Gandini, A. The furan/maleimide Diels–Alder reaction: A versatile click–unclick tool in macromolecular synthesis. *Prog. Polym. Sci.* **2013**, *38*, 1–29. [CrossRef]
24. Fisher, S.A.; Anandakumaran, P.N.; Owen, S.C.; Shoichet, M.S. Tuning the microenvironment: Click-crosslinked hyaluronic acid-based hydrogels provide a platform for studying breast cancer cell invasion. *Adv. Funct. Mater.* **2015**, *25*, 7163–7172. [CrossRef]
25. Yu, F.; Cao, X.; Li, Y.; Chen, X. Diels–Alder click-based hydrogels for direct spatiotemporal postpatterning via photoclick chemistry. *ACS Macro Lett.* **2015**, *4*, 289–292. [CrossRef]
26. Rostovtsev, V.V.; Green, L.G.; Fokin, V.V.; Sharpless, K.B. A stepwise huisgen cycloaddition process: Copper (I)-catalyzed regioselective "ligation" of azides and terminal alkynes. *Angew. Chem. Int. Ed.* **2002**, *41*, 2596–2599. [CrossRef]
27. Pahimanolis, N.; Sorvari, A.; Luong, N.D.; Seppälä, J. Thermoresponsive xylan hydrogels via copper-catalyzed azide-alkyne cycloaddition. *Carbohydr. Polym.* **2014**, *102*, 637–644. [CrossRef] [PubMed]
28. Gong, T.; Adzima, B.J.; Baker, N.H.; Bowman, C.N. Photopolymerization reactions using the photoinitiated Copper (I)-Catalyzed Azide-Alkyne Cycloaddition (CuAAC) reaction. *Adv. Mater.* **2013**, *25*, 2024–2028. [CrossRef] [PubMed]
29. Manzi, G.; Zoratto, N.; Matano, S.; Sabia, R.; Villani, C.; Coviello, T.; Matricardi, P.; Di Meo, C. "Click" hyaluronan based nanohydrogels as multifunctionalizable carriers for hydrophobic drugs. *Carbohydr. Polym.* **2017**, *174*, 706–715. [CrossRef] [PubMed]
30. Laughlin, S.T.; Baskin, J.M.; Amacher, S.L.; Bertozzi, C.R. In vivo imaging of membrane-associated glycans in developing zebrafish. *Science* **2008**, *320*, 664–667. [CrossRef]
31. Fu, S.; Dong, H.; Deng, X.; Zhuo, R.; Zhong, Z. Injectable hyaluronic acid/poly (ethylene glycol) hydrogels crosslinked via strain-promoted azide-alkyne cycloaddition click reaction. *Carbohydr. Polym.* **2017**, *169*, 332–340. [CrossRef]
32. Hoyle, C.E.; Lee, T.Y.; Roper, T. Thiol–enes: Chemistry of the past with promise for the future. *J. Polym. Sci. Part A Polym. Chem.* **2004**, *42*, 5301–5338. [CrossRef]
33. Sawicki, L.A.; Kloxin, A.M. Design of thiol–ene photoclick hydrogels using facile techniques for cell culture applications. *Biomater.Sci.* **2014**, *2*, 1612–1626. [CrossRef]
34. Yang, C.; Mariner, P.D.; Nahreini, J.N.; Anseth, K.S. Cell-mediated delivery of glucocorticoids from thiol-ene hydrogels. *J. Controll. Release* **2012**, *162*, 612–618. [CrossRef]
35. Fairbanks, B.D.; Schwartz, M.P.; Halevi, A.E.; Nuttelman, C.R.; Bowman, C.N.; Anseth, K.S. A versatile synthetic extracellular matrix mimic via thiol-norbornene photopolymerization. *Adv. Mater.* **2009**, *21*, 5005–5010. [CrossRef]
36. Lutolf, M.; Hubbell, J. Synthetic biomaterials as instructive extracellular microenvironments for morphogenesis in tissue engineering. *Nat. Biotechnol.* **2005**, *23*, 47. [CrossRef]
37. Gramlich, W.M.; Kim, I.L.; Burdick, J.A. Synthesis and orthogonal photopatterning of hyaluronic acid hydrogels with thiol-norbornene chemistry. *Biomaterials* **2013**, *34*, 9803–9811. [CrossRef]
38. Khetan, S.; Guvendiren, M.; Legant, W.R.; Cohen, D.M.; Chen, C.S.; Burdick, J.A. Degradation-mediated cellular traction directs stem cell fate in covalently crosslinked three-dimensional hydrogels. *Nat. Mater.* **2013**, *12*, 458. [CrossRef]
39. Yan, S.; Wang, T.; Feng, L.; Zhu, J.; Zhang, K.; Chen, X.; Cui, L.; Yin, J. Injectable in situ self-cross-linking hydrogels based on poly (L-glutamic acid) and alginate for cartilage tissue engineering. *Biomacromolecules* **2014**, *15*, 4495–4508. [CrossRef]
40. Tian, W.; Zhang, C.; Hou, S.; Yu, X.; Cui, F.; Xu, Q.; Sheng, S.; Cui, H.; Li, H. Hyaluronic acid hydrogel as Nogo-66 receptor antibody delivery system for the repairing of injured rat brain: In vitro. *J. Controll. Release* **2005**, *102*, 13–22. [CrossRef]

41. Ito, T.; Fraser, I.P.; Yeo, Y.; Highley, C.B.; Bellas, E.; Kohane, D.S. Anti–inflammatory function of an in situ cross–linkable conjugate hydrogel of hyaluronic acid and dexamethasone. *Biomaterials* **2007**, *28*, 1778–1786. [CrossRef]
42. Chen, F.; Ni, Y.; Liu, B.; Zhou, T.; Yu, C.; Su, Y.; Zhu, X.; Yu, X.; Zhou, Y. Self–crosslinking and injectable hyaluronic acid/RGD–functionalized pectin hydrogel for cartilage tissue engineering. *Carbohydr. Polym.* **2017**, *166*, 31–44. [CrossRef]
43. Wang, H.; Zhu, D.; Paul, A.; Cai, L.; Enejder, A.; Yang, F.; Heilshorn, S.C. Covalently adaptable elastin-like protein–hyaluronic acid (ELP–HA) hybrid hydrogels with secondary thermoresponsive crosslinking for injectable stem cell delivery. *Adv. Funct. Mater.* **2017**, *27*, 1605609. [CrossRef]
44. Kurisawa, M.; Lee, F.; Wang, L.S.; Chung, J.E. Injectable enzymatically crosslinked hydrogel system with independent tuning of mechanical strength and gelation rate for drug delivery and tissue engineering. *J. Mater. Chem.* **2010**, *20*, 5371–5375. [CrossRef]
45. Tran, N.Q.; Joung, Y.K.; Lih, E.; Park, K.M.; Park, K.D. Supramolecular hydrogels exhibiting fast in situ gel forming and adjustable degradation properties. *Biomacromolecules* **2010**, *11*, 617–625. [CrossRef]
46. Roberts, J.J.; Naudiyal, P.; Lim, K.S.; Poole–Warren, L.A.; Martens, P.J. A comparative study of enzyme initiators for crosslinking phenol–functionalized hydrogels for cell encapsulation. *Biomater. Res.* **2016**, *20*, 30. [CrossRef]
47. Rizzuto, F.; Spikes, J.D. The eosin-sensitized photooxidation of substituted phenylalanines and tyrosines. *Photochem. Photobiol.* **1977**, *25*, 465–476. [CrossRef]
48. Xu, K.; Narayanan, K.; Lee, F.; Bae, K.H.; Gao, S.; Kurisawa, M. Enzyme–mediated hyaluronic acid–tyramine hydrogels for the propagation of human embryonic stem cells in 3D. *Acta Biomater.* **2015**, *24*, 159–171. [CrossRef]
49. Raia, N.R.; Partlow, B.P.; McGill, M.; Kimmerling, E.P.; Ghezzi, C.E.; Kaplan, D.L. Enzymatically crosslinked silk–hyaluronic acid hydrogels. *Biomaterials* **2017**, *131*, 58–67. [CrossRef]
50. Su, J. Thiol–mediated chemoselective strategies for in situ formation of hydrogels. *Gels* **2018**, *4*, 72. [CrossRef]
51. Choh, S.-Y.; Cross, D.; Wang, C. Facile synthesis and characterization of disulfide–cross–linked hyaluronic acid hydrogels for protein delivery and cell encapsulation. *Biomacromolecules* **2011**, *12*, 1126–1136. [CrossRef]
52. Bian, S.; He, M.; Sui, J.; Cai, H.; Sun, Y.; Liang, J.; Fan, Y.; Zhang, X. The self–crosslinking smart hyaluronic acid hydrogels as injectable three–dimensional scaffolds for cells culture. *Coll. Surf. B Biointerfaces* **2016**, *140*, 392–402. [CrossRef]
53. Bermejo-Velasco, D.; Azémar, A.; Oommen, O.P.; Hilborn, J.N.; Varghese, O.P. Modulating Thiol pKa promotes disulfide formation at physiological pH: An elegant strategy to design disulfide cross–linked hyaluronic acid hydrogels. *Biomacromolecules* **2019**, *20*, 1412–1420. [CrossRef]
54. Hennink, W.E.; van Nostrum, C.F. Novel crosslinking methods to design hydrogels. *Adv. Drug Deliv. Rev.* **2012**, *64*, 223–236. [CrossRef]
55. Ibrahim, S.; Kothapalli, C.; Kang, Q.; Ramamurthi, A. Characterization of glycidyl methacrylate–crosslinked hyaluronan hydrogel scaffolds incorporating elastogenic hyaluronan oligomers. *Acta Biomater.* **2011**, *7*, 653–665. [CrossRef]
56. Poldervaart, M.T.; Goversen, B.; De Ruijter, M.; Abbadessa, A.; Melchels, F.P.; Öner, F.C.; Dhert, W.J.; Vermonden, T.; Alblas, J. 3D bioprinting of methacrylated hyaluronic acid (MeHA) hydrogel with intrinsic osteogenicity. *PloS ONE* **2017**, *12*, e0177628. [CrossRef]
57. Burdick, J.A.; Chung, C.; Jia, X.; Randolph, M.A.; Langer, R. Controlled degradation and mechanical behavior of photopolymerized hyaluronic acid networks. *Biomacromolecules* **2005**, *6*, 386–391. [CrossRef]
58. Tavsanli, B.; Okay, O. Mechanically robust and stretchable silk/hyaluronic acid hydrogels. *Carbohydr. Polym.* **2019**, *208*, 413–420. [CrossRef]
59. Larrañeta, E.; Henry, M.; Irwin, N.J.; Trotter, J.; Perminova, A.A.; Donnelly, R.F. Synthesis and characterization of hyaluronic acid hydrogels crosslinked using a solvent–free process for potential biomedical applications. *Carbohydr. Polym.* **2018**, *181*, 1194–1205. [CrossRef]
60. Zheng, Z.; Hu, J.; Wang, H.; Huang, J.; Yu, Y.; Zhang, Q.; Cheng, Y. Dynamic softening or stiffening a supramolecular hydrogel by ultraviolet or near–infrared light. *ACS Appl. Mater. Interfaces* **2017**, *9*, 24511–24517. [CrossRef]

61. Rombouts, W.H.; de Kort, D.W.; Pham, T.T.; van Mierlo, C.P.; Werten, M.W.; de Wolf, F.A.; van der Gucht, J. Reversible temperature–switching of hydrogel stiffness of coassembled, silk–collagen–like hydrogels. *Biomacromolecules* **2015**, *16*, 2506–2513. [CrossRef]
62. Chen, G.; Jiang, M. Cyclodextrin–based inclusion complexation bridging supramolecular chemistry and macromolecular self–assembly. *Chem. Soc. Rev.* **2011**, *40*, 2254–2266. [CrossRef]
63. Rodell, C.B.; Kaminski, A.L.; Burdick, J.A. Rational design of network properties in guest–host assembled and shear–thinning hyaluronic acid hydrogels. *Biomacromolecules* **2013**, *14*, 4125–4134. [CrossRef]
64. Rosales, A.M.; Rodell, C.B.; Chen, M.H.; Morrow, M.G.; Anseth, K.S.; Burdick, J.A. Reversible control of network properties in azobenzene–containing hyaluronic acid–based hydrogels. *Bioconj. Chem.* **2018**, *29*, 905–913. [CrossRef]
65. Rowland, M.J.; Atgie, M.; Hoogland, D.; Scherman, O.A. Preparation and supramolecular recognition of multivalent peptide–polysaccharide conjugates by cucurbit [8] uril in hydrogel formation. *Biomacromolecules* **2015**, *16*, 2436–2443. [CrossRef]
66. Montanari, E.; D'arrigo, G.; Di Meo, C.; Virga, A.; Coviello, T.; Passariello, C.; Matricardi, P. Chasing bacteria within the cells using levofloxacin–loaded hyaluronic acid nanohydrogels. *Eur. J. Pharm. Biopharm.* **2014**, *87*, 518–523. [CrossRef]
67. Jung, Y.-S.; Park, W.; Park, H.; Lee, D.-K.; Na, K. Thermo–sensitive injectable hydrogel based on the physical mixing of hyaluronic acid and Pluronic F–127 for sustained NSAID delivery. *Carbohydr. Polym.* **2017**, *156*, 403–408. [CrossRef]
68. Huang, G.; Huang, H. Application of hyaluronic acid as carriers in drug delivery. *Drug Deliv.* **2018**, *25*, 766–772. [CrossRef]
69. Hemshekhar, M.; Thushara, R.M.; Chandranayaka, S.; Sherman, L.S.; Kemparaju, K.; Girish, K.S. Emerging roles of hyaluronic acid bioscaffolds in tissue engineering and regenerative medicine. *Int. J. Biol. Macromol.* **2016**, *86*, 917–928. [CrossRef]
70. Liu, Z.; Tang, M.; Zhao, J.; Chai, R.; Kang, J. Looking into the future: Toward advanced 3D biomaterials for stem-cell-based regenerative medicine. *Adv. Mater.* **2018**, *30*, 1705388. [CrossRef]
71. Dosio, F.; Arpicco, S.; Stella, B.; Fattal, E. Hyaluronic acid for anticancer drug and nucleic acid delivery. *Adv. Drug Deliv. Rev.* **2016**, *97*, 204–236. [CrossRef]
72. Li, J.; Mooney, D.J. Designing hydrogels for controlled drug delivery. *Nat. Rev. Mater.* **2016**, *1*, 16071. [CrossRef]
73. Highley, C.B.; Kim, M.; Lee, D.; Burdick, J.A. Near–infrared light triggered release of molecules from supramolecular hydrogel–nanorod composites. *Nanomedicine* **2016**, *11*, 1579–1590. [CrossRef]
74. Yamaguchi, H.; Kobayashi, Y.; Kobayashi, R.; Takashima, Y.; Hashidzume, A.; Harada, A. Photoswitchable gel assembly based on molecular recognition. *Nat. Commun.* **2012**, *3*, 603. [CrossRef]
75. Kwon, S.S.; Kong, B.J.; Park, S.N. Physicochemical properties of pH–sensitive hydrogels based on hydroxyethyl cellulose–hyaluronic acid and for applications as transdermal delivery systems for skin lesions. *Eur. J. Pharm. Biopharm.* **2015**, *92*, 146–154. [CrossRef]
76. Mattheolabakis, G.; Milane, L.; Singh, A.; Amiji, M.M. Hyaluronic acid targeting of CD44 for cancer therapy: From receptor biology to nanomedicine. *J. Drug Target.* **2015**, *23*, 605–618. [CrossRef]
77. Chen, C.; Zhao, S.; Karnad, A.; Freeman, J.W. The biology and role of CD44 in cancer progression: Therapeutic implications. *J. Hematol. Oncol.* **2018**, *11*, 64. [CrossRef]
78. Rao, N.V.; Yoon, H.Y.; Han, H.S.; Ko, H.; Son, S.; Lee, M.; Lee, H.; Jo, D.-G.; Kang, Y.M.; Park, J.H. Recent developments in hyaluronic acid–based nanomedicine for targeted cancer treatment. *Expert Opin. Drug Deliv.* **2016**, *13*, 239–252. [CrossRef]
79. Choi, K.Y.; Han, H.S.; Lee, E.S.; Shin, J.M.; Almquist, B.D.; Lee, D.S.; Park, J.H. Hyaluronic acid–based activatable nanomaterials for stimuli-responsive imaging and therapeutics: Beyond CD44-mediated drug delivery. *Adv. Mater.* **2019**, 1803549. [CrossRef]
80. Huang, G.; Huang, H. Hyaluronic acid–based biopharmaceutical delivery and tumor–targeted drug delivery system. *J. Controll. Release* **2018**, *278*, 122–126. [CrossRef]
81. Fu, C.; Li, H.; Li, N.; Miao, X.; Xie, M.; Du, W.; Zhang, L.-M. Conjugating an anticancer drug onto thiolated hyaluronic acid by acid liable hydrazone linkage for its gelation and dual stimuli–response release. *Carbohydr. Polym.* **2015**, *128*, 163–170. [CrossRef]

82. Bajaj, G.; Kim, M.R.; Mohammed, S.I.; Yeo, Y. Hyaluronic acid–based hydrogel for regional delivery of paclitaxel to intraperitoneal tumors. *J. Controll. Release* **2012**, *158*, 386–392. [CrossRef]
83. Yang, C.; Wang, X.; Yao, X.; Zhang, Y.; Wu, W.; Jiang, X. Hyaluronic acid nanogels with enzyme–sensitive cross–linking group for drug delivery. *J. Controll. Release* **2015**, *205*, 206–217. [CrossRef]
84. Jhan, H.-J.; Liu, J.-J.; Chen, Y.-C.; Liu, D.-Z.; Sheu, M.-T.; Ho, H.-O. Novel injectable thermosensitive hydrogels for delivering hyaluronic acid–doxorubicin nanocomplexes to locally treat tumors. *Nanomedicine* **2015**, *10*, 1263–1274. [CrossRef]
85. Chen, J.; He, H.; Deng, C.; Yin, L.; Zhong, Z. Saporin–loaded CD44 and EGFR dual–targeted nanogels for potent inhibition of metastatic breast cancer in vivo. *Int. J. Pharm.* **2019**, *560*, 57–64. [CrossRef]
86. Dakwar, G.R.; Shariati, M.; Willaert, W.; Ceelen, W.; De Smedt, S.C.; Remaut, K. Nanomedicine–based intraperitoneal therapy for the treatment of peritoneal carcinomatosis—Mission possible? *Adv. Drug Deliv. Rev.* **2017**, *108*, 13–24. [CrossRef] [PubMed]
87. Cho, E.J.; Sun, B.; Doh, K.-O.; Wilson, E.M.; Torregrosa-Allen, S.; Elzey, B.D.; Yeo, Y. Intraperitoneal delivery of platinum with in–situ crosslinkable hyaluronic acid gel for local therapy of ovarian cancer. *Biomaterials* **2015**, *37*, 312–319. [CrossRef] [PubMed]
88. Qiu, Y.; Park, K. Environment–sensitive hydrogels for drug delivery. *Adv. Drug Deliv. Rev.* **2001**, *53*, 321–339. [CrossRef]
89. Zhang, W.; Jin, X.; Li, H.; Wei, C.-X.; Wu, C.-W. Onion–structure bionic hydrogel capsules based on chitosan for regulating doxorubicin release. *Carbohydr. Polym.* **2019**, *209*, 152–160. [CrossRef]
90. Goldring, M.B.; Berenbaum, F. Emerging targets in osteoarthritis therapy. *Curr. Opin. Pharmacol.* **2015**, *22*, 51–63. [CrossRef] [PubMed]
91. Dougados, M. Sodium hyaluronate therapy in osteoarthritis: Arguments for a potential beneficial structural effect. *Semin. Arthr. Rheum.* **2000**, *30*, 19–25. [CrossRef]
92. Ishida, O.; Tanaka, Y.; Morimoto, I.; Takigawa, M.; Eto, S. Chondrocytes are regulated by cellular adhesion through CD44 and hyaluronic acid pathway. *J. Bone Mineral Res.* **1997**, *12*, 1657–1663. [CrossRef]
93. Cai, Y.; López-Ruiz, E.; Wengel, J.; Creemers, L.B.; Howard, K.A. A hyaluronic acid–based hydrogel enabling CD44–mediated chondrocyte binding and gapmer oligonucleotide release for modulation of gene expression in osteoarthritis. *J. Controll. Release* **2017**, *253*, 153–159. [CrossRef]
94. Garcia, J.P.; Stein, J.; Cai, Y.; Riemers, F.; Wexselblatt, E.; Wengel, J.; Tryfonidou, M.; Yayon, A.; Howard, K.A.; Creemers, L.B. Fibrin–hyaluronic acid hydrogel–based delivery of antisense oligonucleotides for ADAMTS5 inhibition in co–delivered and resident joint cells in osteoarthritis. *J. Controll. Release* **2019**, *294*, 247–258. [CrossRef]
95. Verma, P.; Dalal, K. ADAMTS-4 and ADAMTS-5: Key enzymes in osteoarthritis. *J. Cell. Biochem.* **2011**, *112*, 3507–3514. [CrossRef]

5

Dual Action of the PN159/KLAL/MAP Peptide: Increase of Drug Penetration across Caco-2 Intestinal Barrier Model by Modulation of Tight Junctions and Plasma Membrane Permeability

Alexandra Bocsik [1], Ilona Gróf [1,2], Lóránd Kiss [1,3], Ferenc Ötvös [4], Ottó Zsíros [5], Lejla Daruka [2,6], Lívia Fülöp [7], Monika Vastag [8], Ágnes Kittel [9], Norbert Imre [7], Tamás A. Martinek [7], Csaba Pál [6], Piroska Szabó-Révész [10] and Mária A. Deli [1,*]

1 Institute of Biophysics, Biological Research Centre, Hungarian Academy of Sciences, H-6726 Szeged, Hungary; bocsik.alexandra@brc.mta.hu (A.B.); ilona.grof@brc.mta.hu (I.G.); kiss.lorand@med.u-szeged.hu (L.K.)

2 Doctoral School in Biology, Faculty of Science and Informatics, University of Szeged, H-6726 Szeged, Hungary; daruka.lejla@brc.mta.hu

3 Department of Pathophysiology, University of Szeged, H-6701 Szeged, Hungary

4 Institute of Biochemistry, Biological Research Centre, Hungarian Academy of Sciences, H-6726 Szeged, Hungary; otvos.ferenc@brc.mta.hu

5 Plant Biology, Biological Research Centre, Hungarian Academy of Sciences, H-6726 Szeged, Hungary; zsiros.otto@brc.mta.hu

6 Synthetic and Systems Biology Unit, Institute of Biochemistry, Biological Research Centre, Hungarian Academy of Sciences, H-6726 Szeged, Hungary; pal.csaba@brc.mta.hu

7 Department of Medical Chemistry, University of Szeged, H-6720 Szeged, Hungary; fulop.livia@med.u-szeged.hu (L.F.); imre.norbert@med.u-szeged.hu (N.I.); martinek.tamas@med.u-szeged.hu (T.A.M.)

8 Division of Pharmacology and Drug Safety Research, Gedeon Richter Plc., H-1103 Budapest, Hungary; m.vastag@richter.hu

9 Institute of Experimental Medicine, Hungarian Academy of Sciences, H-1450 Budapest, Hungary; kittel@koki.hu

10 Department of Pharmaceutical Technology, University of Szeged, H-6720 Szeged, Hungary; revesz@pharm.u-szeged.hu

* Correspondence: deli.maria@brc.mta.hu

Abstract: The absorption of drugs is limited by the epithelial barriers of the gastrointestinal tract. One of the strategies to improve drug delivery is the modulation of barrier function by the targeted opening of epithelial tight junctions. In our previous study the 18-mer amphiphilic PN159 peptide was found to be an effective tight junction modulator on intestinal epithelial and blood–brain barrier models. PN159, also known as KLAL or MAP, was described to interact with biological membranes as a cell-penetrating peptide. In the present work we demonstrated that the PN159 peptide as a penetration enhancer has a dual action on intestinal epithelial cells. The peptide safely and reversibly enhanced the permeability of Caco-2 monolayers by opening the intercellular junctions. The penetration of dextran molecules with different size and four efflux pump substrate drugs was increased several folds. We identified claudin-4 and -7 junctional proteins by docking studies as potential binding partners and targets of PN159 in the opening of the paracellular pathway. In addition to the tight junction modulator action, the peptide showed cell membrane permeabilizing and antimicrobial effects. This dual action is not general for cell-penetrating peptides (CPPs), since the other three CPPs tested did not show barrier opening effects.

Keywords: absorption enhancer; antimicrobial peptide; Caco-2; claudin; cell-penetrating peptide (CPP); drug delivery; intestinal epithelial cells; KLAL; PN159; tight junction modulator

1. Introduction

The oral administration of medicines is the most common method in drug therapy because of its easy administration and good patient compliance. However, the absorption of several drugs is limited in the gastrointestinal tract by the barriers composed of epithelial cell layers [1]. Since the non-invasive delivery of orally administered hydrophilic drugs or biopharmaceuticals to the systemic circulation is still a challenge, several strategies and molecules have been investigated as penetration enhancers, including biosurfactants, sucrose esters and peptides [1–3].

Tight junctions (TJs) between epithelial cells form the anatomical basis of the intestinal barrier which is one of the main biological barriers in our organism and the body's largest interface with the external environment [1]. These TJs, located in the apical regions of cells, close the intercellular gap and thus determine the paracellular permeability and the tightness of the epithelial barriers [1, 4]. The absorption level and rate across biological barriers depends on the composition of cellular membranes, the anatomical structures, and the expression pattern of TJ proteins and transporters in the cell membrane [5]. TJs are complex structures composed of integral membrane proteins including among others the occludin protein and the claudin family [6].

One of the basic strategies to improve drug delivery is the modulation of barrier function by the targeted opening of TJs [1] Peptides which act directly on TJs and modulate their permeability are potential candidates to increase the absorption of hydrophilic or large therapeutic molecules in a non-invasive manner [1,7]. In our recent work six TJ modulator peptides acting on different targets were compared using culture models of the intestinal and the blood-brain barriers [8]. All the six peptides induced reversible opening of TJs but barrier selectivity and differences in efficacy were observed. We found the PN159 as the most effective TJ modulator peptide on both barrier models [8]. This peptide was identified as a TJ modulator on cultured human bronchial epithelial cell layers in 2005 [4]. PN159 peptide effectively increased the permeability of respiratory epithelium both in culture and animal experiments [9]. The specific target proteins of the peptide were unknown, but we demonstrated that PN159 interacts with the extracellular loops of integral membrane TJ proteins claudin-1 and -5 [8].

The amino acid sequence of the 18-mer PN159, KLALKLALKALKAALKLA-amide, contains several KLA motifs, and therefore it is also named as KLA or KLAL peptide [10]. The other name of this peptide is MAP, which stands for model amphipathic peptide [11,12]. The structure of the lipid vesicle-bound PN159 peptide is mostly α-helical [10] and strongly interacts with biological membranes [10,13]. Cell-penetrating peptides (CPPs) are a group of short natural or synthetic peptides with 5–30 amino acids, which by crossing cellular membranes can transport into cells a wide range of small and macromolecules, including nucleic acids, proteins, imaging agents [14]. Based on their physical-chemical properties, CPPs can be classified into groups. The most investigated CPPs belong to the amphipathic class. These peptides contain hydrophilic and hydrophobic motifs and are especially rich in lysine, arginine, leucine and alanine. Examples include the PN159 peptide [10,11]; the cyclic φ-peptide [15] and Pep-1 [16]. Among the cationic CPPs penetratin [17] or polyarginine peptides [18] are extensively investigated.

CPPs are structurally similar to antimicrobial peptides, which are important defense elements of the innate immunity, and accordingly, they show an antimicrobial effect against pathogens [19]. Bacterial resistance is a growing clinical problem, as it was highlighted by the Infectious Diseases Society of America publishing the list of ESKAPE pathogens (*Enterobacter species, Staphylococcus aureus, Klebsiella pneumoniae, Acinetobacter baumannii, Pseudomonas aeruginosa* and *Enterococcus faecium*) [20]. This group of microbes causes the large majority of nosocomial infections throughout the world. The combat antibiotic resistance, CPPs can be promising alternative molecules, since increased sensitivity (collateral sensitivity) for antimicrobial peptides were found in antibiotic-resistant *Escherichia coli* strains [21].

As a culture model of the intestinal epithelial barrier, we used in our study the Caco-2 human cell line resembling the epithelium of the small intestine both from structural and functional aspects [22]. The cells have polarized cell morphology, grow in monolayer, possess microvilli, form TJs, express nutrient and efflux transporters, and show good correlation with in vivo data [23,24]. Caco-2 epithelial cells are routinely used in drug permeability studies [24,25].

Crucial parameters for absorption enhancers include their safety, reversibility and efficacy. There are no data available about the effectiveness and safety of PN159 peptide on the intestinal barrier, so our primary goal was to test the TJ modulator peptide for these aspects. Therefore, the aim of the study was to (i) determine the influence of long-time and concentration-dependent effects of treatments with PN159 peptide on intestinal epithelial cell viability, barrier function and recovery; (ii) test the effect of PN159 peptide on drug penetration across the intestinal barrier model; (iii) identify further potential targets of this TJ modulator peptide by molecular modelling; (iv) measure the cell uptake of the PN159 in intestinal epithelial cells and its antimicrobial activity on ESKAPE pathogens; and (iv) test other CPPs for the TJ modulator effect.

2. Materials and Methods

2.1. Materials

All reagents were purchased from Sigma-Aldrich Ltd. (Budapest, Hungary) except for those specifically mentioned.

2.2. Peptide Synthesis

PN159 peptide (KLALKLALKALKAALKLA-amide) [4,10], and Pep-1 (Chariot) peptide (KETWWETWWTEWSQPKKKRKV-amide) were synthesized manually on a 0.5 mmolar scale with the use of standard Fmoc-chemistry on a Rink-amide resin. Couplings were performed in DMF with three-fold excess of DCC, HOBt, and Fmoc-amino acids for 3 h at ambient temperature. In the case of octaarginine (RRRRRRRR-amide, R8) three-fold excess of HATU and six-fold excess of DIPEA was used. Fmoc deprotection was performed in 20% piperidine/DMF mixture for 20 min. The peptides were cleaved from the resin by incubating them with the mixture of TFA/water/triisopropylsilane (48:1:1 volume ratio), precipitated with diethyl-ether and lyophilized. Crude peptides were purified using a Shimadzu semi-preparative high-performance liquid chromatography (HPLC) instrument equipped with a Phenomenex JupiterC18 column, in the following solvent system: (A) 0.1% aqueous TFA and (B) 0.1% TFA in 80% aqueous acetonitrile, in a linear gradient mode. Analysis and purity control were carried out on an analytical HPLC instrument (HP Model 1100 liquid chromatograph equipped with a Phenomenex Jupiter C18 column). Quality control of the peptides was done by performing mass spectrometric measurements on a FinniganTSQ-7000 triple quadrupole mass spectrometer in positive ion mode.

The cyclic φ-peptide (cyclo[CGGFWRRRRGE(εAca)G])was also synthesized manually on a 0.5 mmolar scale with the use of Boc-chemistry on a MBHA-HCl resin, by applying a native chemical ligation strategy. Couplings were performed in DMF with three-fold excess of DIC, HOBt, and Boc-amino acids for 3 h at ambient temperature. Boc deprotection was performed in TFA/DCM (1:1 volume ratio) mixture for 20 min. The peptide was cleaved from the resin by the standard HF method. Native chemical ligation was performed with 2% thiophenol in an ammoniumacetate solution (0.1 M) at room temperature for 12h. Cyclic crude peptide was purified and analyzed as described above.

2.3. Cell Culture

The human Caco-2 intestinal epithelial cell line was purchased from ATCC (cat.no. HTB-37). Caco-2 cells were grown in DMEM/HAM's F-12 culture medium with stable glutamine

(Life Technologies, Gibco, Carlsbad, CA, USA) supplemented with 10% fetal bovine serum (Life Technologies, Gibco, Carlsbad, CA, USA and 50 µg/mL gentamycin in a humidified incubator with 5% CO_2 at 37 °C. All plastic surfaces were coated with 0.05% rat tail collagen in sterile distilled water before cell seeding.

2.4. Peptide Treatment

The PN159 peptide stock solution (5 mM) was prepared freshly in sterile DMSO. Treatment solutions were further diluted in Ringer-Hepes (150 mM NaCl, 6 mM $NaHCO_3$, 5.2 mM KCl, 2.2 mM $CaCl_2$, 0.2 mM $MgCl_2$, 2.8 mM D-glucose, 5 mM Hepes; pH 7.4) or cell culture medium. Final concentrations of the peptide in treatment solutions were as follows: 1, 3, 10, 30 and 100 µM for cell viability assays; 1, 3, 10 and 30 µM for the barrier integrity assays and 10 µM for the recovery measurements.

The stock solutions of the three reference CPPs were the following: Pep-1: 1 mM in distilled water (DW); R8: 1 mM in DW; φ-peptide, 5 mM in DW and 2.5% DMSO. The 100 µM working solutions were dissolved in cell culture medium or Ringer–Hepes buffer. We prepared all solutions freshly in sterile conditions.

2.5. MTT Assay

For the cell viability assays Caco-2 epithelial cells were seeded to 96-well plates at the density of 6×10^3 cells/well (Orange Scientific) and cultured for 3-5 days. Confluent cultures were treated with PN159 peptide (1, 3, 10, 30 and 100 µM) in phenol red free DMEM (Life Technologies, Gibco, Carlsbad, CA, USA) for 1-h. This viability assay was performed at three different time points: (i) immediately after the 1-h treatment, (ii) at one-day recovery, (iii) at one-week recovery. To determine 100% toxicity, cells were incubated with 1 mg/mL Triton X-100 detergent. After treatment the medium was changed and 0.5 mg/mL MTT (3-(4,5-dimethyltiazol-2-yl)-2,5-diphenyltetrazolium bromide) solution was added to the cells for 3 h. During the incubation cells were kept in a CO_2 incubator. The metabolic activity of cells is reflected by the conversion of the yellow MTT dye to purple formazan. Formazan crystals were dissolved in DMSO and the amount of converted dye was determined by measuring absorbance at 595 nm wavelength with a microplate reader (Fluostar Optima, BMG Labtechnologies, Ortenberg, Germany). Cell viability and/or metabolic activity was calculated as percentage of dye conversion by non-treated cells.

2.6. Impedance Measurement

Kinetics of epithelial cell reaction to PN159 peptide treatment was monitored by impedance measurement at 10 kHz (RTCA-SP instrument, ACEA Biosciences, San Diego, CA, USA). Impedance measurement is non-invasive, label-free and real time, and linearly correlates with adherence, growth, number and viability of cells [2,26]. For background measurements 50 µL cell culture medium was added to the wells, then cells were seeded at a density of 6×10^3 cells/well to the coated 96-well plates with integrated gold electrodes (E-plate 96, ACEA Biosciences). Cells were cultured for 5–7 days in a CO_2 incubator at 37 °C and monitored every 10 min until the end of experiments. Cells were treated with PN159 peptide solutions at 1, 3, 10, 30 and 100 µM concentrations at the beginning of the plateau phase of growth and the effects were followed for 1-h or 24 h. To measure cell recovery, peptide solutions were changed to culture medium and the impedance was monitored for one week. Culture medium was changed every 2 days. Caco-2 cells were also treated with the three selected CPPs, Pep-1, R8 and φ-peptide, at 100 µM concentrations at the beginning of the plateau phase of cell growth for 24-h. Triton X-100 detergent (1 mg/mL) was used as a reference compound to induce cell death. Cell index was defined as R_n-R_b at each time point of measurement, where R_n is the cell-electrode impedance of the well when it contains cells and R_b is the background impedance of the well with the medium alone.

2.7. *Measurement of the Electrical Resistance of Caco-2 Cell Layers*

For the measurement of barrier integrity Caco-2 cells were seeded onto culture inserts (Transwell 3460, polyester membrane, 0.4 μm pore size, Corning Costar) and cultured for three weeks [2,24]. Transepithelial electrical resistance (TEER) reflects the tightness of the intercellular junctions. TEER was measured by an EVOM volt-ohmmeter (World Precision Instruments, Sarasota, FL, USA) combined with STX-2 electrodes, and was expressed relative to the surface area of the monolayers ($\Omega \times cm^2$). Resistance of cell-free inserts ($130\ \Omega \times cm^2$) was subtracted from the measured values. TEER values were measured before and right after permeability experiments). TEER values indicated the integrity and paracellular permeability of cell layers for ions. The TEER of Caco-2 monolayers was $1302 \pm 49\ \Omega \times cm^2$ (mean ± SD; $n = 46$) after 3 weeks culturing. For the recovery experiment, after changing the 10 μM peptide solutions to culture medium, TEER was monitored for one day.

2.8. *Penetration of Marker and Drug Molecules across Caco-2 Cell Layers*

In the permeability experiments inserts with Caco-2 cell layers grown for 3 weeks were transferred to 12-well plates containing 1.5 mL Ringer–Hepes buffer in the lower (basal or acceptor) compartments. In the upper or apical compartments culture medium was replaced by 0.5 mL buffer containing peptide solutions: PN159 peptide at 1, 3, 10 and 30 μM concentrations and CPPs at 100 μM concentration. Permeability marker molecules albumin (1 mg/mL; *Mw*: 65 kDa) labeled with Evans blue (167.5 μg/mL) and fluorescein (10 μg/mL; *Mw*: 376 Da) were added 30 min later. The incubation with permeability markers in the presence of PN159 peptide lasted for 30 min. In case of CPPs the incubation time with fluorescein was 1-h. Samples were collected from both compartments and the concentrations of the marker molecules were determined by a fluorescence multi-well plate reader (Fluostar Optima; excitation wavelength: 485 nm, emission wavelength: 535 nm in the case of fluorescein and excitation wavelength: 584 nm, emission wavelength: 680 nm in the case of Evans-blue labeled albumin). Fluorescein isothiocyanate (FITC)-labelled dextran marker molecules (Table 1) were used at 1 mM concentrations, and fluorescence intensities of collected samples were measured using a Fluorolog FL3-22 (Horiba Jobin Yvon, Paris, France) spectrofluorometer using 492 nm excitation wavelength, 515 nm emission wavelength, and 0.5 s integration time. Drugs were used at 10 μM concentrations and samples were measured by HPLC as described below. The apparent permeability coefficients (P_{app}) were calculated as described previously [8,24]. Briefly, cleared volume was calculated from the concentration difference of the tracer in the basal compartments ($\Delta[C]_B$) after 30 min and apical compartments at 0 h ($[C]_A$), the volume of the basal compartment (V_B; 1.5 mL) and the surface area available for permeability (A; 1.1 cm^2).

Table 1. The amino acid sequences of the tested cell-penetrating peptides.

CPPs	Amino Acid Sequence	References
PN159 (KLAL/MAP)	KLALKLALKALKAALKLA-amide	[4,10]
Pep-1	KETWWETWWTEWSQPKKKRKV-amide	[16]
R8	RRRRRRRR-amide	[18]
φ-peptide	cyclo[CGGFWRRRRGE(εAca)G]	[15]

2.9. *High-Performance Liquid Chromatography (HPLC)Analytical Procedures*

Analytical measurements were performed on a Merck-Hitachi LaChrom HPLC system equipped with an ultraviolet (UV) and fluorescence detector (Merck, Darmstadt, Germany). All reagents used were of analytical reagent grade. Atenolol and verapamil were determined by using a Gemini C18 column (150 × 3 mm, 5 μm, 110 Å; Phenomenex Inc., Torrance, CA, USA) operated at 0.5 mL/min flow rate, maintained at 35°C. For atenolol measurements isocratic elution was applied with a mixture of 300 mL methanol, 400 mL 100 mM ammonium acetate, 20 mL 10% ammonium-hydroxide and 2 mL 0.1 M ethylenediaminetetraacetic acid. The mobile phase for verapamil consisted of 350 mL methanol with 250 mL 20 mM ammonium acetate and 2 mL 10% trifluoroacetic acid with isocratic elution, at 0.5 mL/min flow rate. UV detection for atenolol was performed at 270 nm while for verapamil the 230 nm wavelength was adjusted. The calibration curve was linear (r^2 = 0.9999) over a range of 0.01–1.5 μM for atenolol. The calibration curve for verapamil also showed a good linearity within the examined concentration range of 0.01–1 μM (r^2 = 0.9952). In both cases 10μL sample was injected into the chromatographic system. Samples at higher than 1 μM atenolol and verapamil concentrations were 10× diluted with Ringer–Hepes solution.

HPLC measurement of quinidine was performed using a YMC Pack Pro C18 column (RS 150 × 2.1 mm, 5 μm, 80 Å; YMC America Inc., Allentown, PA, USA) equipped with a guard column operated at 0.2 mL/min flow rate. The chromatographic column was maintained at 40 °C and the 5 μL sample was injected onto the column. The elution of quinidine was performed with a buffer containing a mixture of 100 mL methanol, 250 mL 0.1% ammonium acetate, and 4 mL 10% trifluoroacetic acid. Quinidine was quantified at 250/430 nm excitation/emission wavelengths. The calibration curve was linear over the quantitation range of 0.01–1 μM (r^2 = 0.9984).

HPLC measurement of cimetidine was performed using a Gemini NX column (150 × 4.6 mm, 3 μM) equipped with a guard column operated at 0.8 mL/min flow rate. The column temperature was maintained at 40 °C and a 20 μL sample was injected onto the chromatographic system. A buffer comprising of 15% acetonitrile and 85% 100 mM ammonium acetate was utilized for the isocratic elution of cimetidine. UV detection was set at 228 nm. The calibration curve was linear (r^2 = 0.9999) over the range of 0.01–10 μM.

2.10. Electron Microscopy

Cells grown on culture inserts were treated with 10 μM PN159 peptide for 30 min and fixed immediately after treatment or after a 1-day recovery. Cells were briefly washed with phosphate-buffered saline (PBS) and fixed with 3% paraformaldehyde containing 0.5% glutaraldehyde in cacodylate buffer (pH 7.4) for 30 min at 4 °C. After washing with the buffer several times, cells were postfixed in 1% OsO_4 for 20 min. Following a rinse with distilled water, the cells were block stained with 1% uranyl acetate in 50% ethanol for 20 min, dehydrated in graded ethanol and after the last step of dehydration inserts were placed in the 1:1 mixture of ethanol and Taab 812 (Taab; Aldermaston, Berks, UK) for 10 min at 30°C. Finally, the membranes of the culture inserts with the cells were removed from their support and embedded in Taab 812. Polymerization was performed overnight at 60°C. Ultrathin sections were cut perpendicularly for the membrane using a Leica EM UC6 ultramicrotome (Nussloch, Germany) and picked up on formvar-coated single-slot copper grids. The sections were examined using a Hitachi 7100 transmission electron microscope (Hitachi Ltd., Tokyo, Japan) and a side-mounted Veleta CCD camera (Olympus Soft Imaging Solutions). Altogether, 105 non-overlapping images from the 3 groups at the same magnification were analyzed for the presence or absence of tight junctions (control group n = 28; PN159 group n = 42; recovery group n = 35).

2.11. Immunohistochemistry

Morphological changes in interepithelial junctions after treatment with different concentrations of CPPs (100 μM) and PN159 peptide (1, 3, 10, 30 and 100 μM) were followed by immunostaining for claudin-1 integral membrane tight junction protein, β-catenin and zonula occludens protein-1 (ZO-1) cytoplasmic linker proteins. F-actin was stained by fluorescently labeled phalloidin. Treatments lasted for 1 h. After peptide treatment cell layers were washed with PBS and fixed with a 1:1 mixture of ice cold acetone and methanol for 2 min. Cells were blocked with 3% bovine serum albumin in PBS and incubated with primary antibodies mouse anti-claudin-1 and -4, rabbit anti-ZO-1 and rabbit anti-β-catenin (Life Technologies, Carlsbad, CA, USA) overnight. Fluorescent Atto 647N-phalloidin (ATTO-TEC GmbH, Germany) lasted for 1 h. Incubation with Alexa Fluor-488-labeled anti-mouse and anti-rabbit secondary antibodies (Life Technologies, Invitrogen, USA) lasted for 1 h. Bis-benzimide dye (Hoechst 33342) was used to stain cell nuclei. After mounting (Fluoromount-G; Southern Biotech,

Birmingham, AL, USA) the samples staining was visualized by a Leica TCS SP5 confocal laser scanning microscope (Leica Microsystems GmbH, Wetzlar, Germany) and Visitron spinning disk confocal system (Visitron Systems GmbH, Puchheim, Germany).

2.12. Circular Dichroism (CD) Spectroscopy

Far-UV circular dichroism (CD) spectra of the peptides were recorded at 25°C temperature on a J-810 spectropolarimeter (JASCO International Co. Ltd., Tokyo, Japan). The CD spectra were measured between 260 nm and 185 nm with an optical pathlength of 1 mm, at a peptide concentration of 0.1 mg/mL in Milli-Q water diluted directly from powder. The bandwidth was 2 nm and data pitch 0.5 nm, the scan speed was set to 100 nm/min and the integration time was 1 sec. Ten spectra were accumulated and plotted. The data were analyzed by CDSSTR method [27]. To test the thermostability of the peptide structure the CD spectra were recorded between 25 °C and 55 °C temperature with a ramp rate of 5 °C/min on a JASCO J-810 spectropolarimeter by using a Peltier sample holder. The CD spectra were measured immediately between 260 and 185 nm with an optical pathlength of 1 mm, the peptide concentration was 0.1 mg/mL in Milli-Q water. The bandwidth was 2 nm and data pitch 1 nm, the scan speed was set to 100 nm/min, and the integration time was 1 sec. Five spectra were accumulated and plotted.

2.13. Molecular Modelling

Protein structures were obtained by homology modeling using the MODELLER program package [28]. First, the structure of mouse claudin-15 was completed by homology modelling because its X-ray structure file is lacking the fragment of residues from 34 to 41 [29]. Human claudins 1, 4 and 7 were homology modeled using the completed mouse claudin-15 as a template. The protein homology models were further relaxed by a short (400 ns) molecular dynamics simulation in which the proteins were embedded in a 95 by 95 Å POPC bilayer-water system containing 150 mM NaCl. Molecular dynamics simulations were performed by the program NAMD [30], using the CHARMM27 molecular force field with CMAP correction. The results were visualized by VMD v1.9.1. [31]. The docking studies were performed by the CABS docking server [32] and the resulting C-alpha traces were reconstructed by MODELLER using the python script supplied by the server homepage.

2.14. Visualization of the Uptake of PN159 Peptide in Caco-2 Cells

The Caco-2 cells were grown on glass bottomed petri dishes coated with collagen to visualize the cellular uptake of the Bodipy FL maleimide labeled (BODIPY FL *N*-(2-aminoethyl) maleimide, Thermo Fischer, Waltham, MA, USA) PN159 peptide. The cells were treated with peptide at concentrations of 1, 3 and 10 μM for 5 min. To stain the cell nuclei the H33342dye (1 μg/mL) was used before peptide treatment for 10 min. After peptide incubation the living cells were washed three times with Ringer–Hepes buffer supplemented with 1%fetal bovine serum (FBS) and examined immediately with a Visitron spinning disk confocal system.

In the case of the co-localization analysis the labeled PN159 peptide was used in 10 μM for 5 min. Then the cellular uptake cells were fixed and immunohistochemistry was performed for claudin-4. The samples were mounted and visualized by a Leica TCS SP5 confocal laser-scanning microscope.

2.15. Determination of Minimum Inhibitory Concentration (MIC) on Microbial Pathogens

We tested the spectrum of activity of PN159 on a set of five sensitive ESKAPE pathogens: *Staphylococcus aureus* (ATCC 29213), *Klebsiella pneumoniae* (ATCC 10031), *Acinetobacter baumannii* (ATCC

17978), *Pseudomonas aeruginosa* (ATCC 27853), *Enterobacter cloacae spp. cloacae* (ATCC 13047); and one vancomycin resistant ESKAPE pathogen, *Enterococcus faecium* (ATCC 700221). The MIC of PN159 on the 6 sensitive and resistant ESKAPE pathogenic strains was determined in cation-adjusted Muller–Hinton broth. For *Enterococcus faecium*, which does not grow in Muller-Hinton broth, Brain-Heart-Infusion broth was used. Minimum inhibitory concentrations (MICs) were determined by using a standard serial broth dilution technique [33]. Briefly, 11-step serial dilutions were prepared in 96-well microtiter plates with three biological replicates per strain. Pathogens were inoculated into each well at a density of 5×10^5 bacteria/mL, and the plates were incubated at 37 °C. Plates were shaken at 300 rpm during incubation for 18 h. Cell growth was monitored by measuring the optical density (OD600 value, Synergy 2 microplate reader BioTek Instruments Inc, Winooski, VT, USA). MIC was defined as complete growth inhibition (i.e., OD600 < 0.05). As reference compounds we tested the antimicrobial activity of three bactericidal drugs with different modes of action. Cefoxitin inhibits the cell wall synthesis, gentamicin (Applichem GmbH, Darmstadt, Germany) is a 30S ribosomal subunit inhibitor, while ciprofloxacin is a gyrase inhibitor. The highest tested concentrations were 100 μg/mL in the case of cefoxitin and gentamicin, and 10 μg/mL for ciprofloxacin.

2.16. Statistical Analysis

For statistical analysis Graph Pad Prism 5.0 software (Graph Pad Software Inc., San Diego, CA, USA) was used. All data presented are means ± SD. Values were compared using analysis of variance followed by Dunnett's test. Changes were considered statistically significant at $p < 0.05$. All measurements were repeated three times and the number of parallel samples was minimum three.

3. Results

3.1. Concentration-Dependent Effect of PN159 Peptide on Epithelial Cell Viability

The colorimetric endpoint MTT test was performed after a 1-h treatment with different PN159 peptide concentrations at three different time points: (i) immediately after the 1-h treatment, (ii) at one-day recovery and (iii) at one-week recovery (Figure 1A). Low concentrations of the peptide (1–10 μM) did not decrease cell viability, while cell damage was found at higher, 30 and 100 μM concentrations. The cytotoxic effect of PN159 at 100 μM concentration was not reversible after one day or even one week. The kinetics of PN159 effects on Caco-2 cells were followed by real-time impedance measurements after 1-h (Figure 1B) or one-day treatment (Figure 1C). In both conditions only the two highest peptide concentrations decreased the cell impedance indicating cell damage, similarly to the results of the MTT assay.

Based on both tests, PN159 peptide treatment for 1-h was non-toxic at 10 μM or lower concentrations, reversible at 30 μM and toxic at the highest 100 μM concentration. The results obtained by MTT test and impedance measurement on Caco-2 cells were similar (Figure 1) and indicated that all the used concentrations of PN159 peptide were safe, except the 100 μM. Because of its toxicity, the 100 μM concentration was not used in further experiments.

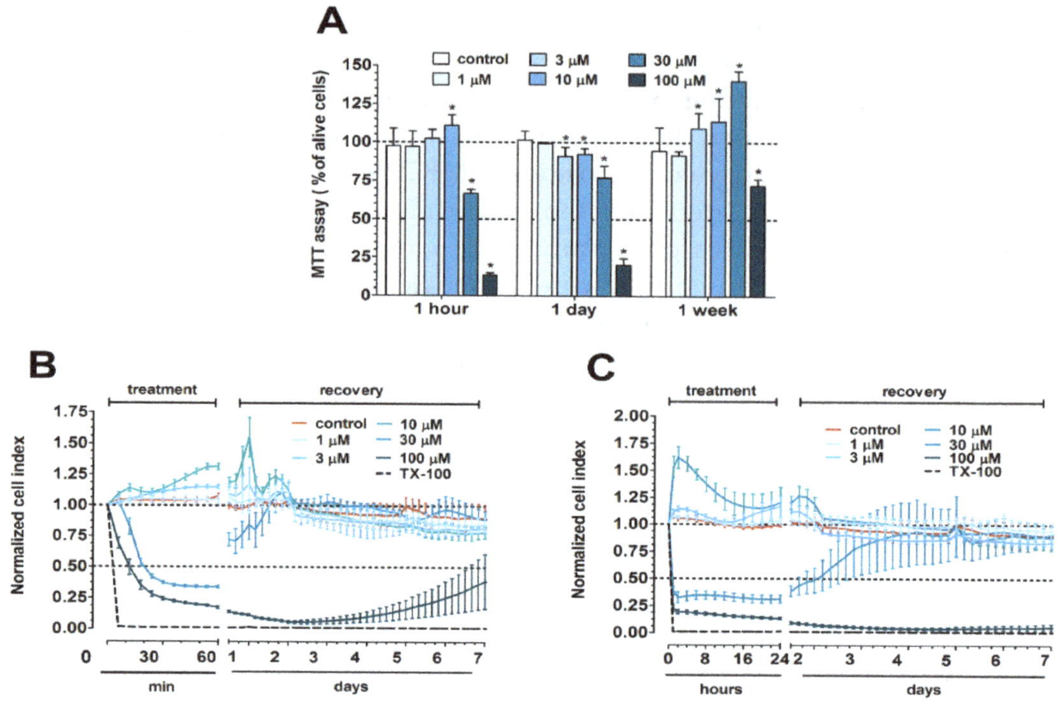

Figure 1. (**A**) MTT assay after 1-h treatment with PN159 peptide on Caco-2 cells followed by 1-h, 1-day or 1-week recovery. The MTT values are given as percent of the control group (100% viability). Values are presented as means ± SD, $n = 3–8$. Statistical analysis: analysis of variance (ANOVA) followed by Dunnett test, $p < 0.05$ as compared with the control groups. (**B**) Impedance measurements after 1-h treatment and (**C**) 1-day treatment followed by a recovery phase of 1-week. The effects of PN159 peptide on the impedance were shown as normalized cell index. Values are presented as means ± SD, $n = 3–8$.

3.2. Concentration-Dependent Effect of PN159 Peptide on Intestinal Epithelial Barrier Integrity

All tested concentrations of the PN159 peptide significantly decreased the resistance of epithelial cell layers after a 1-h treatment (Figure 2A). The two highest concentrations, 10 and 30 μM, opened the paracellular barrier the most, causing 80–90% decrease in TEER. In concordance, these two highest concentrations of PN159 showed the most effective permeability enhancer activity for both fluorescein and albumin (Figure 2B). Because the peptide was safe for the cells but effectively opened the barrier at 10 μM, this concentration was selected to reveal the kinetics of the reversibility of barrier opening, and to investigate its effects on drug penetration.

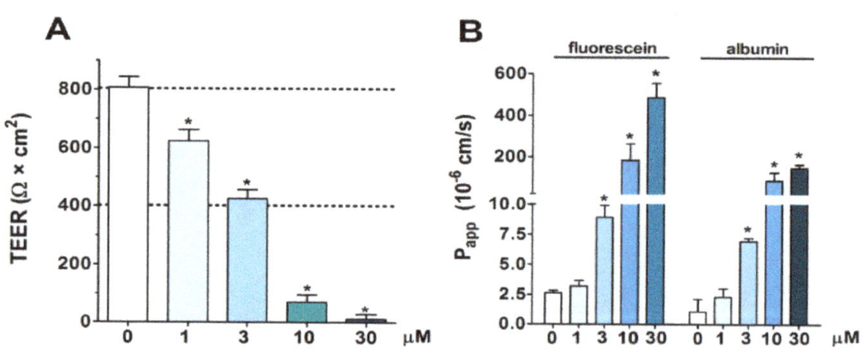

Figure 2. Effect of 1-h PN159 treatment on barrier integrity of Caco-2 cell layers. (**A**) Transepithelial electrical resistance (TEER). (**B**) Permeability for fluorescein and albumin marker molecules (P_{app} A-B 10^{-6} cm/s). Values are presented as means ± SD, $n = 3–8$. Statistical analysis: ANOVA followed by Dunnett's test, $p < 0.05$ as compared with the control groups.

3.3. *Reversible Effect of PN159 Peptide on the Opening of the Paracellular Cleft*

The effect of PN159 peptide was very rapid, the electrical resistance dropped already to 42% of the control value after 1-min treatment (Figure 3A). The decrease of TEER continued until the end of the 30-min treatment (5 min: 16%, 15 min: 2.7%, 30 min: 1.4% of the control value). After the removal of the peptide the barrier function of Caco-2 cells was restored about 44% of the control value at six hours and a complete recovery could be observed at the 20 h timepoint. Intact TJs providing the morphological basis of barrier functions were visualized between Caco-2 epithelial cells in the control group by transmission electron microscopy, but no junctions were observed following treatment with PN159 peptide (Figure 3B). The disappearance of intercellular TJs was reversible, because after 1-day recovery the ultrastructure of epithelial junctions became similar to control cells. No open TJs were observed in the control or recovery groups by checking the electron micrographs (28–42 images/groups).

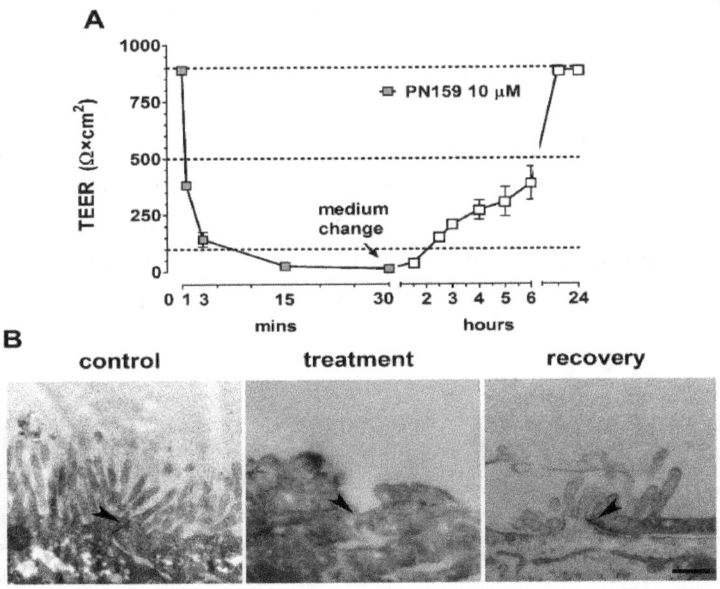

Figure 3. Reversible effect of PN159 peptide (10 μM, 30-min treatment, 24-h recovery) on Caco-2 cells. (**A**) Kinetic analysis of transepithelial electrical resistance (TEER) after PN159 peptide treatment. (**B**) Transmission electron micrographs of cell–cell connections (arrowheads); bar = 400 nm.

3.4. *Effects of PN159 Peptide on the Penetration of Dextran Marker Molecules and Drugs*

All these previous functional and morphological results pointed to the TJ opening effect of PN159 in Caco-2 cells which potentially can be exploited to increase drug penetration across the intestinal barrier. The permeability of Caco-2 monolayers was measured in the apical to basal (intestine to blood) direction for four water-soluble dextran marker molecules of different sizes (4–40 kDa) and four drugs, the hydrophilic atenolol and cimetidine, and the lipophilic quinidine and verapamil (Table 2). All four drugs are substrates of active efflux transporters [24]. The apparent permeability coefficients of the large fluorescein isothiocyanate-labeled dextran (FD) macromolecules were very low in control conditions but they were elevated by 159-400 fold following PN159 treatment. The highest increase was measured in the case of FD-40, the largest macromolecule. In control conditions the permeability of atenolol and cimetidine was the lowest from the tested molecules, while the highest penetration was measured for quinidine and verapamil on Caco-2 cells. PN159 treatment caused more than 30-fold change for atenolol and cimetidine which penetrate slowly across the cells layers. The peptide increased about 2 fold the permeability of the intestinal culture model for the lipophilic quinidine and verapamil, which already showed a good penetration.

Table 2. Apparent permeability coefficients of dextran marker molecules and drugs in the apical-basal direction (P_{app} A-B, 10^{-6} cm/s) in control and PN159 treated cultures. The differences between control and treated groups were expressed in fold changes. FD, fluorescein isothiocyanate-labeled dextran.

Markers and Drug	Control	PN159	Fold Change
FD-4	0.021 ± 0.001	4.2 ± 0.1	200.0
FD-10	0.025 ± 0.010	4.8 ± 0.7	192.0
FD-20	0.022 ± 0.002	3.5 ± 1.0	159.0
FD-40	0.015 ± 0.003	6.0 ± 0.3	400.0
atenolol	1.2 ± 0.3	36.3 ± 1.9	30.0
cimetidine	0.9 ± 0.2	34.5 ± 4.5	38.3
quinidine	45.0 ± 13.3	72.6 ± 2.4	1.6
verapamil	46.2 ± 3.9	86.7 ± 18.8	1.9

3.5. The Effect of PN159 Peptide on the Staining of Junctional Proteins and F-Actin

The concentration-dependent effects of the peptide on epithelial barrier integrity in Caco-2 cells were confirmed by the immunostaining of junctional proteins claudin-1, ZO-1 and β-catenin, and the labeling of the actin cytoskeleton (F-actin) (Figure 4). The 1 μM concentration of the peptide caused a slight effect on cell morphology. At higher than 3 μM concentrations significant changes were observed both in the junctional protein pattern and in the actin cytoskeleton organization. Claudin-1 was the junctional protein most sensitive to the peptide treatment. PN159 at a concentration of 10 μM caused a drastic change in actin cytoskeleton and epithelial junctional morphology, with a visible opening of intercellular junctions.

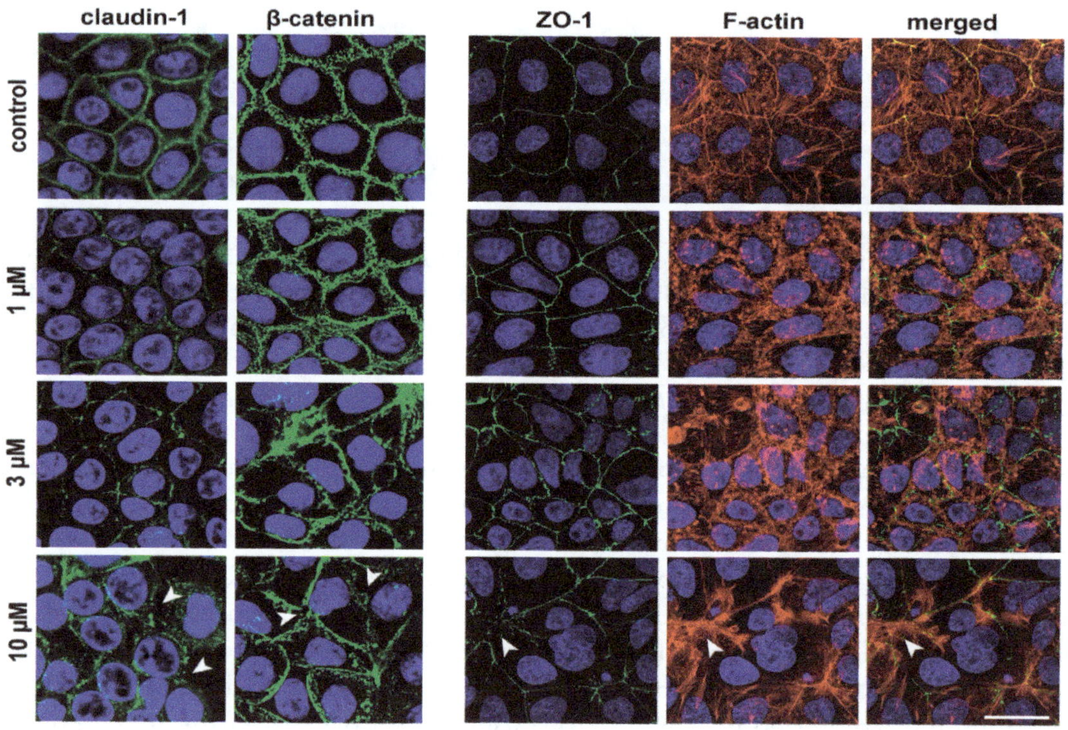

Figure 4. Effects of PN159 peptide on junctional morphology of Caco-2 cells. Immunostaining for claudin-1, β-catenin and zonula occludens-1 (ZO-1) junctional proteins and fluorescent staining for F-actin are shown in control conditions or after 1-hour peptide treatment. Green color: immunostaining for ZO-1, β-catenin and claudin-1. Blue color: staining of cell nuclei. Red color staining of F-actin. Bar = 20 μm. Arrowheads indicate the opened junctions between the cells.

3.6. *Molecular Modeling of Human Claudin Proteins and Docking of PN159 Peptide*

According to the CD spectra obtained, the secondary structure of PN159 peptide contains 11% α-helix, 31% β-sheet, 24% turns and 34% unordered structure (Figure 5A). This secondary structure of PN159 peptide was stable between 25 and 55 °C (Figure 5B). In concordance with the result of CD spectra, similar secondary structure motifs were found by molecular modeling (Figure 5C).

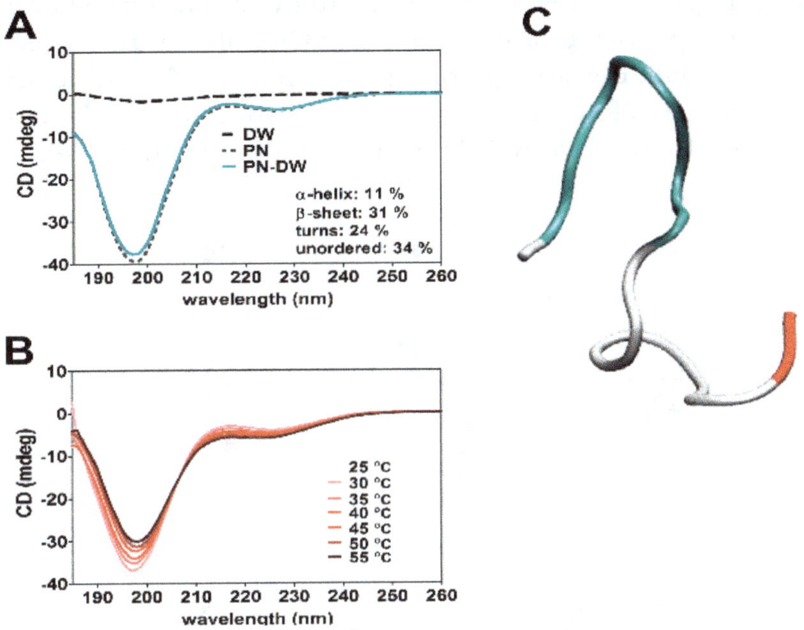

Figure 5. (**A**) Circular dichroism (CD) spectroscopy of PN159 peptide at 25 °C. (**B**) Thermostability measurement of the peptide structure. (**C**) Structure of PN159 by molecular modeling. Blue color: turn motifs; White color: coil-coil motifs; Red color: C-terminal region.

Claudin protein structures were obtained by homology modeling using the MODELLER program package (Figure 6A). Docking of PN159 peptide to full length homology modeled human claudin-1, -3, -4, and -7 monomers, highly expressed in Caco-2 cells [34] was performed on the CABS server (Figure 6B). Favorable docking poses located around extracellular loops ECL1 and ECL2 were sought by both energetic and geometric considerations and analyzed in all docking trajectories. Docking energies ("total energy") were decomposed to "ligand energy", "interaction energy" and "receptor energy" parts (Table 3). Correct docking poses were expected to have low values not only for the total energies, but as low as possible for all energy components simultaneously. Thus, the "ligand energy", "interaction energy" and "total energy" values were investigated. Based on the modeling, energetically highly favorable interactions were found between PN159 and the ECLs of claudin-1, -4 and -7, but not for claudin-3 (Table 3). Docked poses of PN159 with ECLs of claudin-1, -4 and -7 are shown on Figure 6B.

Table 3. Docking energy components of PN159 to selected human claudin monomers. E_{tot}, total energy; E_{lig}, ligand energy; E_{int}, interaction energy.

Energy	Claudin-1	Claudin-3	Claudin-4	Claudin-7
E_{lig}	−34	−17	−61	−32
E_{int}	−63	−59	−79	−186
E_{tot}	−1228	−1163	−1229	−1798

The amino acid sequence of ECL1 and ECL2 of the three claudins which showed interaction with the TJ modulator peptide were compared and the most important amino acids which interact with PN159 were identified (Figure 6C). Four residues in ECL1, the polar Q44 and S/N/D53, the hydrophobic V55 and L71, and in ECL2 the polar N/Q156 participate in major interactions with the peptide. Q44 and V55 residues of claudin-1 and -7 form a binding pocket for L11 of the peptide, and the same two residues of claudin-4 bind L6 and K9 (Figure 6C). The polar S/N/D53 and L71 of claudin-4 and -7 interact with K5, while the same amino acids of claudin-1 bind K12. The N/Q156 amino acid of ECL2 of all three claudins interacts with lysine: in the case of claudin-1 this is L17 of PN159, for claudin-4 L2, and for claudin-7 L6, L8, L15, L17. Based on the docking results, lysine, especially K1 and K5 and leucine L6 and L17 of PN159 interact with all three claudins examined (Figure 6D). After docking of the peptide disappearance of β-strands in ECLs of claudins was observed (Figure 6B), which seems to be correlated with the strength of interaction (Table 3). Comparing the docking energy values of PN159 to claudins the following rank order in the strength of interaction can be established: claudin-3 < claudin-1 < claudin-4< claudin-7. The energy values from modeling are shown in Table 3.

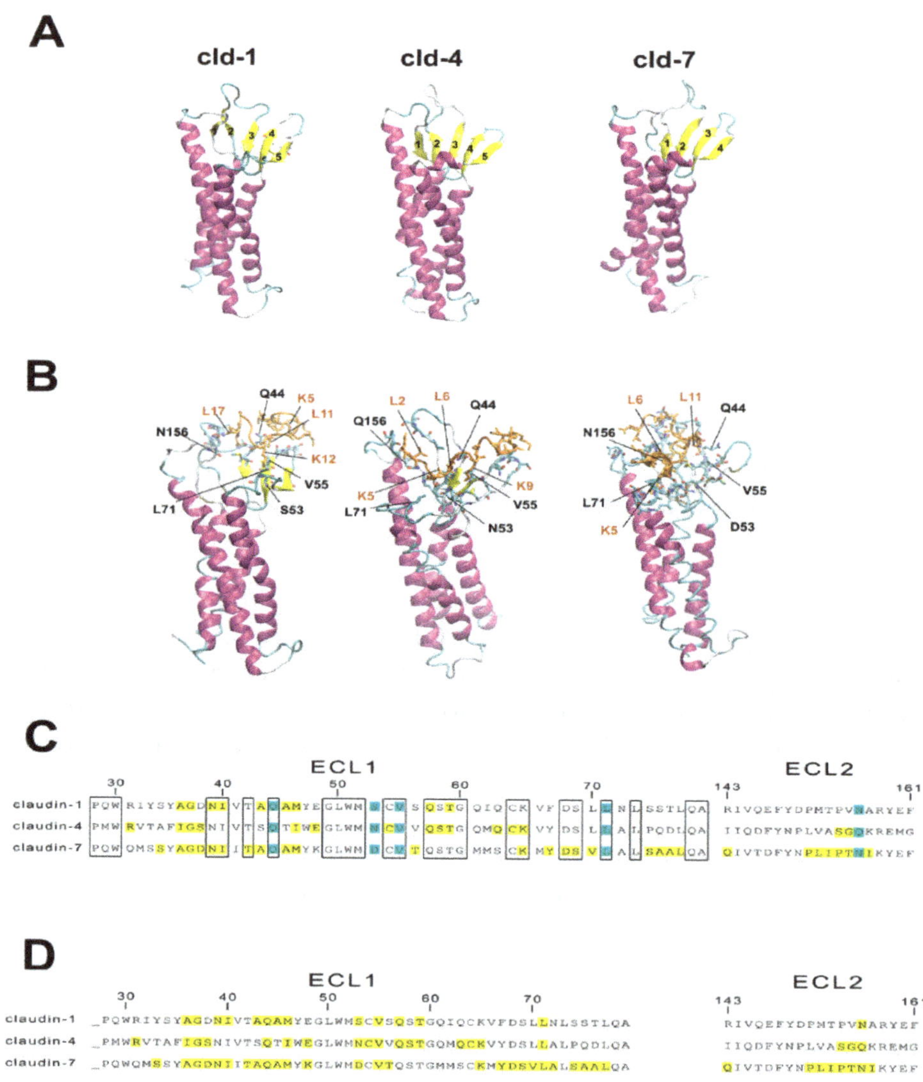

Figure 6. (**A**) Modeling human claudin-1, -4, -7 proteins. (**B**) Docking of PN159 peptide to claudin proteins. Interacting residues are shown as sticks. Orange color: PN159 peptide; Yellow color: β-strands; purple color: α-helices of claudins. (**C**) Amino acid sequence of ECL1 and ECL2 of human claudin monomers 1, 4 and 7. Conserved amino acids are indicated in the boxes. The amino acids which interact with PN159 according to docking studies are marked by yellow and light blue. Blue color indicates interaction between the amino acids of claudins and PN159 peptide at the same position in all three claudins. ECL: extracellular loop. (**D**) Interaction between PN159 peptide and human claudin monomers 1, 4 and 7. Amino acids of PN159 peptide which interact with the claudins according to docking.

3.7. Cell-Penetrating Effect and Uptake of PN159 Peptide in Epithelial Cells

Besides the junctional effects, changes in the cell membrane integrity were also examined by ethidium homodimer-1 (856.77 Da) staining of Caco-2 epithelial cells after 24-h treatments in the concentration range of 1 to 10 μM. Only the highest PN159 concentration caused plasma membrane entry of the red fluorescent dye, which stained cell nuclei (Figure 7A).

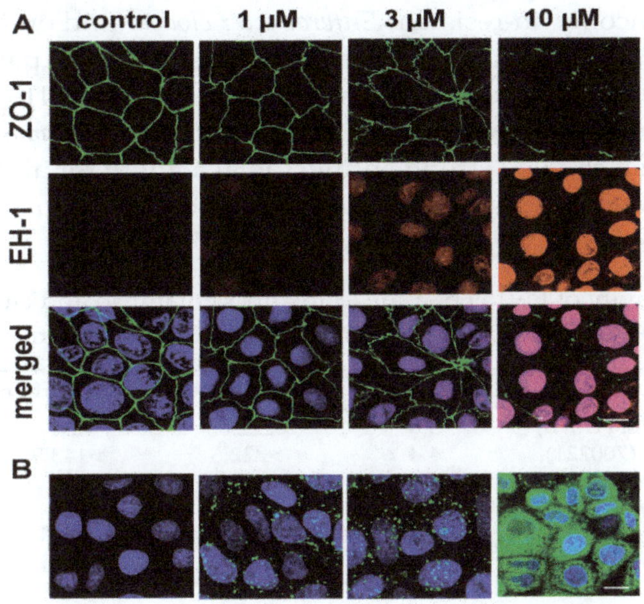

Figure 7. (**A**) Fluorescent staining of juntional protein zonula occludens-1 and double staining of cell nuclei in Caco-2 cells after 1-h treatment with PN159 peptide. Green color: immunostaining for ZO-1. Red color: staining by ethidium homodimer-1 (EH-1), indicating increased membrane permeability.Blue color: staining of all cell nuclei by H33342. Bar = 10 μm. (**B**) Confocal microscopy images of living Caco-2 epithelial cells incubated with Bodipy FL labeled PN159 peptide in different concentrations for 5 min at 37°C. Green color: BodipyFL-PN159 peptide. Blue color: staining of cell nuclei. Bar = 10 μm.

The uptake of the fluorescently labeled PN159 peptide, reflected by the green fluorescent signal, was visualized by confocal microscopy (Figure 7B). In Caco-2 cells treated with 1 and 3 μM concentrations, the peptide was detectable in the cytoplasm as green dots. The cellular uptake of the peptide in cells incubated with 10 μM concentration was more pronounced.

We confirmed the interaction of PN159 peptide with claudin-4 junctional protein by a co-localization analysis. The labeled peptide was visible in the cytoplasm and also in the cell membrane at the level of intercellular junctions immunolabeled for claudin-4 (Figure 8).

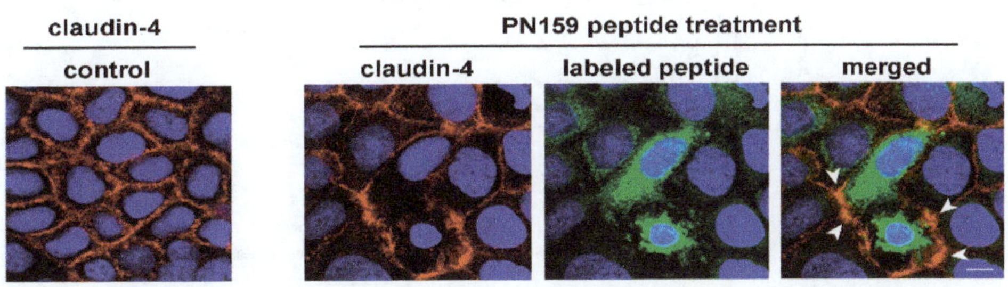

Figure 8. Caco-2 cells were treated with Bodipy FL labeled PN159 peptide (5 min), then fluorescent immunostaining of junctional protein claudin-4 and staining of cell nuclei were performed. Red color: immunostaining for claudin-4. Green color: Bodipy FL labeled PN159 peptide. Blue color: staining of cell nuclei by H33342. Bar = 10 μm. Arrowheads indicate co-localization of claudin-4 and the labeled PN159 peptide.

3.8. Antimicrobial Effect of PN159

We tested the antimicrobial activity of PN159 peptide on six ESKAPE pathogens (Table 4) at a wide range of concentration (0.8 to 70 μM). Among the tested bacteria *Acinetobacter baumannii* and *Enterococcus faecium* were the two most sensitive strains with MIC values below 5 μM. The concentration of PN159 to inhibit the growth of *Staphylococcus aureus* and *Klebsiella pneumoniae* was around 10 μM, which was in similar range where peptide effects were seen on human epithelial cells. The peptide was still effective on the vancomycin-resistant *Enterobacter cloacae* and on *Pseudomonas aeruginosa*, but at 10-times higher concentrations than in the case of the most sensitive pathogens.

As compared to the reference bactericidal antibiotic cefoxitin, PN159 was more effective in the case of *Acinetobacter baumannii*, *Enterococcus faecium*, *Enterobacter cloacae* and *Pseudomonas aeruginosa*. Gentamicin and ciprofloxacin showed strong antimicrobial activity for all ESKAPE pathogens, except *Enterococcus faecium*. This strain was resistant for all investigated antibiotics, however, PN159 efficiently inhibited its growth (Table 4).

Table 4. Antibacterial activity of PN159 peptide, cefoxitin, gentamicin and ciprofloxacin antibiotics on ESKAPE pathogens. ATCC numbers are added in brackets. MIC (μM), minimal inhibitory concentration.

ESKAPE Pethogens (ATCC)	PN159	Cefoxitin	Gentamicin	Ciprofloxacin
Acinetobacter baumannii (17978)	3.6	222.6	0.6	0.94
Enterococcus faecium (700221)	4.4	>222.6	>143.9	>30.18
Staphylococcus aureus (29213)	9.2	6.9	1.1	1.89
Klebsiella pneumonia (10031)	13.8	3.5	0.6	0.06
Enterobacter cloacae (13047)	31.0	>222.6	1.1	0.06
Pseudomonas aeruginosa (27853)	46.4	>222.6	2.3	1.89

3.9. The Effect of Cell-Penetrating Peptides on Intestinal Barrier Integrity

The kinetics of the effects of three other CPPs on Caco-2 cells were followed by real-time impedance measurements (Figure 9A). The R8 and φ-peptides decreased the cell impedance during the 24-h monitoring which indicates a cell reaction. Changes in cell index without cytotoxic effects most probably are caused by an increase in plasma membrane ionic permeability. There was no major influence of CPPs on barrier integrity (Figure 9B,C) as compared to the effect of PN159. We observed a slightly decreased TEER in the case of R8 and φ-peptide and only the φ-peptide caused an elevated permeability for the fluorescein marker molecule. Based on these results the investigated CPPs have no significant opening effect on the intercellular junctions, which was also verified by immunostaining for junctional proteins (Figure 9D).

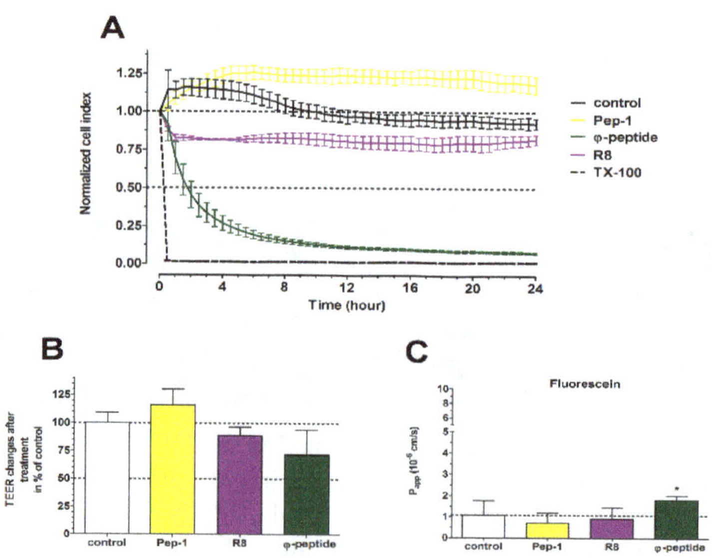

Figure 9. *Cont.*

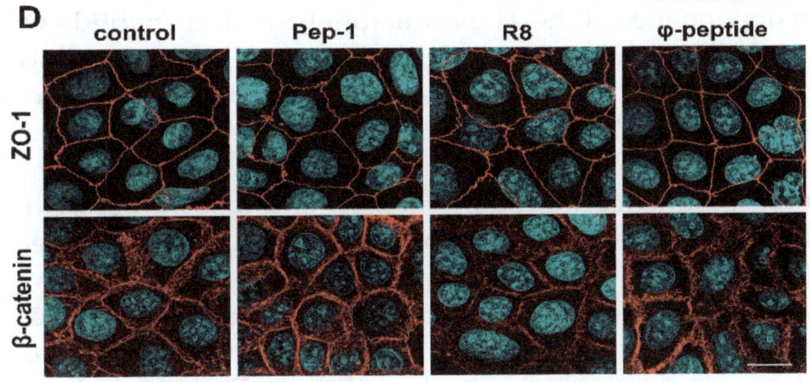

Figure 9. (**A**) Effects of different cell-penetrating peptides (CPPs; 100 μM, 24 h) on Caco-2 cells followed by impedance measurements. The effects of peptides on the impedance were shown as normalized cell index. Values are presented as means ± SD, $n = 3-8$. (**B**) Evaluation of barrier integrity on Caco-2 cell layers by measurement of transepithelial electrical resistance (TEER) after 1-h CPP treatment. (**C**) Caco-2 cell layer permeability for fluorescein marker molecule (P_{app} A-B 10^{-6} cm/s) after 1-h CPP treatment. (**D**) Effects of CPPs on junctional morphology of Caco-2 cells. Immunostaining for zonula occludens-1 (ZO-1) and β-catenin junctional proteins in control conditions and after 1-h peptide treatment. Red color: immunostaining for ZO-1 and β-catenin. Blue color: staining of cell nuclei. Bar = 20 μm.

4. Discussion

We investigated for the first time the dual, TJ modulator and cell membrane actions of the PN159 peptide. PN159 was described as a TJ modulator and permeability-enhancing peptide on airway epithelial cell layers in vitro and in vivo [4], and in our previous comparative work we found it also very effective on culture models of the blood–brain and intestinal barriers [8]. The same peptide, known also as KLAL or MAP was extensively studied for its cell membrane action as a CPP [10–12,35]. However, the identity of the differently named molecule was not previously known for the researchers of the two fields. We demonstrated, that beside the cell-penetrating and antimicrobial effects, PN159 is a TJ modulator on intestinal epithelial cells and by molecular modeling new members of the claudin family were identified as its potential targets.

4.1. TJ Modulator Effect of PN159: Safety, Concentration Dependence and Reversibility

All the presented functional and morphological results point to the safe, concentration-dependent and reversible TJ opening effect of PN159 in Caco-2 cells. The effect of the peptide on epithelial cell viability was investigated for one and 24 h. We found that the peptide has no effect on cell metabolism measured by MTT test or on impedance kinetics and can be considered as safe up to 10 μM. The changes seen after higher, 30 μM concentration were fully reversible. The 100 μM concentration of PN159 caused irreversible changes in both parameters on intestinal epithelial cells after either 1-h or one-day treatment. Using respiratory epithelial tissue (EpiAirway model) and MTT assay, PN159 was found to be safe at concentrations up to 100 μM for a 1-h treatment [9]. The difference between the sensitivity of the epithelial models and also the sensitivity of the applied methods may explain the dissimilarity of these data.

We found a marked concentration-dependence of the TJ modulator effect. With the most sensitive method, TEER, we could determine that 1 μM PN159 already opened the paracellular cleft for ions, while higher concentrations gradually decreased TEER. This TJ modulation by the effective but safe 10 μM concentration of the peptide was fast, within minutes, but after removal of the peptide a full recovery was seen. This opening and complete recovery of the intestinal TJ structure was verified by electron microscopy in the present study and by immunohistochemistry for TJ proteins both in this and our previous work [8]. A similar concentration-dependent and reversible effect of PN159 on TEER was found on airway epithelial tissue, too [4].

The concentration dependence of the TJ modulator effect of the peptide was also detected in the permeability assay for a small and a large hydrophilic marker, fluorescein and albumin. A similarly high permeability increase with a full reversibility was measured for the same markers on both Caco-2 and blood–brain barrier culture models with the 10 μM concentration of PN159 peptide [8]. This action of the peptide was verified by the immunostaining of junctional proteins with higher concentrations causing bigger alterations in junctional protein intensity and distribution. Other claudin-specific TJ modulator peptides act similarly on junctional protein staining as well as on permeability of epithelial and endothelial cells [36,37].

In addition, the opening of the paracellular pathway in Caco-2 monolayers was measured by four dextran markers with size between 4 and 40 kDa. The apparent permeability coefficients of the large dextran macromolecules were very low in control conditions. PN159 treatment (10 μM) elevated the dextran penetration by 159- to 400-fold. The highest increase was measured in the case of the largest, FD-40 marker. The concentration dependency of the permeability increasing effect of PN159 was also observed on the EpiAirway model, but in the concentration range of 25 to 100 μM. The elevation of the permeability was 10- to 30-fold for FD-4 [4] and for peptide hormones with the same size [9].

To study the effect of PN159 on drug penetration, we tested two hydrophilic and two lipophilic drugs, which are substrates of active efflux transporters [24,38]. The permeability of hydrophilic atenolol and cimetidine was very low, while high penetration was measured for the lipophilic quinidine and verapamil on Caco-2 cells in agreement with our previous study [24]. PN159 treatment caused more than 30-fold permeability elevation for atenolol and cimetidine which penetrate slowly across the cell's layers. The peptide increased about 2-fold the permeability of the intestinal culture model for the lipophilic quinidine and verapamil, which already showed a high penetration. The permeability of the slightly lipophilic plant alkaloid, galantamine (287 Da), a substrate of P-glycoprotein, was also increased 2 to 3-fold by PN159 in airway epithelial tissue model [9] confirming the peptide's penetration enhancer effect.

4.2. Tight Junction (TJ)Modulator Effect of PN159: Interaction with Claudins

In our previous study, binding of PN159 in the micromolar range to epithelial claudin-1 and endothelial claudin-5 was demonstrated by affinity measurements and confirmed by docking studies [8]. In this report we describe an additional two intestinal epithelial junctional proteins, claudin-4 and -7 which are highly expressed in Caco-2 cells [34], as potential targets of the peptide by molecular docking. All these results suggest that PN159 peptide may open cell–cell junctions by acting on claudins, the most prominent family of integral membrane junctional proteins. C-CPE and C1C2 tight junction modulator peptides were also described to target claudins. C-CPE is a fragment of *Clostridium perfringens* enterotoxin which directly binds claudin subtypes including claudin-3 and -4 and induces disintegration of tight junctions [39]. The peptidomimetic C1C2 which contains the C-terminal half of ECL1 of claudin-1 predominantly binds to claudin-1 and -5, opens the paracellular barrier in cultured cells and causes cytosolic distribution of claudin-1, -2, -3, -4, and -5 [36]. What is common in the action of these three TJ modulator peptides is that they have specific interactions with conserved amino acids of claudins [8,40], however, these peptides do not share any similarity in their amino acid sequence. The secondary structure of C1C2 consists of β-sheet stabilized by α-helix [40], the claudin-binding domain of C-CPE is a nine-stranded β-sandwich [41], while according to our CD measurements and molecular modelling PN159 also contains β-sheet in addition to α-helix. This structural similarity between the three different but claudin-targeting peptides may be linked to the TJ modulator effect.

4.3. Cell Penetration and Antimicrobial Effect of PN159

We observed a concentration-dependent cellular uptake of PN159 on intestinal barrier cells as reflected in the confocal microscope images. PN159 has a fast uptake in human melanoma cells, treatment with 1 μM concentration already causing detectable entry of the peptide into the cells, in concordance with our results [12]. The cellular uptake of PN159 was also verified on other four cell lines [42]. After treatment with a concentration of 10 μM, the peptide entered the cytoplasm of cells without cytotoxic effects, similar to our data.

Most of the CPPs have antimicrobial activity due to their structural properties, especially the cationic and the amphipathic membrane active peptides [13]. Based on literature data the amphipathic PN159 effectively inhibited the growth of different microorganisms, like *Escherichia coli, Staphylococcus epidermidis, Bacillus megaterium, Saccharomyces cerevisiae* [10,19,43]. In this study we demonstrated the antimicrobial activity of PN159 peptide in the concentration range of 3–46 μM on clinically relevant ESKAPE pathogens. As compared to the reference antibiotics, PN159 was more effective in the inhibition of the growth of *Acinetobacter baumannii, Enterococcus faecium, Enterobacter cloacae* and *Pseudomonas aeruginosa*. (Table 4).

Comparing our results with data from the literature, another amphipathic antimicrobial peptide, melittin, inhibited the growth of *Escherichia coli* and *Micrococcus luteus* [44] and was also tested against three of the ESKAPE pathogens. *Acinetobacter baumannii* and *Pseudomonas aeruginosa* were more sensitive for melittin treatment, than *Klebsiella pneumoniae:* for the inhibition of growth of *Klebsiella pneumoniae* more than 100 μM melittin was needed [45], while in our study around 10 μM PN159 was already effective.

PN159, as a model amphipathic CPP peptide, strongly interacts with biological membranes due to its physical-chemical properties. As a CPP, PN159 enters epithelial cells [42], enhances the membrane penetration of molecules and exerts antimicrobial effects [10,11]. Because PN159 binds different claudins and interacts specifically with their conserved amino acids, it acts as a TJ modulator [8]. It is an open question, however, if the plasma membrane and the TJ modulator actions of PN159 are connected or not.

4.4. TJ Modulator Effect of Other CPPs?

Based on these results we asked the question whether this TJ modulator ability is a unique effect of PN159 among the CPPs or not. Therefore, we have tested two other amphipathic CPPs, the widely used Pep-1 [16] and the cyclic φ-peptide [15], and one cationic CPP, R8 peptide [18] on the barrier integrity of Caco-2 monolayers. None of the tested CPPs had a TJ modulator effect similar to PN159. There was no change in the TEER values and only the φ-peptide increased the permeability of fluorescein. Since no effect was seen on junctional staining in epithelial cells treated with φ-peptide, the increase in permeability and decrease in the cell layer impedance may be linked to the cell membrane action of this CPP [15]. As we demonstrated by our modeling results, PN159 peptide interacts with conserved residues of the claudins investigated (Figure 6) suggesting its ability for specific interactions [8]. The amino acid sequence of PN159 results in an amphipathic helix structure [10], which is not characteristic of the other CPPs investigated in our paper. From the other three investigated peptides, R8 and φ-peptide have positively charged arginine clusters (Table 1) and are considered as clearly cationic CPPs [17]. Pep-1 also contains a positively charged amino acid cluster and is rich in tryptophan repeats (Table 1). Neither PN159 contains clusters of arginine or positively charged amino acids, nor tryptophan (Table 1). While we have not found a CPP with a TJ modulator effect in the current study, we cannot exclude that other membrane active peptides can have such dual action. The amphipathic antimicrobial peptide melittin enhanced the paracellular permeability for dextran marker molecules on Caco-2 cells [46]. The opening of TJs by melittin was mediated, at least partially, by the prostaglandin signaling pathway [46].

5. Conclusions

We demonstrated that PN159 (KLAL/MAP) peptide as a penetration enhancer has a dual action on intestinal epithelial cells. The peptide safely and reversibly enhances the permeability of model molecules and drugs through intestinal epithelial cell layers by opening the intercellular junctions. We identified claudin-4 and -7 junctional proteins by docking studies as potential binding partners and targets of the peptide in the opening of the paracellular pathway. In addition to the tight junction modulator action, the peptide has a concentration-dependent cellular uptake and cell membrane permeabilizing effect, which can also contribute to its penetration-enhancing effect. This dual action is not general for cell-penetrating peptides, since the other three CPPs tested did not show barrier opening effects. Therefore, we propose the investigation of CPPs for testing their effect on paracellular permeability.

Author Contributions: Conceptualization, M.A.D., A.B. and T.A.M.; methodology, A.B., I.G. and L.K.; formal analysis, A.B. and F.Ö.; investigation, A.B., I.G., L.K., O.Z., L.D., M.V. and Á.K.; resources, L.F., N.I., T.A.M., C.P., P.S.-R. and M.A.D.; data curation, A.B. and I.G.; writing—original draft preparation, A.B., M.A.D.; writing—review and editing, A.B., I.G., L.K., F.Ö., O.Z., L.D., L.F., M.V., Á.K., N.I., T.A.M., C.P., P.S.-R. and M.A.D.; visualization, A.B., Á.K. and F.Ö.; supervision, M.A.D., P.S.-R., T.A.M., and C.P.; funding acquisition, M.A.D., T.A.M., M.V. and C.P.

Acknowledgments: The help of Zoltán Kóta during the experiments is gratefully acknowledged. We are grateful to Zsombor Kapás for his help in the preparation of the figures. The European Research Council H2020-ERC-2014-CoG 648364—Resistance Evolution (C.P.).

References

1. Deli, M.A. Potential use of tight junction modulators to reversibly open membranous barriers and improve drug delivery. A review. *Biochim. Biophys. Acta* **2009**, *1788*, 892–910. [CrossRef] [PubMed]
2. Kiss, L.; Hellinger, É.; Pilbat, A.M.; Kittel, Á.; Török, Z.; Füredi, A.; Szakács, G.; Veszelka, S.; Sipos, P.; Ózsvári, B.; et al. Sucrose esters increase drug penetration, but do not inhibit p-glycoprotein in caco-2 intestinal epithelial cells. *J. Pharm. Sci.* **2014**, *103*, 3107–3119. [CrossRef] [PubMed]
3. Perinelli, D.R.; Vllasaliu, D.; Bonacucina, G.; Come, B.; Pucciarelli, S.; Ricciutelli, M.; Cespi, M.; Itri, R.; Spinozzi, F.; Palmieri, G.F.; et al. Rhamnolipids as epithelial permeability enhancers for macromolecular therapeutics. *Eur. J. Pharm. Biopharm.* **2017**, *119*, 419–425. [CrossRef] [PubMed]
4. Johnson, P.H.; Quay, S.C. Advances in nasal drug delivery through tight junction technology. A review. *Expert. Opin. Drug Deliv.* **2005**, *2*, 281–298. [CrossRef] [PubMed]
5. Chiba, H.; Osanai, M.; Murata, M.; Kojima, T.; Sawada, N. Transmembrane proteins of tight junctions. A review. *Biochim. Biophys. Acta* **2008**, *1778*, 588–600. [CrossRef] [PubMed]
6. Krause, G.; Winkler, L.; Mueller, S.L.; Haseloff, R.F.; Piontek, J.; Blasig, I.E. Structure and function of claudins. A review. *Biochim. Biophys. Acta* **2008**, *1778*, 631–645. [CrossRef] [PubMed]
7. Tscheik, C.; Blasig, I.E.; Winkler, L. Trends in drug delivery through tissue barriers containing tight junctions. *Tissue Barriers* **2013**, *1*, e24565. [CrossRef] [PubMed]
8. Bocsik, A.; Walter, R.F.; Gyebrovszki, A.; Fülöp, L.; Blasig, I.; Dabrowski, S.; Ötvös, F.; Tóth, A.; Rákhely, G.; Veszelka, S.; et al. Reversible opening of intercellular junctions of intestinal epithelial and brain endothelial cells with tight junction modulator peptides. *J. Pharm. Sci.* **2016**, *105*, 754–765. [CrossRef] [PubMed]
9. Chen, S.C.; Eiting, K.; Cui, K.; Leonard, A.K.; Morris, D.; Li, C.Y.; Farber, K.; Sileno, A.P.; Houston, M.E., Jr.; Johnson, P.H.; et al. Therapeutic utility of a novel tight junction modulating peptide for enhancing intranasal drug delivery. *J. Pharm. Sci.* **2006**, *95*, 1364–1371. [CrossRef] [PubMed]
10. Dathe, M.; Schümann, M.; Wieprecht, T.; Winkler, A.; Beyermann, M.; Krause, E.; Matsuzaki, K.; Murase, O.; Bienert, M. Peptide helicity and membrane surface charge modulate the balance of electrostatic and hydrophobic interactions with lipid bilayers and biological membranes. *Biochemistry* **1996**, *35*, 12612–12622. [CrossRef]
11. Oehlke, J.; Scheller, A.; Wiesner, B.; Krause, E.; Beyermann, M.; Klauschenz, E.; Melzig, M.; Bienert, M. Cellular uptake of an alpha-helical amphipathic model peptide with the potential to deliver polar compounds into the cell interiornon-endocytically. *Biochim. Biophys. Acta* **1998**, *1414*, 127–139. [CrossRef]
12. Hällbrink, M.; Florén, A.; Elmquist, A.; Pooga, M.; Bartfai, T.; Langel, U. Cargo delivery kinetics of cell-penetrating peptides. *Biochim. Biophys. Acta* **2001**, *1515*, 101–109. [CrossRef]
13. Arouri, A.; Dathe, M.; Blume, A. The helical propensity of KLA amphipathic peptides enhances their binding to gel-state lipid membranes. *Biophys. Chem.* **2013**, *180–181*, 10–21. [CrossRef] [PubMed]

14. Copolovici, D.M.; Langel, K.; Eriste, E.; Langel, Ü. Cell-penetrating peptides: Design, synthesis, and applications. A review. *ACS Nano* **2014**, *8*, 1972–1994. [CrossRef] [PubMed]
15. Qian, Z.; LaRochelle, J.R.; Jiang, B.; Lian, W.; Hard, R.L.; Selner, N.G.; Luechapanichkul, R.; Barrios, A.M.; Pei, D. Early endosomal escape of a cyclic cell-penetrating peptide allows effective cytosolic cargo delivery. *Biochemistry* **2014**, *53*, 4034–4046. [CrossRef]
16. Morris, M.C.; Deshayes, S.; Heitz, F.; Divita, G. Cell-penetrating peptides: From molecular mechanisms to therapeutics. A review. *Biol. Cell* **2008**, *100*, 201–217. [CrossRef]
17. Guidotti, G.; Brambilla, L.; Rossi, D. Cell-Penetrating Peptides: From Basic Research to Clinics. A review. *Trends Pharmacol. Sci.* **2017**, *38*, 406–424. [CrossRef]
18. He, L.; Sayers, E.J.; Watson, P.; Jones, A.T. Contrasting roles for actin in the cellular uptake of cell penetrating peptide conjugates. *Sci. Rep.* **2018**, *8*, 7318. [CrossRef]
19. Palm, C.; Netzereab, S.; Hällbrink, M. Quantitatively determined uptake of cell-penetrating peptides in non-mammalian cells with an evaluation of degradation and antimicrobial effects. *Peptides* **2006**, *27*, 1710–1716. [CrossRef]
20. Boucher, H.W.; Talbot, G.H.; Bradley, J.S.; Edwards, J.E.; Gilbert, D.; Rice, L.B.; Scheld, M.; Spellberg, B.; Bartlett, J. Bad bugs, no drugs: No ESKAPE! An update from the Infectious Diseases Society of America. A review. *Clin. Infect. Dis.* **2009**, *48*, 1–12. [CrossRef]
21. Lázár, V.; Martins, A.; Spohn, R.; Daruka, L.; Grézal, G.; Fekete, G.; Számel, M.; Jangir, P.K.; Kintses, B.; Csörgő, B.; et al. Antibiotic-resistant bacteria show widespread collateral sensitivity to antimicrobial peptides. *Nat. Microbiol.* **2018**, *3*, 718–731. [CrossRef] [PubMed]
22. Artursson, P.; Palm, K.; Luthman, K. Caco-2 monolayers in experimental and theoretical predictions of drug transport. *Adv. Drug Deliv. Rev.* **2001**, *46*, 27–43. [CrossRef]
23. Hubatsch, I.; Ragnarsson, E.G.; Artursson, P. Determination of drug permeability and prediction of drug absorption in Caco-2 monolayers. *Nat. Protoc.* **2007**, *2*, 2111–2119. [CrossRef] [PubMed]
24. Hellinger, E.; Veszelka, S.; Tóth, A.E.; Walter, F.; Kittel, A.; Bakk, M.L.; Tihanyi, K.; Háda, V.; Nakagawa, S.; Duy, T.D.; Niwa, M.; et al. Comparison of brain capillary endothelial cell-based and epithelial (MDCK-MDR1, Caco-2, and VB-Caco-2) cell-based surrogate blood-brain barrier penetration models. *Eur. J. Pharm. Biopharm.* **2012**, *82*, 340–351. [CrossRef] [PubMed]
25. Roka, E.; Vecsernyes, M.; Bacskay, I.; Félix, C.; Rhimi, M.; Coleman, A.W.; Perret, F. para-Sulphonato-calix[n]arenes as selective activators for the passage of molecules across the Caco-2 model intestinal membrane. *Chem. Commun.* **2015**, *51*, 9374–9376. [CrossRef] [PubMed]
26. Kürti, L.; Veszelka, S.; Bocsik, A.; Dung, N.T.; Ozsvári, B.; Puskás, L.G.; Kittel, A.; Szabó-Révész, P.; Deli, M.A. The effect of sucrose esters on a culture model of thenasal barrier. *Toxicol. In Vitro* **2012**, *26*, 445–454. [CrossRef] [PubMed]
27. Dichroweb, on-line Analysis for Protein Circular Dichroism spectra. Available online: dichroweb.cryst.bbk.ac.uk/html/home.shtml (accessed on 10 December 2015).
28. Sali, A.; Blundell, T.L. Comparative protein modelling by satisfaction of spatial restraints. *J. Mol. Biol.* **1993**, *234*, 779–815. [CrossRef] [PubMed]
29. Suzuki, H.; Nishizawa, T.; Tani, K.; Yamazaki, Y.; Tamura, A.; Ishitani, R.; Dohmae, N.; Tsukita, S.; Nureki, O.; Fujiyoshi, Y. Crystal structure of a claudin provides insight into the architecture of tight junctions. *Science* **2014**, *344*, 304–307. [CrossRef]
30. Phillips, J.C.; Braun, R.; Wang, W.; Gumbart, J.; Tajkhorshid, E.; Villa, E.; Chipot, C.; Skeel, R.D.; Kalé, L.; Schulten, K. Scalable molecular dynamics with NAMD. *J. Comput. Chem.* **2005**, *26*, 1781–1802. [CrossRef]
31. Humphrey, W.; Dalke, A.; Schulten, K. VMD: Visual molecular dynamics. *J. Mol. Graph.* **1996**, *14*, 33–38. [CrossRef]
32. Kurcinski, M.; Jamroz, M.; Blaszczyk, M.; Kolinski, A.; Kmiecik, S. CABS-dock web server for the flexible docking of peptides to proteins without prior knowledge of the binding site. *Nucleic. Acids. Res.* **2015**, *43*, W419–W424. [CrossRef] [PubMed]
33. Wiegand, I.; Hilpert, K.; Hancock, R.E. Agar and broth dilution methods to determine the minimal inhibitory concentration (MIC) of antimicrobial substances. *Nat. Protoc.* **2008**, *3*, 163–175. [CrossRef] [PubMed]
34. Veszelka, S.; Tóth, A.; Walter, F.R.; Tóth, A.E.; Gróf, I.; Mészáros, M.; Bocsik, A.; Hellinger, É.; Vastag, M.; Rákhely, G.; Deli, M.A. Comparison of a Rat Primary Cell-Based Blood-Brain Barrier Model With Epithelial

and Brain Endothelial Cell Lines: Gene Expression and Drug Transport. *Front. Mol. Neurosci.* **2018**, *11*, 166. [CrossRef] [PubMed]

35. Erbe, A.; Kerth, A.; Dathe, M.; Blume, A. Interactions of KLA amphipathic model peptides with lipid monolayers. *ChemBioChem* **2009**, *10*, 2884–2892. [CrossRef] [PubMed]
36. Staat, C.; Coisne, C.; Dabrowski, S.; Stamatovic, S.M.; Andjelkovic, A.V.; Wolburg, H.; Engelhardt, B.; Blasig, I.E. Mode of action of claudin peptidomimetics in the transient opening of cellular tight junction barriers. *Biomaterials* **2015**, *54*, 9–20. [CrossRef] [PubMed]
37. Dithmer, S.; Staat, C.; Müller, C.; Ku, M.C.; Pohlmann, A.; Niendorf, T.; Gehne, N.; Fallier-Becker, P.; Kittel, Á.; Walter, F.R.; Veszelka, S.; et al. Claudin peptidomimetics modulate tissue barriers for enhanced drug delivery. *Ann. N. Y. Acad. Sci.* **2017**, *1397*, 169–184. [CrossRef] [PubMed]
38. Hellinger, E.; Bakk, M.L.; Pócza, P.; Tihanyi, K.; Vastag, M. Drug penetration model of vinblastine-treated Caco-2 cultures. *Eur. J. Pharm. Sci.* **2010**, *41*, 96–106. [CrossRef] [PubMed]
39. Sonoda, N.; Furuse, M.; Sasaki, H.; Yonemura, S.; Katahira, J.; Horiguchi, Y.; Tsukita, S. Clostridium perfringens enterotoxin fragment removes specific claudins from tight junction strands: Evidence for direct involvement of claudins in tight junction barrier. *J. Cell Biol.* **1999**, *147*, 195–204. [CrossRef]
40. Dabrowski, S.; Staat, C.; Zwanziger, D.; Sauer, R.S.; Bellmann, C.; Günther, R.; Krause, E.; Haseloff, R.F.; Rittner, H.; Blasig, I.E. Redox-sensitive structure and function of the first extracellular loop of the cell-cell contact protein claudin-1: Lessons from molecular structure to animals. *Antioxid. Redox. Signal* **2015**, *22*, 1–14. [CrossRef]
41. Veshnyakova, A.; Piontek, J.; Protze, J.; Waziri, N.; Heise, I.; Krause, G. Mechanism of Clostridium perfringens enterotoxin interaction with claudin-3/-4 protein suggests structural modifications of the toxin to target specific claudins. *J. Biol. Chem.* **2012**, *287*, 1698–1708. [CrossRef]
42. Mueller, J.; Kretzschmar, I.; Volkmer, R.; Boisguerin, P. Comparison of cellular uptake using 22 CPPs in 4 different cell lines. *Bioconjug. Chem.* **2008**, *19*, 2363–2374. [CrossRef] [PubMed]
43. Bagheri, M.; Beyermann, M.; Dathe, M. Immobilization reduces the activity of surface-bound cationic antimicrobial peptides with no influence upon the activity spectrum. *Antimicrob. Agents Chemother.* **2009**, *53*, 1132–1141. [CrossRef] [PubMed]
44. Maher, S.; McClean, S. Investigation of the cytotoxicity of eukaryotic and prokaryotic antimicrobial peptides in intestinal epithelial cells in vitro. *Biochem. Pharmacol.* **2006**, *71*, 1289–1298. [CrossRef] [PubMed]
45. Lam, S.J.; O'Brien-Simpson, N.M.; Pantarat, N.; Sulistio, A.; Wong, E.H.; Chen, Y.Y.; Lenzo, J.C.; Holden, J.A.; Blencowe, A.; Reynolds, E.C.; et al. Combating multidrug-resistant Gram-negative bacteria with structurally nanoengineered antimicrobial peptide polymers. *Nat. Microbiol.* **2016**, *1*, 16162. [CrossRef] [PubMed]
46. Maher, S.; Feighery, L.; Brayden, D.J.; McClean, S. Melittin as an epithelial permeability enhancer I: Investigation of its mechanism of action in Caco-2 monolayers. *Pharm. Res.* **2007**, *24*, 1336–1345. [CrossRef] [PubMed]

6

Enhanced Transepithelial Permeation of Gallic Acid and (−)-Epigallocatechin Gallate across Human Intestinal Caco-2 Cells Using Electrospun Xanthan Nanofibers

Adele Faralli, Elhamalsadat Shekarforoush, Ana C. Mendes and Ioannis S. Chronakis *

Nano-BioScience Research Group, DTU-Food, Technical University of Denmark, Kemitorvet, B202, 2800 Kgs. Lyngby, Denmark; adele.faralli@gmail.com (A.F.); elham.shekar@gmail.com (E.S.); anac@food.dtu.dk (A.C.M.)

* Correspondence: ioach@food.dtu.dk

Abstract: Electrospun xanthan polysaccharide nanofibers (X) were developed as an encapsulation and delivery system of the poorly absorbed polyphenol compounds, gallic acid (GA) and (−)-epigallocatechin gallate (EGCG). Scanning electron microscopy was used to characterize the electrospun nanofibers, and controlled release studies were performed at pH 6.5 and 7.4 in saline buffer, suggesting that the release of polyphenols from xanthan nanofibers follows a non-Fickian mechanism. Furthermore, the X-GA and X-EGCG nanofibers were incubated with Caco-2 cells, and the cell viability, transepithelial transport, and permeability properties across cell monolayers were investigated. Increases of GA and EGCG permeabilities were observed when the polyphenols were loaded into xanthan nanofibers, compared to the free compounds. The observed in vitro permeability enhancement of GA and EGCG was induced by the presence of the polysaccharide nanofibers, which successfully inhibited efflux transporters, as well as by opening tight junctions.

Keywords: xanthan gum; electrospinning; gallic acid; (−)-epigallocatechin gallate; permeability

1. Introduction

Polyphenols are the most abundant antioxidants in our diet and they are receiving increasing interest due to the established association between the intake of a polyphenol-rich diet and the prevention of various diseases [1,2]. Because of their antioxidant [3], antimutagenic [4], and anticarcinogenic properties [5,6], polyphenols have recently attracted research interest towards the study of their metabolism and absorption mechanisms across the gut barrier [7].

Polyphenols are categorized according to the chemical structure of their carbon skeleton, and the most abundant classes in our diet are phenolic acids and flavonoids. The most encountered phenolic acids are caffeic acid, ferulic acid, and gallic acid (GA). The latter, also known as 3,4,5-trihydroxybenzoic acid, is one of the main endogenous phenolic acids found in plants, mostly in tea leaves [8]. GA, also found in vegetables, grapes, and pomegranates, is a potent non-enzymatic antioxidant and has a natural antitumor activity against lung, prostate, colon, gastric, and breast cancer and human pre-myelocytic leukemia [9–12]. It has been reported that the in vitro treatment of lung and human cervical cancer cells with GA concentrations in the micromolar range induces cell death associated with the depletion of glutathione (GSH) as well as reactive oxygen species (ROS) level changes [13,14]. The physiological impact and efficiency of GA is strictly dependent on its bioavailability, biochemical integrity, and successful interaction with target tissues. Many studies have demonstrated that only small amounts of orally administered GA are absorbed through the intestine due to its low permeability, poor water solubility, and chemical instability. The GA instability in the gastrointestinal tract is promoted by endogenous enzymes, interfering nutrients, and oxidative reactions that lead to a considerable loss in its activity [15]. It is also reported that the phenol concentrations needed to result in an in vitro efficiency are higher than the moderate in vivo levels, and gastrointestinal permeation is supported only by passive diffusion [15]. Moreover, previous studies found that after oral administration of *Phyllanthi* tannin fraction at a dose of 6 g/kg in rats, the maximum concentration of absorbed GA was less than 10.47 μg/mL [16]. In vitro investigations have also been conducted with Caco-2 cell monolayers, in order to evaluate the transepithelial transport of pure GA across the cellular barrier, and the apparent permeability coefficient, P_{app}, under a proton gradient was about 0.20×10^{-6} cm/s [8].

Flavonoids, the most abundant polyphenols in our diet together with phenolic acids, can be divided into several classes, and catechins are the main flavonols found in tea [1]. The major tea catechins are (−)-epigallocatechin gallate (EGCG), (−)-epicatechin gallate (ECG), (−)-epicatechin (EC), and (−)-epigallocatechin (EGC) [17]. These natural compounds have demonstrated various health-beneficial properties, including antioxidant, anti-inflammatory, and anticancer effects, both in animals and humans [18,19]. Indeed, an inverse association between tea consumption and colorectal cancer frequency as well as gastric cancer has been identified [20,21]. An increasing interest towards EGCG has led to an extensive investigation of the beneficial properties of this natural molecule in the cosmetic, nutritional, and pharmaceutical fields. However, like GA, EGCG has a poor oral bioavailability and poor biochemical stability. In fact, EGCG has a low lipophilicity (octanol/water partition coefficient of 0.86 ± 0.03), thus limiting its intrinsic permeability across the intestinal epithelium [19]. Several studies have instead demonstrated a high and specific accumulation of tea flavonoids in epithelial Caco-2 cells or epithelial cells along the aerodigestive tract [17,22,23], which have been recognized as major sites for biological activity of flavonoids. In the Caco-2 cell model, apical uptake transporters and efflux pumps, such as the multidrug resistance-associated proteins, MRP1 and MRP2, and P-glycoprotein have been identified to play a major role in cellular accumulation of catechins [17,19,24,25].

In the light of these considerations, the oral administration of GA and EGCG requires a formulation strategy able to protect and maintain their structural integrity, increase their bioavailability and water solubility, and deliver them to target tissues. Among the existing delivery and stabilization approaches, the encapsulation of sensitive compounds is considered the most effective strategy for improving the oral bioavailability and shelf-life of compounds [15,26,27]. Nowadays, a plethora of encapsulation techniques are commonly used in oral delivery systems, and carrier systems for phenolic acids and flavonoids encapsulation have found feasible approaches to overcome both enzymatic degradation and membrane permeation issues [7,19]. The encapsulation of EGCG in a niosomal formulation results in a significantly enhanced bioactive absorption, stronger chemical stability, and lower toxicity compared with the free EGCG [19]. The in vitro apparent permeability, P_{app}, of EGCG niosome across Caco-2 cell monolayers was found to be $1.42 \pm 0.24 \times 10^{-6}$ cm/s, almost 2-fold more as free EGCG ($P_{app} = 0.88 \pm 0.09 \times 10^{-6}$ cm/s). Furthermore, GA-loaded mesoporous silica nanoparticles (MSNs-GA) were easily internalized into Caco-2 cells without any deleterious effect on cell viability, and preserving the same antitumor properties of free GA [7]. In addition, the topical and transdermal delivery of GA loaded into poly(ʟ-lactic acid) fiber mats resulted in a preserved radical scavenging activity of the released phenolic acid [28]. GA has also been encapsulated within electrospun fibers as delivery carriers using the protein zein [29], cellulose acetate [30], and polylactic acid (PLA) nanofibers, including GA-cyclodextrin complexes [31]. The encapsulation and release of EGCG loaded into electrospun nanofibers has also been investigated using zein nanofibers [32], hyaluronic acid/ lactic-*co*-glycolic acid fibers (HA/PLGA, core/shell) [33], PLGA nanofibers [34,35], cellulose electrospun nanofibrous mats coated with bilayers of chitosan and EGCG [36], and electrospun hydroxypropyl methylcellulose nanofibers [37].

In our previous study, electrospun xanthan-chitosan nanofibers loaded with curcumin, as a model hydrophobic bioactive, were incubated with Caco-2 cells and the transepithelial transport and permeability properties across cell monolayers were assessed. A 3.4-fold increase of curcumin permeability was detected in the presence of xanthan-chitosan nanofibers, in comparison with free-curcumin [38,39]. Moreover, electrospun xanthan nanofibers developed from a solution of xanthan dissolved in formic acid, remained intact and morphologically stable over a wide pH range in saline buffers [40]. In the present study, electrospun xanthan nanofibers were assessed as an encapsulation and delivery system of the two polyphenols, GA and EGCG. The xanthan-GA and xanthan-EGCG loaded nanofibers were incubated with Caco-2 cells, and the transepithelial transport and permeability of GA and EGCG across the cell monolayers were investigated.

2. Materials and Methods

2.1. Materials

The human colon adenocarcinoma cell line, Caco-2 [Caco-2] (ATCC® HTB-37™), was obtained from the American Type Culture Collection (Rockville, MD, USA). Dulbecco's modified Eagle's medium (DMEM) high glucose (4.5 g/L), L-glutamine (200 mM), nonessential amino acids (100X), penicillin-streptomycin (10,000 U/mL and 10 mg/mL in 0.9% sodium chloride, respectively), trypsin-EDTA (10X), Dulbecco's Phosphate Buffered Saline 1X without calcium chloride and magnesium chloride (indicated in the text as PBS), fluorescein sodium salt (FLUO), lucifer yellow dilithium salt (LY), methanesulfonic acid, MES (1 M; pH 5.5–6.7), 4-(2-hydroxyethyl)-1-piperazineethanesulfonic acid solution, HEPES (1 M; pH 7.0–7.6), gallic acid (GA), and (−)-epigallocatechin gallate (EGCG) were purchased from Sigma Aldrich (Brøndby, Denmark). Tissue culture 12-well plates and 12-mm polycarbonate cell culture inserts with an area of 1.12 cm^2 and a pore size of 0.4 μm were purchased from Corning Costar® Corporation. Fetal bovine serum (FBS) and Hanks' balanced salt solution (HBSS) with calcium and magnesium and without phenol red were obtained from Thermo Fisher Scientific (Roskilde, Denmark). CellTiter 96® AQueous One Solution Cell Proliferation Assay (MTS) was purchased from Promega Biotech AB (Nacka, Sweden). Xanthan gum (Cosphaderm X-34) from *Xanthomonas campestris* was kindly provided by Cosphatec GmbH (Drehbahn, Hamburg, Germany) [40].

2.2. Fabrication of Electrospun Nanofibers

Xanthan was dissolved in formic acid at a final concentration of 2.5% *w/v* under vigorous stirring overnight at room temperature. Subsequently, GA and EGCG were added to the polysaccharide solution and further stirred for 30 min. The electrospinning setup consisted of a high voltage generator (ES50P-10W, Gamma High Voltage Research, Inc., Ormond Beach, FL, USA) to provide a voltage of 20 kV, and a syringe pump (New Era Pump Systems, Inc., Farmingdale, NY, USA) to feed the xanthan solution at a flow rate of 0.01 mL/min using a 21 G needle gauge. Xanthan fibers were collected on a steel plate covered with an aluminum foil perpendicularly placed at 8 cm from the end of the needle. The electrospinning process was carried out at ambient conditions (20°C and around 20% relative humidity).

2.3. Morphology and FTIR Characterisation of the Nanofibers

The morphology of electrospun X, X-GA, and X-EGCG nanofibers was studied using a Phenom Pro scanning electron microscope (SEM) (Phenom World, Thermo Fisher Scientific, Eindhoven, The Netherlands). For SEM analysis, a small piece of nanofibers web was attached on SEM specimen stubs by a double-sided adhesive tape. The average fiber diameter of nanofibers was calculated using image J analysis software (National Institutes of Health, Bethesda, MD, USA) measured at 100 different points for each image.

Fourier transform infrared (FTIR) spectroscopy analysis of X, X-GA, X-EGCG nanofibers, GA, and EGCG was analyzed using a Perkin Elmer Spectrum 100 spectrometer (Perkin Elmer, Waltham, MA, USA) based on a universal attenuated total reflectance (ATR) sensor. Four scans for each sample were accumulated at 20 °C at a resolution of 1 cm^{-1}. The infrared peaks were identified with a Spectrum™ 10 software using a 1% transmittance (T) peak threshold.

2.4. *In Vitro Release of Gallic Acid and (−)-Epigallocatechin Gallate from Electrospun Nanofibers*

The amount of GA and EGCG loaded into xanthan nanofibers was evaluated by immersing the nanofibers in equal volumes of complete growth medium (DMEM-FBS) or HBSS at pH 6.5 or pH 7.4. Briefly, 1.0 mg of X-GA and X-EGCG fibers were immersed in 2 mL pre-warmed medium in a 48-well plate, and the release of molecules from nanofibers was conducted at 37 °C for 8 h. The withdrawn aliquots were analyzed by RP-HPLC with detection of GA and EGCG at 255 nm and 270 nm, respectively (see also Section 2.10). The cumulative amount of each compound released from nanofibers was then considered as the maximum releasable GA and EGCG from the nanofiber formulation under those conditions. All data are expressed as mean ± SD of three independent experiments.

2.5. *Caco-2 Cell Culture and Subculture*

Caco-2 cells were routinely seeded at a concentration of 1.0×10^5 cells/mL in T-75 cm^2 flasks and incubated at 37 °C in a humidified atmosphere of 5% CO_2. The complete cell medium, here indicated as DMEM-FBS, consisted of high glucose DMEM containing 10% heat-inactivated FBS, 2 mM L-glutamine, 1% nonessential amino acids, 100 U/mL penicillin, and 100 µg/mL streptomycin. The medium was renewed every second day until cells reached approximately 90% confluence. Cells were passaged at a subcultivation ratio of 1:4 by treatment with 0.25% trypsin—0.53 mM EDTA solution for 10 min at 37 °C. After trypsinization, the cells were suspended in complete growth medium and centrifuged for 5 min at 1000 rpm. After supernatant removal, the pellet was suspended in the growth medium and cell concentration was determined with an ORFLO Moxi Z Mini Automated Cell Counter using Type S cassette (Biofrontier Technology, Bukit, Singapore). All Caco-2 cells were used between passages 9–15.

2.6. *Compounds and Electrospun Nanofibers Tested with Caco-2 Cell Monolayers*

Xanthan (X), gallic acid-loaded xanthan (X-GA), and (−)-epigallocatechin gallate-loaded xanthan (X-EGCG) nanofibers were produced by electrospinning a solution of the mixed compounds dissolved in formic acid. These nanofibers were tested with Caco-2 cell monolayers to evaluate their toxicity and apparent permeability coefficient (P_{app}) after GA and EGCG release from nanofibers and as free compounds. Before testing nanofiber mats with Caco-2 cells, the collected fibers were kept under an air stream for 3 days allowing complete formic acid evaporation. Besides GA and EGCG, the transepithelial transport of fluorescein (FLUO) and Lucifer yellow (LY) across Caco-2 cell monolayers were also investigated as markers for intestinal epithelial permeability and integrity.

2.7. *Caco-2 Cell Viability Assay*

The in vitro Caco-2 cell viability after treatment with free GA, free EGCG, xanthan nanofibers (X), GA-loaded xanthan nanofibers (X-GA), and EGCG-loaded xanthan nanofibers was evaluated by using the MTS [3-(4,5-dimethylthiazol-2-yl)-5-(3-carboxymethoxyphenyl)-2-(4-sulfophenyl)-2H-tetrazolium inner salt] colorimetric bioassay. Different concentrations of free GA and EGCG ranging from 1 µM to 1 mM were prepared in PBS and sterile-filtered with a 0.22 µm pore size. Furthermore, increasing amounts of dried X, X-GA, and X-EGCG nanofibers were peeled off from the aluminum foils and incubated with cells. In a 48-well plate, 1.5×10^5 cells/mL were seeded in a complete growth medium and incubated for 2 days at 37 °C in a humidified atmosphere of 5% CO_2. Then, the monolayers were washed with PBS and the complete medium was renewed. Caco-2 cells were incubated with free GA and free EGCG solutions, X nanofibers, X-GA nanofibers, X-EGCG nanofibers, and PBS as a control. The plates were incubated for 24 h at 37 °C in a humidified atmosphere of 5% CO_2. The following day, all supernatants, including those with suspended nanofibers, were removed, cells were washed with PBS, and the medium was renewed. 40 µL of pre-warmed MTS solution was added to each well under dark conditions. After 3 h incubation at 37 °C, the absorbance of the reduced MTS (formazan product) was recorded at 490 nm through a well plate reader (Wallac 1420 Victor2 Multilabel Counter, Perkin Elmer, Waltham, MA, USA).

2.8. Transepithelial Transport

The transepithelial transport of free fluorescein (FLUO), free lucifer yellow (LY), free gallic acid (GA), free (−)-epigallocatechin gallate (EGCG), free gallic acid in the presence of empty xanthan nanofibers (X + GA), free (−)-epigallocatechin gallate in the presence of empty xanthan nanofibers (X + EGCG), gallic acid-loaded xanthan nanofibers (X-GA), and (−)-epigallocatechin gallate-loaded xanthan nanofibers (X-EGCG) across Caco-2 cell monolayers were investigated according to the protocol reported by Hubatsch et al. [41]. The transport experiments were performed in both apical-to-basolateral (AB, absorptive) and basolateral-to-apical (BA, secretory) directions, under a proton gradient. In fact, to mimic the acidic microclimate of the small intestine, apical and basolateral pH of around 6.5 and 7.4 were used, respectively. Briefly, 1.0×10^5 cells/insert were seeded onto pre-wetted 12-mm polycarbonate cell culture inserts with an area of 1.12 cm^2 and a pore size of 0.4 μm. The apical and basolateral compartments were filled with 0.5 mL and 1.5 mL complete medium, respectively. The Caco-2 cells were incubated onto the filters overnight at 37 °C in a humidified atmosphere of 5% CO_2. The day after, the growth medium was replaced in both compartments and the plates were incubated for 21 days at 37 °C in a humidified atmosphere of 5% CO_2, renewing the complete growth medium every second day. For the AB transport experiments, donor solutions of FLUO, LY, GA, and EGCG at a concentration of 11 mM, 9.57 mM, 1.1 mM, and 1.1 mM, respectively, were prepared in sterile-filter HBSS at pH 6.5 buffered with 10 mM MES. Again, donor solutions of FLUO, LY, GA, and EGCG at a concentration of 10.3 mM, 9 mM, 1.03 mM, and 1.03 mM, respectively, were prepared in sterile-filter HBSS at pH 7.4 buffered with 25 mM HEPES to evaluate their BA transport. A volume of 50 μL of each stock solution was added to the donor chamber (0.55 mL and 1.55 mL were the total volumes in A and B, respectively). The transport of GA and EGCG released from nanofibers and as free compounds in the presence of empty X nanofibers was also investigated. For the AB transport, 0.2 mg X-GA, 1.0 mg X-EGCG, 0.2 mg, and 1.0 mg X were used, and accordingly, 0.6 mg X-GA, 3.0 mg X-EGCG, 0.6 mg, and 3.0 mg X were incubated with cell monolayers to evaluate their BA transport. Prior to incubation of the nanofibers, the mats were peeled off from the aluminum foil and kept under an air stream for 3 days. After 21 days of cell growth, the complete DMEM medium was removed from the cell monolayers and replaced with HBSS at pH 6.5 and pH 7.4 at the apical and basolateral compartments, respectively. For the AB transport studies, 1.5 mL HBSS was used in the basolateral side and 0.55 mL of each donor solution and/or nanofibers were added to the apical side. Immediately, 200 μL aliquots were withdrawn from each donor compartment (time = 0). Aliquots from the acceptor side were then withdrawn at different time intervals, and the volume was replaced with fresh HBSS at pH 7.4 maintaining the well plates at 37 °C in a humidified atmosphere of 5% CO_2. A final aliquot from the donor chamber was taken as the last time point. BA transport studies were conducted using the same procedure and incubating 0.5 mL HBSS at pH 6.5 in the apical side and 1.55 mL of donor solution and/or nanofibers in the basolateral chamber. During the transport experiments, all cell media were pre-warmed at 37 °C. Each transport experiment was performed for a time interval of 8 h in triplicate ($n = 3$). After 8 h of transport studies and TEER measurements, both apical and basolateral chambers were washed twice with PBS and cell monolayers were detached from the insert membrane with 0.25% trypsin-0.53 mM EDTA solution for 10 min at 37 °C. The collected Caco-2 cell lysates were centrifuged for 5 min at 1000 rpm and supernatants were discarded. Furthermore, the semipermeable membranes were carefully removed from the insert using a scalpel and collected into Eppendorf tubes in 500 μL HBSS at pH 6.5 (apical conditions). Cell pellets were re-suspended in 500 μL HBSS at pH 6.5 and both cells and membranes were sonicated for 3 h using an ultrasonic bath (Branson Ultrasonic Corp., VWR, Søborg, Denmark). The collected samples were then centrifuged for 15 min at 10,000 rpm and supernatants were analyzed by HPLC (Thermo Fisher Scientific, Roskilde, Denmark). The same procedure was used to quantify the compound amounts adsorbed (X + GA and X + EGCG) or remaining encapsulated (X-GA and X-EGCG) in the nanofibers at the end of the transport experiments. The tested nanofibers were removed from the donor chamber and suspended in 500 μL of HBSS (pH 6.5 for AB transport and pH 7.4 for BA transport). After sonication and centrifugation, the molecules in the supernatants were quantified by HPLC.

2.9. Measurement of Transepithelial Electrical Resistance (TEER)

The transepithelial electrical resistance (TEER) was measured at 20 °C before and after permeability experiments with an epithelial volt-ohmmeter equipped with STX2 "chopstick" electrodes (EVOM2™, World Precision Instruments, Sarasota, FL, USA). Before measuring the resistance values of each well, the cell monolayers and the basolateral chamber were washed twice with pre-warmed HBSS at pH 6.5 and HBSS at pH 7.4, respectively. The resistance values of the semipermeable membrane without cells (R_{BLANK}) were recorded and subtracted from the resistance values obtained from the measurement of each cellular monolayer onto the semipermeable membrane (R_{TOTAL}). The specific cell resistance values (R_{TISSUE}) were calculated by:

$$R_{TISSUE}\ (\Omega) = R_{TOTAL}\ (\Omega) - R_{BLANK}\ (\Omega) \quad (1)$$

TEER values of cellular monolayers were expressed in $\Omega \times cm^2$ and calculated by:

$$TEER_{TISSUE}\ (\Omega\ cm^2) = R_{TISSUE}\ (\Omega) \times A_{MEMBRANE}\ (cm^2) \quad (2)$$

2.10. Quantification of Compounds

Donor solutions of FLUO, LY, GA, and EGCG were prepared and sterile-filtered in HBSS at pH 6.5 and pH 7.4 to perform transepithelial studies. Standard curves of GA and EGCG dissolved in HBSS at pH 6.5 and pH 7.4 were obtained by HPLC analysis. 200 µL samples withdrawn from the donor and acceptor compartments during transport experiments across cell monolayers were quantitatively analyzed using RP-HPLC (Thermo Fisher Scientific, Denmark). A C18 column (3.0 × 100 mm) and 0.5 mL/min flow rate were used. GA and EGCG were quantified with detection at 255 nm and 270 nm, respectively. FLUO and LY aliquots were instead analyzed by UV-vis spectrometry (Nanodrop One^C, Thermo Fisher Scientific, Denmark), recording their absorbance at 490 nm and 430 nm, respectively. The amount of each compound transported across the cell monolayers within a time interval of 8 h was calculated for both apical-to-basolateral (AB) and basolateral-to-apical (BA) directions. FLUO, LY, GA, and EGCG that remained entrapped within the cell monolayers, insert membranes and nanofibers were likewise quantified at the end of the permeability studies.

2.11. FLUO, LY, GA, and EGCG Distribution after Transport Experiments and Mass Balance

After transport experiments in both AB and BA directions, the amount of each compound collected at the apical and basolateral chambers was quantified. Donor concentrations at time = 0 ($C_{D,t=0\ h}$), donor and acceptor concentrations at time = 8 h ($C_{D,t=8\ h}$ and $C_{A,t=8\ h}$), compound concentrations remaining inside the cell monolayer at time = 8 h ($C_{Caco\text{-}2,t=8\ h}$), within membrane filters at time = 8 h ($C_{insert,t=8\ h}$), and adsorbed or remaining encapsulated in nanofibers at time = 8 h ($C_{fibers,t=8\ h}$) were experimentally measured. The mass balance of each compound was calculated as follows:

$$C_{D,t=0\ h} = C_{D,t=8\ h} + C_{A,t\ =\ 8\ h} + C_{Caco-2,t=8\ h} + C_{insert,t=8\ h} + (C_{fibers,t=8\ h}) \quad (3)$$

Mass balance values of >90% were found for all tested compounds.

2.12. Calculation of the Apparent Permeability Coefficients, $P_{app,AB}$ and $P_{app,BA}$

The absorptive apparent permeability coefficient ($P_{app,AB}$) and the secretory apparent permeability coefficient ($P_{app,BA}$) were calculated by:

$$P_{app} = \frac{dC}{dt} * \frac{V}{A * C_0} \quad (4)$$

where, *dC/dt* (µM/s) is the rate of change in concentration on the acceptor chamber over time; *V* (cm^3) is the volume of the solution in the acceptor compartment; *A* (cm^2) is the area of the semipermeable membrane; and C_0 (μM) is the initial concentration in the donor chamber. The results of this study are expressed as mean ± SD of three independent experiments. Permeability directional ratio (PDR) is a measure of the compound polarization in Caco-2 cell monolayers, and was calculated by:

$$PDR = \frac{P_{app,BA}}{P_{app,AB}} \quad (5)$$

3. Results

3.1. Morphological and FTIR Characterization of Nanofibers

Uniform and randomly oriented xanthan nanofibers, with average diameters of 235 ± 49 nm, were obtained by electrospinning a 2.5% *w/v* xanthan solution in formic acid (Figure 1). The average diameter of electrospun X-GA and X-EGCG nanofibers was slightly increased to 327 ± 119 nm and 270 ± 95 nm, respectively, with the encapsulation of 2 mM of phenolic compounds.

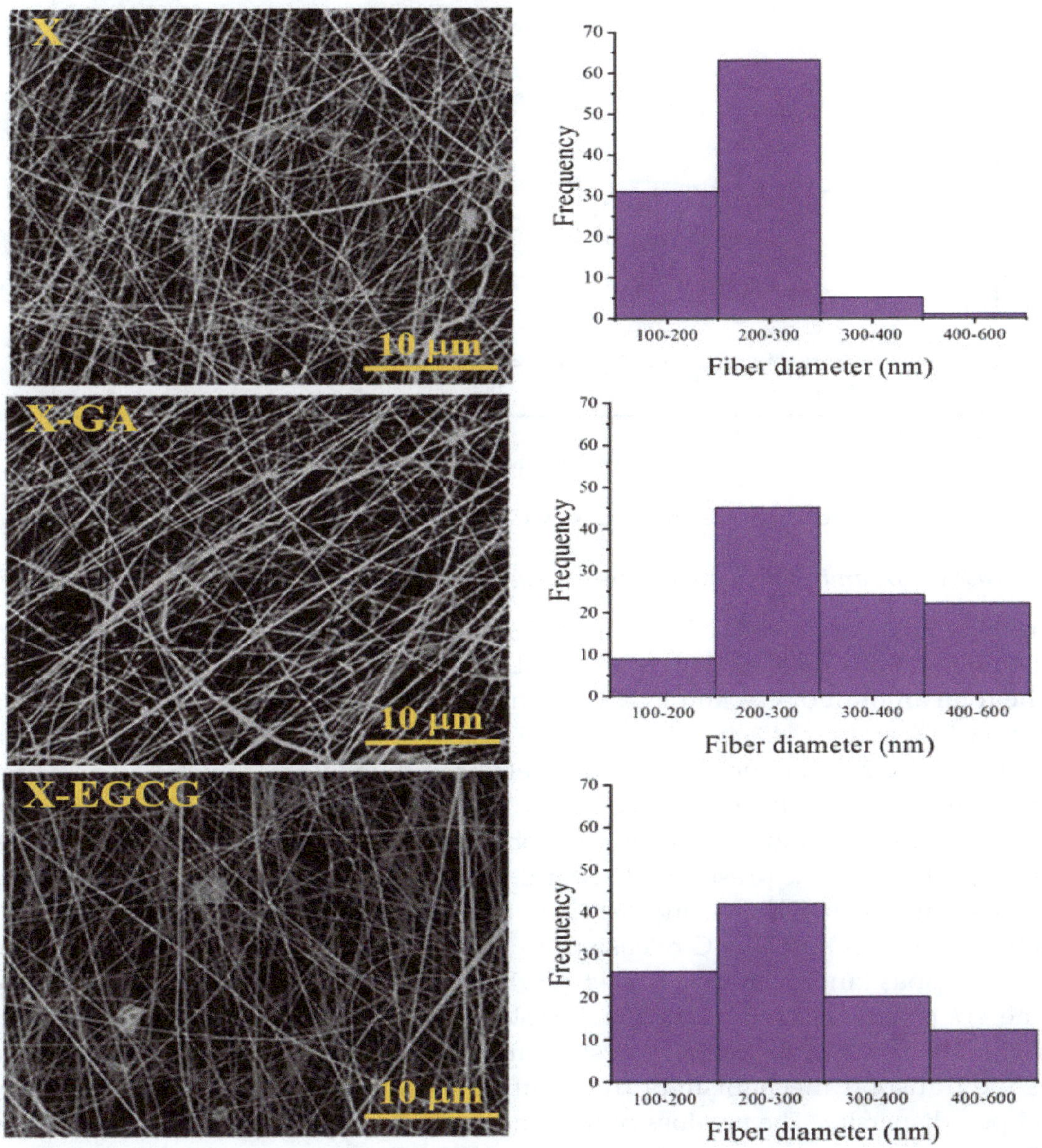

Figure 1. Morphological analysis by scanning electron microscopy (SEM) and average fiber diameter distributions of electrospun (upper) X nanofibers, (middle) X-GA, and (lower) X-EGCG nanofibers.

The FTIR spectra of X nanofibers, X-GA nanofibers, X-EGCG nanofibers, and GA and EGCG powders are shown in Figure 2. The FTIR spectrum of X nanofibers showed a characteristic broad peak in the region of 3500–3000 cm^{-1} due to O-H stretching, and a peak at around 2900 cm^{-1} due to the axial deformation of CH and CH_2 groups. In the region between 1800–1700 cm^{-1}, the stretching vibration of C=O was observed. In the region of 1200–1000 cm^{-1}, the O–H, C–O–C stretching of tertiary alcohols and esters, as well as the O–H stretching of primary alcohols was distinguished [40]. As discussed in the study by Shekarforoush et al. [40], the FTIR studies confirmed that an esterification reaction had taken place, where formic acid reacted with the pyruvic acid groups of xanthan. Hence, the esterification of pyruvic acid to pyruvyl formate induced a decrease of the negative charges of xanthan and stabilized the helical conformation of xanthan. Moreover, the FTIR spectra of X-GA and X-EGCG nanofibers are comparable to those of X without the bioactives. It is concluded that there are no physical or chemical interactions between the encapsulated GA, EGCG, and the X nanofibers matrix.

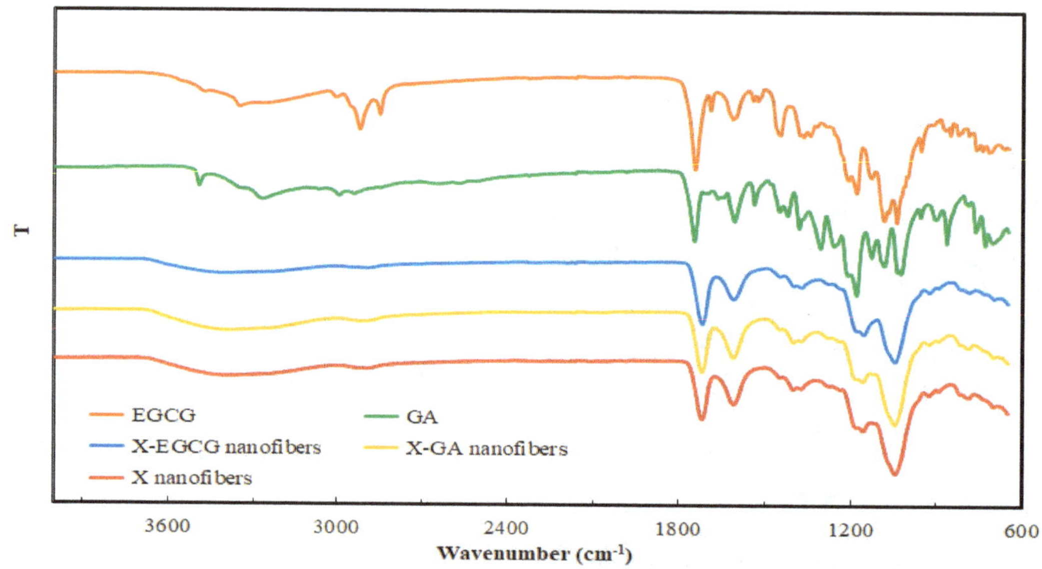

Figure 2. FTIR spectra of electrospun X, X-GA, X-EGCG nanofibers, GA, and EGCG.

3.2. *In Vitro Release of GA and EGCG from Xanthan Nanofibers*

The cumulative in vitro release of GA and EGCG from xanthan nanofibers was investigated by immersing the fibers in complete growth medium (DMEM-FBS), HBSS at pH 6.5 and HBSS at pH 7.4 (Figure 3). The total amount of GA and EGCG released from fibers was 69.01% and 70.53% in HBSS at pH 6.5, and 58.47% and 83.44% in HBSS at pH 7.4, respectively. Slightly different release values emerged from the immersion of fibers in the complete growth medium, which had an experimentally measured pH value of 7.28. Electrospun X, X-GA, and X-EGCG nanofibers remained intact in all release media and no morphological changes were observed during the experimental studies (data not shown). It is suggested that the presence of several salts in both DMEM-FBS and HBSS successfully prevented the dissolution of X, X-GA, and X-EGCG nanofibers.

The mechanism of GA and EGCG release from X nanofibers in pH 6.5 and 7.4 media were fitted by a Korsmeyer-Peppas kinetic model ($C = kt^n$), where, C is the amount of the compound released within the time, t; k is the rate constant; and n the release exponent. The constant value of k is usually related to the characteristics of the delivery system and drug; while n is the diffusion exponent, which characterizes the transport mechanism of the compound, and it depends on the type of transport, geometry, and polydispersity. The n values of the kinetic model in pH 6.5 and 7.4 media for the release of GA were 0.85 and 0.83, respectively. In the case of EGCG release, the n values in pH 6.5 and 7.4 media were 0.84 and 0.77, respectively. These results confirm that the release of the studied phenolic compounds is governed by the non-Fickian mechanism.

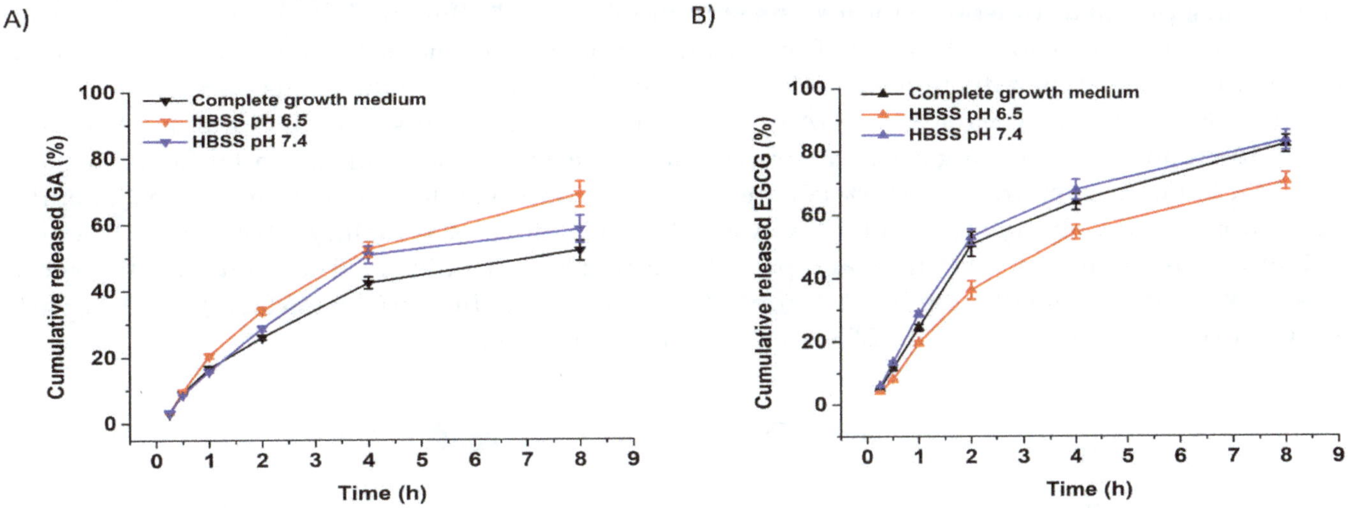

Figure 3. Cumulative in vitro release of GA (**A**) and EGCG (**B**) from xanthan nanofibers. All data were the mean ± SD of three independent experiments.

3.3. Effect of GA, EGCG, and Their Nanofiber Forms on Caco-2 Cell Viability

The viability of Caco-2 cells after 24 h treatment with free GA, EGCG, and PBS as the control was evaluated through MTS bioassay (Figure 4).

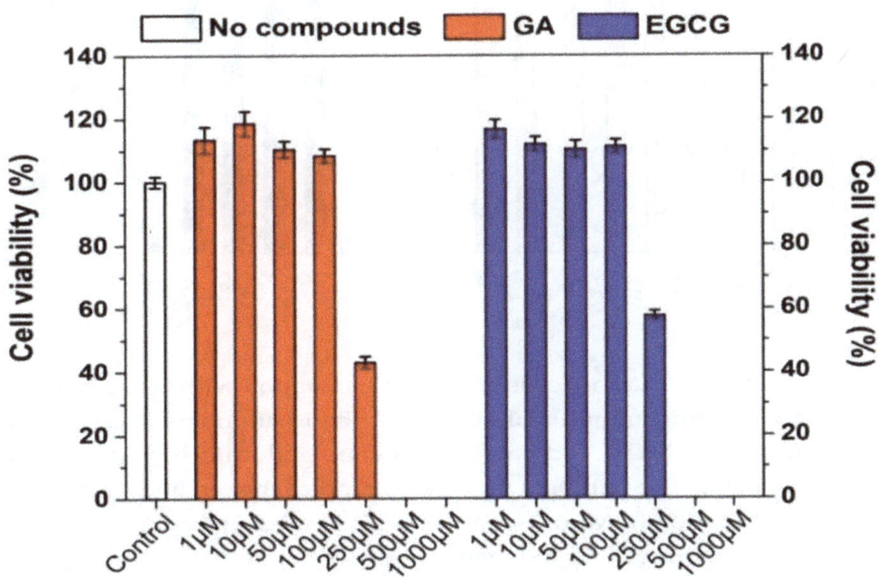

Figure 4. Viability bioassay of Caco-2 cells incubated with PBS (control, white bar) and increasing concentrations of free GA (red bars) and free EGCG (blue bars) diluted in PBS ranging from 1 μM to 1 mM. Data were the mean ± SD of four independent experiments.

When Caco-2 cells were incubated with free GA or EGCG in the concentration range between 1–100 μM, an increase in the cell viability was observed. By contrast, concentrations above 100 μM resulted in a drastically decreased cell viability, with a 50% or even higher cell mortality. The IC_{50} of free GA after 24 h incubation was estimated to be around 180 μM [7]. The concentration-dependent toxic effect of GA and EGCG was fundamental to perform transepithelial transport studies across proliferating cell monolayers. Indeed, the amount of X-GA and X-EGCG fibers was accordingly selected to obtain a final released GA and EGCG concentration lower or equal to 100 μM.

The viability of Caco-2 cells after 24 h treatment with increasing amounts of empty X, X-GA, and X-EGCG nanofibers was also investigated to establish the amount of fibers (in milligrams) to be used for transepithelial transport studies. As shown in Figure 5, the incubation of empty X fibers induced a directly proportional decrease of cell viability, reaching around 60% cell viability for 10 mg X nanofibers. However, this reduction was found to be more pronounced when cells were treated with X-GA and X-EGCG fibers. The release of GA from 2.0 mg X-GA fibers caused a cell mortality of around 70% and down until 98% for 5 mg X-GA fibers. The same effect was also confirmed after EGCG release from X-EGCG fibers, even though a 95% cell mortality was observed for 10 mg fibers. Consequently, the reduction of cell viability induced by X-GA and X-EGCG fibers was mainly attributed to GA and EGCG release, as confirmed in Figure 4, and partially caused by X nanofibers. Transepithelial transport studies were conducted incubating in 0.4 mg/mL X-GA (corresponding to 0.15 mM GA) and 1 mg/mL X-EGCG (corresponding to 0.051mM EGCG) in the donor chamber.

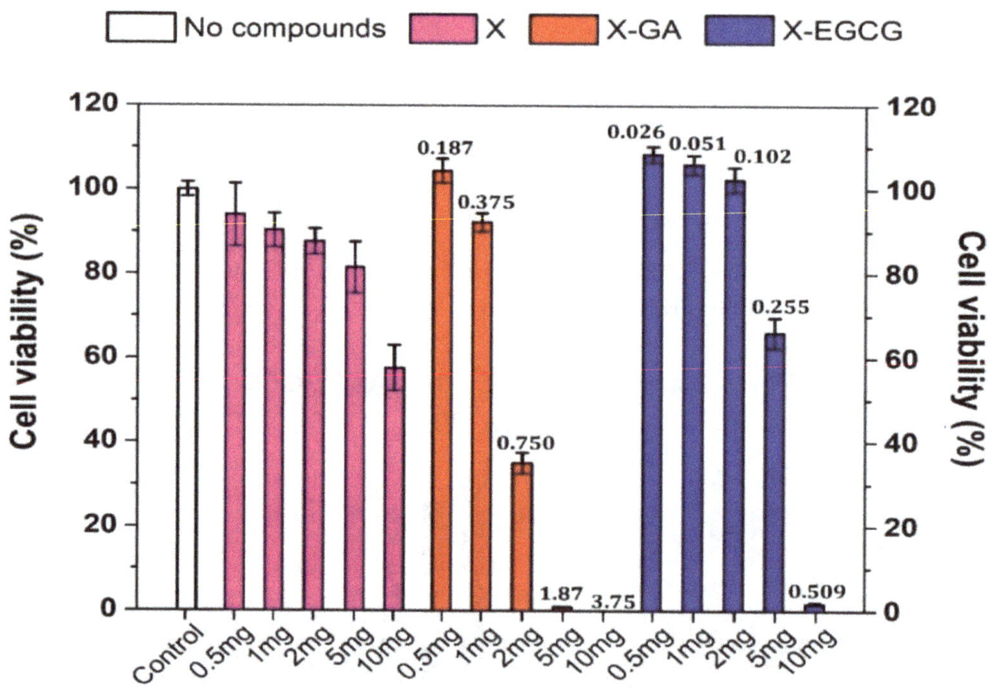

Figure 5. MTS viability bioassay of Caco-2 cells after 24 h incubation with complete growth medium (control, white bar) and increasing amounts of empty xanthan nanofibers (X, magenta bars), gallic acid-loaded xanthan nanofibers (X-GA, red bars), and (−)-epigallocatechin gallate-loaded xanthan nanofibers (X-EGCG, blue bars). The numbers reported on top of the red and blue bars represent the maximum releasable concentration (mM) of GA and EGCG in a 1.2 mL volume of complete growth medium. Data were the mean ± SD of four independent experiments.

3.4. *Assessment of Cell Monolayers' Integrity*

The cell monolayers' integrity is a fundamental determinant for the study of compound transport across the intestinal barrier, especially when passive transport through tight junctions is involved [42]. To ensure reliable in vitro permeability experiments across Caco-2 cell monolayers, the transport of non-radiolabeled markers, fluorescein (FLUO) and lucifer yellow (LY), and transepithelial electrical resistance measurement were conducted to quantitatively investigate the integrity of monolayers after 21 days growth on 12-mm polycarbonate inserts. The average TEER value for Caco-2 cell monolayers randomly chosen for transport studies was 370.74 ± 15.81 Ω cm^2. The TEER values of monolayers before and after transport of FLUO and LY were found in the range of 300–500 Ω cm^2 (Figure 6), indicating an "intermediate" tightness of the gastrointestinal epithelium [43].

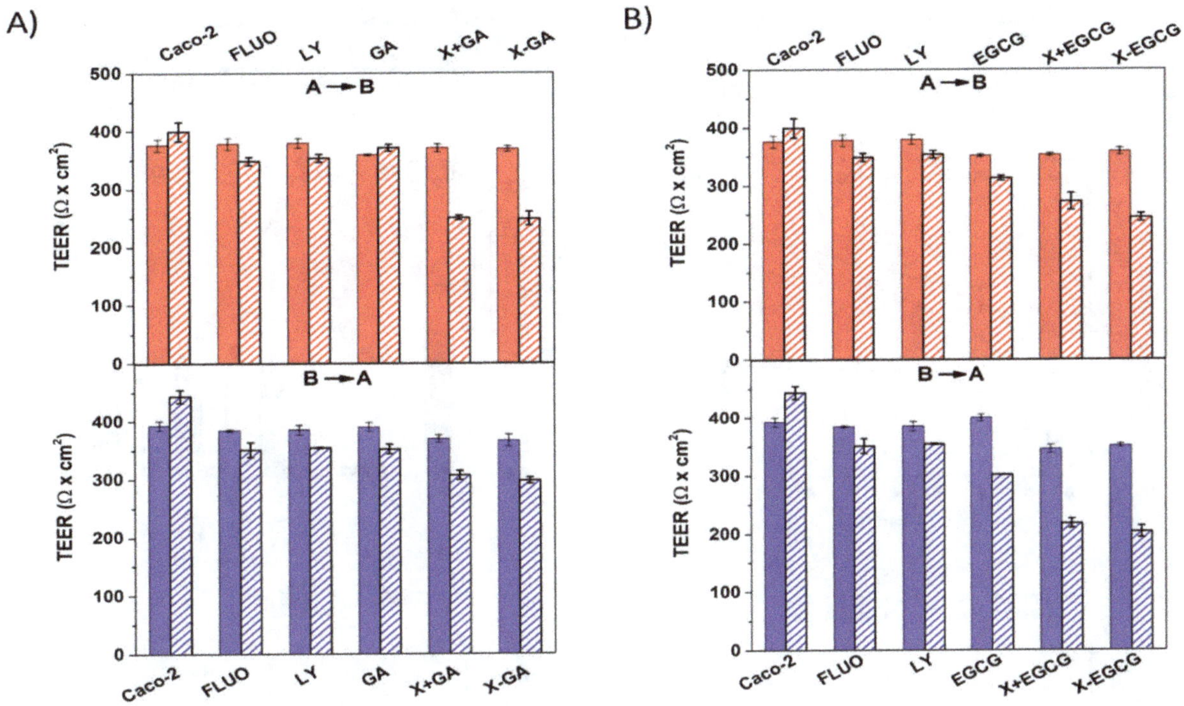

Figure 6. Transepithelial electrical resistance (TEER) measurements of cell monolayers before (full colored bars) and after (patterned bars) apical-to-basolateral (AB) and basolateral-to-apical (BA) studies for a time interval of 8 h. TEER values were recorded for GA, X + GA, and X-GA (**A**) and EGCG, X + EGCG, and X-EGCG (**B**). All data were the mean ± SD of three independent experiments.

The AB and BA transepithelial transports of FLUO and LY across Caco-2 monolayers under a proton gradient were investigated, resulting in a pH-dependent transport of FLUO. The apparent permeability coefficients of FLUO were $P_{app,AB} = 3.31 \times 10^{-6}$ cm/s and $P_{app,BA} = 2.01 \times 10^{-6}$ cm/s, whereas much lower values were observed from the LY transport: $P_{app,AB} = 1.13 \times 10^{-7}$ cm/s and $P_{app,BA} = 1.21 \times 10^{-7}$ cm/s (Figure 7C). Due to the lipoid nature of polarized epithelial cell layers, the transport of ions and hydrophilic compounds is restricted through the membrane. Indeed, hydrophilic LY was transported across epithelial cells solely via tight junctions, whereas the lipophilic FLUO permeated through transcellular transport [44–46]. Thus, from the TEER and permeability observations it was concluded that the integrity and tightness of epithelial cell monolayers were maintained after 21 days culturing.

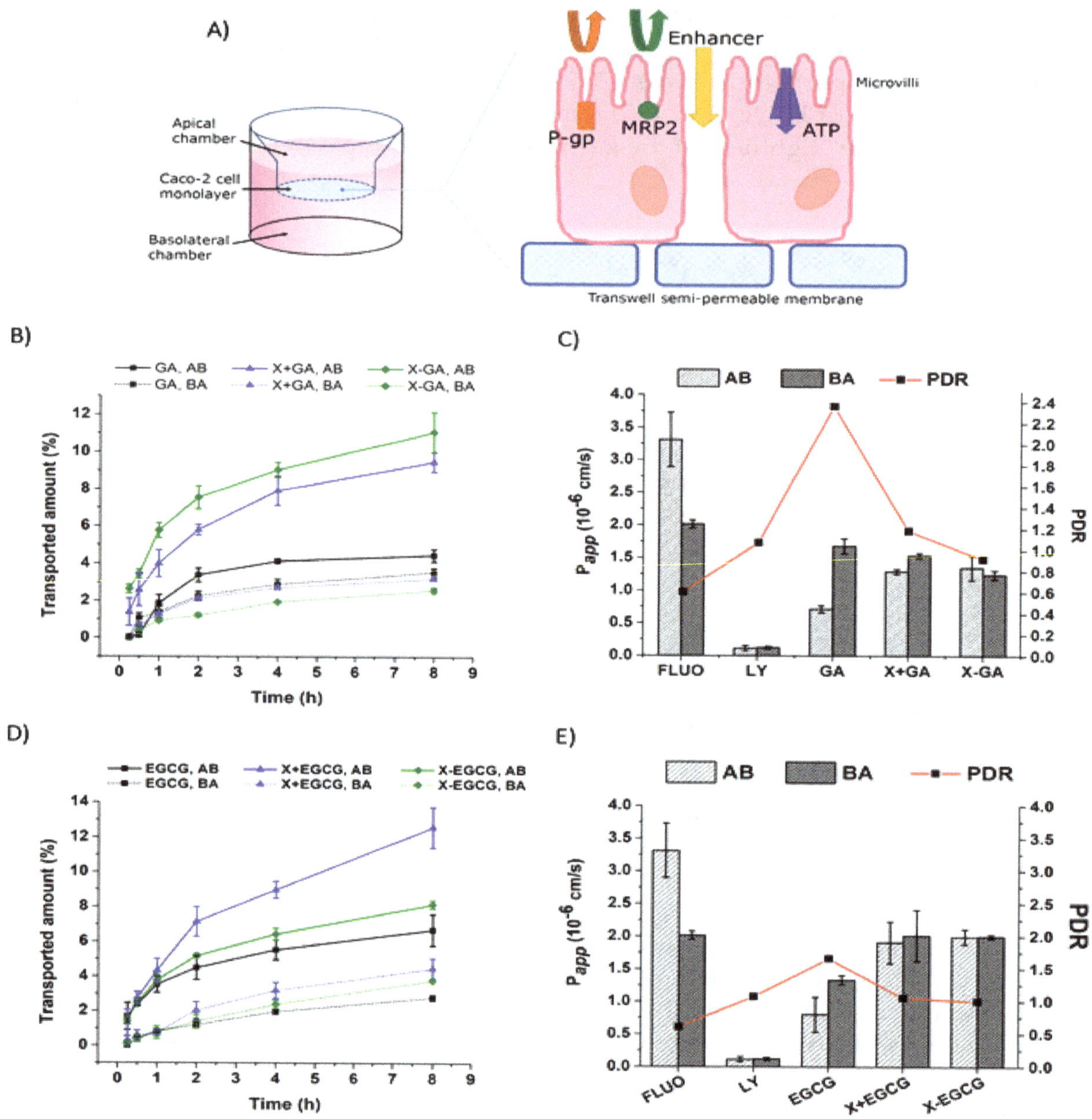

Figure 7. Transepithelial transport of GA and EGCG across Caco-2 monolayers. Illustration of the efflux transporters expressed on the apical membrane of epithelial cells (**A**). Transported amount of GA, X + GA, and X-GA (**B**), and EGCG, X + EGCG, and X-EGCG (**D**) in both AB and BA directions. Apparent permeability coefficient, P_{app}, and PDR of GA, X + GA and X-GA (**C**), and EGCG, X + EGCG, and X-EGCG (**E**). All data were the mean ± SD of three independent experiments.

3.5. Transepithelial Transport and Distribution of Free GA, EGCG, and Their Nanofiber Forms

The transported amounts of GA and EGCG, their apparent permeability coefficient, and their permeability directional ratio were assessed for both the AB and BA directions under a proton gradient. In addition, the compounds were incubated at the donor chamber in a free form (GA and EGCG), in a free form in the presence of empty xanthan nanofibers (X + GA and X + EGCG), and in the nanofiber forms (X-GA and X-EGCG). Figure 7 summarizes all the above-mentioned parameters. Firstly, the amounts of molecules transported in the acceptor chamber were higher in the AB direction than in the BA. Secondly, the addition of empty or loaded xanthan nanofibers enhanced the transport of GA and EGCG in the AB direction (Figure 7B–D). Indeed, the permeated amount of GA in the X + GA and X-GA formulations was 2-fold and 2.5-fold higher than that of free GA. The same results were obtained for the transported EGCG in the AB direction, but on the contrary, the X + EGCG form was the most effective (1.9-fold increase over the free EGCG). These results suggested that the permeation of the compounds was greatly enhanced by the presence of xanthan nanofibers, either as empty nanostructures or loaded with polyphenols. Accordingly, the apparent permeability coefficients of GA and EGCG incubated with nanofibers were at least 2-fold higher than those of the free compounds. Indeed, the GA and X-GA permeability values in the AB direction were $P_{app,AB} = 7.12 \times 10^{-7}$ cm/s and $P_{app,AB} = 1.96 \times 10^{-6}$ cm/s, respectively (Figure 7C). The same increase in permeability was detected also for the EGCG nanofiber form, where EGCG and X-EGCG had a $P_{app,AB} = 7.99 \times 10^{-7}$ cm/s and $P_{app,AB} = 1.99 \times 10^{-6}$ cm/s, respectively (Figure 7E). An increment of the apparent permeability coefficient values was also found in the BA direction, even though this was less pronounced than in the AB direction.

The fate of GA and EGCG during 8 h transepithelial transport in both AB and BA directions, was monitored by quantifying their concentration in the donor and acceptor compartments, in the cell lysate, insert membrane (filter), and within xanthan nanofibers (adsorbed or unreleased). Figure 8 shows the distribution of the tested compounds in the above-mentioned compartments. After 8 h experiment, most of the incubated compounds were still found in the donor chamber (≥60% of the concentration at time = 0 h), and only less than 20% were detected in the acceptor side. However, the yields of GA and EGCG recorded in A were higher when incubated with xanthan nanofibers than in its absence. Small amounts of GA and EGCG were also detected inside the epithelial monolayers (3% and 1.3%, respectively), and adsorbed to or unreleased from xanthan nanofibers (29% and 21%, respectively).

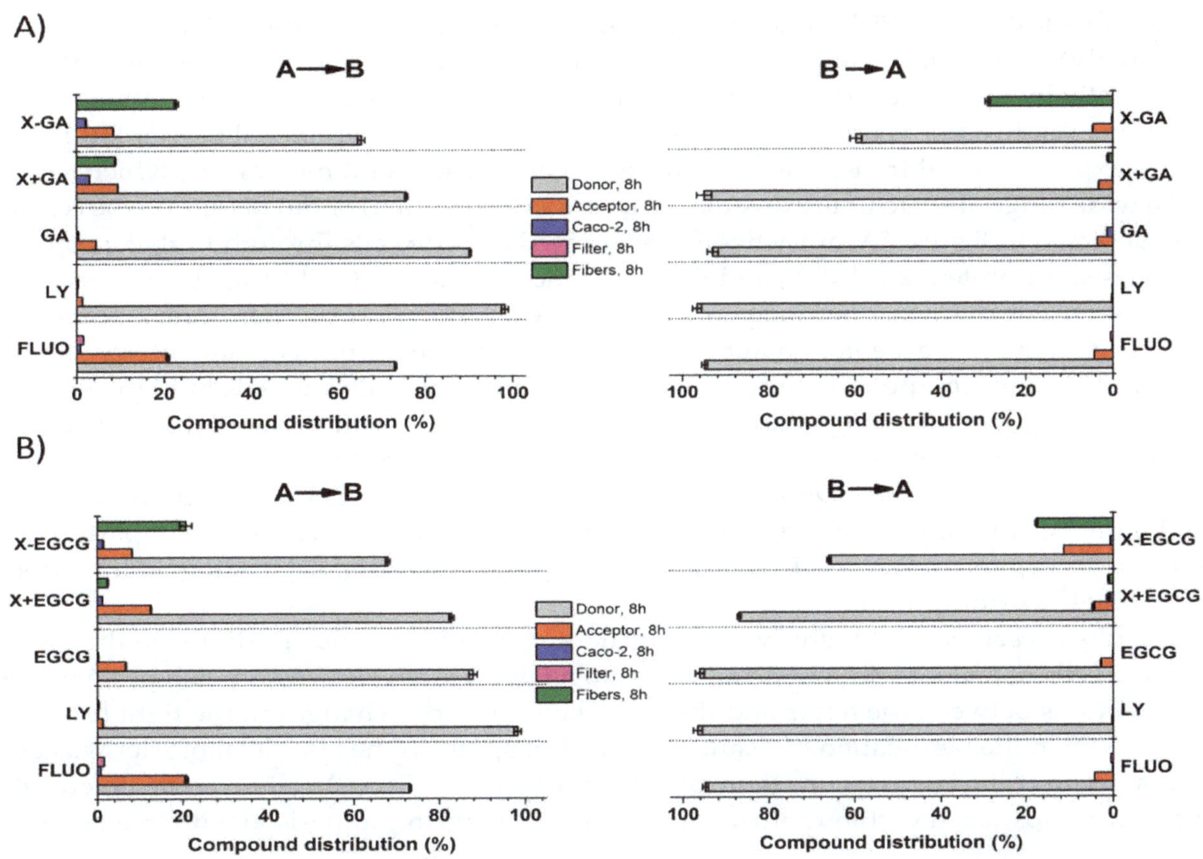

Figure 8. Quantification of GA (**A**) and EGCG (**B**) distribution in the donor side, acceptor side, cell lysate, membrane insert, and fibers after 8 h transepithelial transport in both AB and BA directions. All data are the mean ± SD of three independent experiments.

4. Discussion

In this study, human differentiated epithelial Caco-2 cells were chosen as an established in vitro cell model for the prediction of bioactive compounds' absorption and transport mechanism [47]. The Caco-2 cells possess many features, among which are their ability to slowly differentiate into monolayers forming microvilli and tight junctions at the apical side, and to express brush-border transporters and enzymes involved in the metabolism and transport of several substrates [41,48,49]. Therefore, transepithelial transport studies of GA and EGCG were performed across Caco-2 monolayers in the apical-to-basolateral and basolateral-to-apical directions under a proton gradient. The two polyphenols investigated in this study are characterized by a poor intestinal absorption due to their high hydrophilicity; in fact, they can hardly penetrate the cell membrane and only passive diffusion seems to be involved in their permeation [19].

The incubation of nanofibers with Caco-2 cells (24 h) revealed a proliferative effect in cell viability for amounts lower or equal to 0.5 mg X-GA and 2.0 mg X-EGCG; a drastic cell mortality was observed for doses above this range. In addition, the treatment of Caco-2 cells with increasing amounts of empty xanthan nanofibers resulted in a dose-dependent reduction of cell viability, close to 60% viability for 10.0 mg X incubated. However, the observed reduction in cell viability was expected to be less pronounced for transepithelial transport studies, since the cell monolayers were exposed to X, X-GA, and X-EGCG for 8 h rather than 24 h. The transepithelial transport of GA and EGCG in the acceptor compartment was successfully enhanced by the presence of xanthan, both as an empty nanostructure and as a nanocarrier, and the permeability coefficients were higher than those calculated for free compounds. In addition, the PDR values of free GA and free EGCG were both higher than 1.5 (2.4 and 1.7, respectively), suggesting that their transport is modulated by an active transport pathway, and more specifically by efflux. Several studies have described the mechanism and the efflux transporters involved in the unidirectional transport of GA and EGCG across the epithelial barrier [16,17,19,50,51]. Enterocytes express several transporters on the apical and basolateral membrane, which can actively transport a wide range of structurally diverse compounds into (influx) or out of (efflux) the cell. GA and EGCG, as depicted in Figure 7A, are actively transported outside cells through P-glycoprotein (P-gp), multidrug resistant protein 2 (MRP2), and the ATP binding cassette (ATP) transporters expressed on the apical membrane of Caco-2 monolayers [49,51]. These efflux pumps, therefore, restrict the influx of GA and EGCG into the acceptor chamber, rather promoting their efflux from enterocytes. Several efflux pump inhibitory compounds, such as indomethacin, verapamil, and MK-571 [16,19], have been thoroughly investigated, resulting in an increase in oral absorption. In this study, the calculated PDR values obtained for free GA and free EGCG transport were higher than 1.5, confirming their efflux from monolayers. However, the PDR values of X + GA, X-GA, X + EGCG, and X-EGCG were all lower than 1.5 (Figure 7C–E). Hence, the incubation of xanthan nanofibers in the donor compartment greatly improved the absorption of GA and EGCG across the epithelial barrier, suggesting an inhibitory effect of xanthan on efflux transporters.

The results presented in this study are congruent with our previous findings on the permeation across Caco-2 cells of a model protein (insulin) encapsulated within electrospun fish protein fibers [52]. Direct interactions between the fibers and the monolayer induced changes in the tight junctions, and thus, an increase in the permeation of insulin at local hot spots on the epithelial barrier was observed. Similarly, a 3.4-fold increase of curcumin permeability across Caco-2 cells was detected when the bioactive was encapsulated within xanthan-chitosan nanofibers, in comparison with free-curcumin [39].

5. Conclusions

Encapsulation and release of two poorly absorbed polyphenol compounds, GA and EGCG, using electrospun xanthan nanofibers were investigated. It was found that X, X-GA, and X-EGCG nanofibers remained stable in aqueous HBSS medium at different pH (6.5 and pH 7.4). The total amount of GA and EGCG released from xanthan nanofibers was 69.01% and 70.53% in HBSS at pH 6.5, and 58.47% and 83.44% in HBSS at pH 7.4, respectively. Moreover, the nanofibers were incubated with Caco-2 cells and the cell viability, transepithelial transport, and GA and EGCG permeability properties across cell monolayers were investigated. At least a 2-fold increase of GA and EGCG permeability was observed in the presence of X-GA and X-EGCG nanofibers, in comparison with the free-phenolic compounds. Indeed, the polysaccharide nanofibers enhanced the GA and EGCG permeability by opening the tight junctions of Caco-2 monolayers, as well as inhibiting the efflux transporters. These findings are relevant for promoting the delivery not only of polyphenols, but also of other poorly absorbable bioactives and drugs.

Author Contributions: A.F. designed the experiments, A.F. and E.S. performed the experiments, A.F., A.C.M., I.S.C. analyzed the data and wrote the manuscript.

Acknowledgments: The project was also supported by a PhD stipend (to Elhamalsadat Shekarforoush) from the Technical University of Denmark.

References

1. Scalbert, A.; Williamson, G. Dietary intake and bioavailability of polyphenols. *J. Nutr.* **2000**, *130*, 2073S–2085S. [CrossRef] [PubMed]
2. Kühnau, J. The flavonoids. A class of semi-essential food components: Their role in human nutrition. *World Rev. Nutr. Diet.* **1976**, *24*, 117–191.
3. Inoue, M.; Suzuki, R.; Koide, T.; Sakaguchi, N.; Ogihara, Y.; Yabu, Y. Antioxidant, gallic acid, induces apoptosis in HL-60RG cells. *Biochem. Biophys. Res. Commun.* **1994**, *204*, 898–904. [CrossRef] [PubMed]
4. Inoue, M.; Suzuki, R.; Sakaguchi, N.; Li, Z.; Takeda, T.; Ogihara, Y.; Jiang, B.Y.; Chen, Y. Selective induction of cell death in cancer cells by gallic acid. *Biol. Pharm. Bull.* **1995**, *18*, 1526–1530. [CrossRef]
5. Gali, H.U.; Perchellet, E.M.; Perchellet, J.P. Inhibition of tumor promoter-induced ornithine decarboxylase activity by tannic acid and other polyphenols in mouse epidermis in vivo. *Cancer Res.* **1991**, *51*, 2820–2825.
6. Gali, H.U.; Perchellet, E.M.; Klish, D.S.; Johnson, J.M.; Perchellet, J.P. Antitumor-promoting activities of hydrolyzable tannins in mouse skin. *Carcinogenesis* **1992**, *13*, 715–718. [CrossRef]
7. Rashidi, L.; Vasheghani-Farahani, E.; Soleimani, M.; Atashi, A.; Rostami, K.; Gangi, F.; Fallahpour, M.; Tahouri, M.T. A cellular uptake and cytotoxicity properties study of gallic acid-loaded mesoporous silica nanoparticles on Caco-2 cells. *J. Nanoparticle Res.* **2014**, *16*, 2285. [CrossRef]
8. Konishi, Y.; Kobayashi, S.; Shimizu, M. Transepithelial transport of *p*-coumaric acid and gallic acid in Caco-2 cell monolayers. *Biosci. Biotechnol. Biochem.* **2003**, *67*, 2317–2324. [CrossRef]
9. Huang, P.-J.; Hseu, Y.-C.; Lee, M.-S.; Senthil Kumar, K.J.; Wu, C.-R.; Hsu, L.-S.; Liao, J.-W.; Cheng, I.-S.; Kuo, Y.-T.; Huang, S.-Y.; et al. In vitro and in vivo activity of gallic acid and toona sinensis leaf extracts against HL-60 human premyelocytic leukemia. *Food Chem. Toxicol.* **2012**, *50*, 3489–3497. [CrossRef]
10. Inoue, M.; Sakaguchi, N.; Isuzugawa, K.; Tani, H.; Ogihara, Y. Role of reactive oxygen species in gallic acid-induced apoptosis. *Biol. Pharm. Bull.* **2000**, *23*, 1153–1157. [CrossRef]
11. Kaur, M.; Velmurugan, B.; Rajamanickam, S.; Agarwal, R.; Agarwal, C. Gallic acid, an active constituent of grape seed extract, exhibits anti-proliferative, pro-apoptotic and anti-tumorigenic effects against prostate carcinoma xenograft growth in nude mice. *Pharm. Res.* **2009**, *26*, 2133–2140. [CrossRef] [PubMed]
12. Pal, C.; Bindu, S.; Dey, S.; Alam, A.; Goyal, M.; Iqbal, M.S.; Maity, P.; Adhikari, S.S.; Bandyopadhyay, U. Gallic acid prevents nonsteroidal anti-inflammatory drug-induced gastropathy in rat by blocking oxidative stress and apoptosis. *Free Radic. Biol. Med.* **2010**, *49*, 258–267. [CrossRef]
13. You, B.R.; Park, W.H. Gallic acid-induced lung cancer cell death is related to glutathione depletion as well as reactive oxygen species increase. *Toxicol. Vitr.* **2010**, *24*, 1356–1362. [CrossRef]
14. You, B.R.; Moon, H.J.; Han, Y.H.; Park, W.H. Gallic acid inhibits the growth of HeLa cervical cancer cells via apoptosis and/or necrosis. *Food Chem. Toxicol.* **2010**, *48*, 1334–1340. [CrossRef] [PubMed]
15. Munin, A.; Edwards-Lévy, F. Encapsulation of natural polyphenolic compounds; a review. *Pharmaceutics* **2011**, *3*, 793–829. [CrossRef] [PubMed]
16. Mao, X.; Wu, L.-F.; Zhao, H.-J.; Liang, W.-Y.; Chen, W.-J.; Han, S.-X.; Qi, Q.; Cui, Y.-P.; Li, S.; Yang, G.-H.; et al. Transport of corilagin, gallic acid, and ellagic acid from fructus phyllanthi tannin fraction in Caco-2 cell monolayers. *Evid.-Based Complement. Alternat. Med.* **2016**, *2016*, 9205379. [CrossRef]

17. Vaidyanathan, J.B.; Walle, T. Cellular uptake and efflux of the tea flavonoid (−)epicatechin-3-gallate in the human intestinal cell line Caco-2. *J. Pharmacol. Exp. Ther.* **2003**, *307*, 745–752. [CrossRef]
18. Katiyar, S.; Mukhtar, H. Tea in chemoprevention of cancer. *Int. J. Oncol.* **1996**, *8*, 221–238. [CrossRef] [PubMed]
19. Song, Q.; Li, D.; Zhou, Y.; Yang, J.; Yang, W.; Zhou, G.; Wen, J. Enhanced uptake and transport of (+)-catechin and (−)-epigallocatechin gallate in niosomal formulation by human intestinal Caco-2 cells. *Int. J. Nanomed.* **2014**, *9*, 2157. [CrossRef]
20. Ji, B.T.; Chow, W.H.; Hsing, A.W.; McLaughlin, J.K.; Dai, Q.; Gao, Y.T.; Blot, W.J.; Fraumeni, J.F. Green tea consumption and the risk of pancreatic and colorectal cancers. *Int. J. Cancer* **1997**, *70*, 255–258. [CrossRef]
21. Su, J.; Arab, L. Tea consumption and the reduced risk of colon cancer—results from a national prospective cohort study. *Public Health Nutr.* **2002**, *5*, 419–425. [CrossRef] [PubMed]
22. Chow, H.H.; Cai, Y.; Alberts, D.S.; Hakim, I.; Dorr, R.; Shahi, F.; Crowell, J.A.; Yang, C.S.; Hara, Y. Phase I pharmacokinetic study of tea polyphenols following single-dose administration of epigallocatechin gallate and polyphenon E. *Cancer Epidemiol. Biomark. Prev.* **2001**, *10*, 53–58.
23. Warden, B.A.; Smith, L.S.; Beecher, G.R.; Balentine, D.A.; Clevidence, B.A. Catechins are bioavailable in men and women drinking black tea throughout the day. *J. Nutr.* **2001**, *131*, 1731–1737. [CrossRef]
24. Teng, Z.; Yuan, C.; Zhang, F.; Huan, M.; Cao, W.; Li, K.; Yang, J.; Cao, D.; Zhou, S.; Mei, Q. Intestinal absorption and first-pass metabolism of polyphenol compounds in rat and their transport dynamics in Caco-2 cells. *PLoS ONE* **2012**, *7*, e29647. [CrossRef] [PubMed]
25. Liu, L.; Guo, L.; Zhao, C.; Wu, X.; Wang, R.; Liu, C. Characterization of the intestinal absorption of seven flavonoids from the flowers of trollius chinensis using the Caco-2 cell monolayer model. *PLoS ONE* **2015**, *10*, e0119263. [CrossRef] [PubMed]
26. Dube, A.; Ng, K.; Nicolazzo, J.A.; Larson, I. Effective use of reducing agents and nanoparticle encapsulation in stabilizing catechins in alkaline solution. *Food Chem.* **2010**, *122*, 662–667. [CrossRef]
27. Caddeo, C.; Teskač, K.; Sinico, C.; Kristl, J. Effect of resveratrol incorporated in liposomes on proliferation and UV-B protection of cells. *Int. J. Pharm.* **2008**, *363*, 183–191. [CrossRef] [PubMed]
28. Chuysinuan, P.; Chimnoi, N.; Techasakul, S.; Supaphol, P. Gallic acid-loaded electrospun poly(L-lactic acid) fiber mats and their release characteristic. *Macromol. Chem. Phys.* **2009**, *210*, 814–822. [CrossRef]
29. Neo, Y.P.; Ray, S.; Jin, J.; Gizdavic-Nikolaidis, M.; Nieuwoudt, M.K.; Liu, D.; Quek, S.Y. Encapsulation of food grade antioxidant in natural biopolymer by electrospinning technique: A physicochemical study based on zein-gallic acid system. *Food Chem.* **2013**, *136*, 1013–1021. [CrossRef]
30. Phiriyawirut, M.; Phaechamud, T. Gallic acid-loaded cellulose acetate electrospun nanofibers: Thermal properties, mechanical properties, and drug release behavior. *Open J. Polym. Chem.* **2012**, *02*, 21–29. [CrossRef]
31. Aytac, Z.; Kusku, S.I.; Durgun, E.; Uyar, T. Encapsulation of gallic acid/cyclodextrin inclusion complex in electrospun polylactic acid nanofibers: Release behavior and antioxidant activity of gallic acid. *Mater. Sci. Eng. C* **2016**, *63*, 231–239. [CrossRef] [PubMed]
32. Li, Y.; Lim, L.-T.; Kakuda, Y. Electrospun zein fibers as carriers to stabilize (−)-epigallocatechin gallate. *J. Food Sci.* **2009**, *74*, C233–C240. [CrossRef]
33. Lee, E.J.; Lee, J.H.; Jin, L.; Jin, O.S.; Shin, Y.C.; Sang, J.O.; Lee, J.; Hyon, S.-H.; Han, D.-W. Hyaluronic acid/poly(lactic-*co*-glycolic acid) core/shell fiber meshes loaded with epigallocatechin-3-*O*-gallate as skin tissue engineering scaffolds. *J. Nanosci. Nanotechnol.* **2014**, *14*, 8458–8463. [CrossRef] [PubMed]
34. Lee, M.H.; Kwon, B.-J.; Koo, M.-A.; Jang, E.H.; Seon, G.M.; Park, J.-C. Exovascular application of epigallocatechin-3-*O*-gallate-releasing electrospun poly(L-lactide glycolic acid) fiber sheets to reduce intimal hyperplasia in injured abdominal aorta. *Biomed. Mater.* **2015**, *10*, 055010. [CrossRef]
35. Ho, L.J.; Cheol, S.Y.; Jun, Y.W.; Chul, P.J.; Hyu, H.S.; Wook, H.D. Epigallocatechin-3-*O*-gallate-loaded poly(lactic-*co*-glycolic acid) fibrous sheets as anti-adhesion barriers. *J. Biomed. Nanotechnol.* **2014**, *11*, 1461–1471. [CrossRef]
36. Tian, J.; Tu, H.; Shi, X.; Wang, X.; Deng, H.; Li, B.; Du, Y. Antimicrobial application of nanofibrous mats self-assembled with chitosan and epigallocatechin gallate. *Colloids Surf. B Biointerfaces* **2016**, *145*, 643–652. [CrossRef]
37. Ayca, A.; Gulum, S.; Serpil, S. Fabrication of gallic acid loaded hydroxypropyl methylcellulose nanofibers by electrospinning technique as active packaging material. *Carbohydr. Polym.* **2019**, *208*, 241–250. [CrossRef]

38. Shekarforoush, E.; Ajalloueian, F.; Zeng, G.; Mendes, A.C.; Chronakis, I.S. Electrospun xanthan-chitosan nanofibers as delivery carrier of hydrophobic bioactives. *Mater. Lett.* **2018**, *228*, 322–326. [CrossRef]
39. Faralli, A.; Shekarforoush, E.; Ajalloueian, F.; Mendes, A.C.; Chronakis, I.S. In vitro permeability enhancement of curcumin across Caco-2 cells monolayers using electrospun xanthan-chitosan nanofibers. *Carbohydr. Polym.* **2019**, *206*, 38–47. [CrossRef]
40. Shekarforoush, E.; Faralli, A.; Ndoni, S.; Mendes, A.C.; Chronakis, I.S. Electrospinning of xanthan polysaccharide. *Macromol. Mater. Eng.* **2017**, *302*, 1700067. [CrossRef]
41. Hubatsch, I.; Ragnarsson, E.G.E.; Artursson, P. Determination of drug permeability and prediction of drug absorption in Caco-2 monolayers. *Nat. Protoc.* **2007**, *2*, 2111–2119. [CrossRef] [PubMed]
42. Srinivasan, B.; Kolli, A.R.; Esch, M.B.; Abaci, H.E.; Shuler, M.L.; Hickman, J.J. TEER measurement techniques for in vitro barrier model systems. *J. Lab. Autom.* **2015**, *20*, 107–126. [CrossRef] [PubMed]
43. Amidon, G.L.; Lee, P.I.; Topp, E.M. *Transport Processes in Pharmaceutical Systems*; M. Dekker: New York, NY, USA, 2000; ISBN 9780824766108.
44. Högerle, M.L.; Winne, D. Drug absorption by the rat jejunum perfused in situ. Dissociation from the pH-partition theory and role of microclimate-pH and unstirred layer. *Naunyn. Schmiedebergs. Arch. Pharmacol.* **1983**, *322*, 249–255.
45. Bock, U.; Kolac, C.; Borchard, G.; Koch, K.; Fuchs, R.; Streichhan, P.; Lehr, C.M. Transport of proteolytic enzymes across Caco-2 cell monolayers. *Pharm. Res.* **1998**, *15*, 1393–1400. [CrossRef] [PubMed]
46. Konishi, Y.; Hagiwara, K.; Shimizu, M. Transepithelial transport of fluorescein in Caco-2 Cell monolayers and use of such transport in in vitro evaluation of phenolic acid availability. *Biosci. Biotechnol. Biochem.* **2002**, *66*, 2449–2457. [CrossRef] [PubMed]
47. Artursson, P.; Palm, K.; Luthman, K. Caco-2 monolayers in experimental and theoretical predictions of drug transport. *Adv. Drug Deliv. Rev.* **2001**, *46*, 27–43. [CrossRef]
48. Yee, S. In vitro permeability across Caco-2 cells (colonic) can predict in vivo (small intestinal) absorption in man—Fact or myth. *Pharm. Res.* **1997**, *14*, 763–766. [CrossRef] [PubMed]
49. Naruhashi, K.; Kurahashi, Y.; Fujita, Y.; Kawakita, E.; Yamasaki, Y.; Hattori, K.; Nishimura, A.; Shibata, N. Comparison of the expression and function of ATP binding cassette transporters in Caco-2 and T84 cells on stimulation by selected endogenous compounds and xenobiotics. *Drug Metab. Pharmacokinet.* **2011**, *26*, 145–153. [CrossRef] [PubMed]
50. Hoosain, F.G.; Choonara, Y.E.; Tomar, L.K.; Kumar, P.; Tyagi, C.; du Toit, L.C.; Pillay, V. Bypassing P-glycoprotein drug efflux mechanisms: Possible applications in pharmacoresistant schizophrenia therapy. *BioMed Res. Int.* **2015**, 484963. [CrossRef] [PubMed]
51. Werle, M. Expert review. Natural and synthetic polymers as inhibitors of drug efflux pumps. *Pharm. Res.* **2007**, *25*, 500–511. [CrossRef]
52. Stephansen, K.; García-Díaz, M.; Jessen, F.; Chronakis, I.S.; Nielsen, H.M. Bioactive protein-based nanofibers interact with intestinal biological components resulting in transepithelial permeation of a therapeutic protein. *Int. J. Pharm.* **2015**, *495*, 58–66. [CrossRef] [PubMed]

7

Poloxamer Hydrogels for Biomedical Applications

Eleonora Russo * and Carla Villa

Department of Pharmacy, University of Genoa, Viale Benedetto XV, 16132 Genova, Italy; villa@difar.unige.it
* Correspondence: russo@difar.unige.it

Abstract: This review article focuses on thermoresponsive hydrogels consisting of poloxamers which are of high interest for biomedical application especially in drug delivery for ophthalmic, injectable, transdermal, and vaginal administration. These hydrogels remain fluid at room temperature but become more viscous gel once they are exposed to body temperature. In this way, the gelling system remains at the topical level for a long time and the drug release is controlled and prolonged. Poloxamers are synthetic triblock copolymers of poly(ethylene oxide)-b-poly(propylene oxide)-b-poly(ethylene oxide) (PEO-PPO-PEO), also commercially known as Pluronics®, Synperonics® or Lutrol®. The different poloxamers cover a range of liquids, pastes, and solids, with molecular weights and ethylene oxide–propylene oxide weight ratios varying from 1100 to 14,000 and 1:9 to 8:2, respectively. Concentrated aqueous solutions of poloxamers form thermoreversible gels. In recent years this type of gel has arouse interest for tissue engineering. Finally, the use of poloxamers as biosurfactants is evaluated since they are able to form micelles in an aqueous environment above a concentration threshold known as critical micelle concentration (CMC). This property is exploited for drug delivery and different therapeutic applications.

Keywords: poloxamer; hydrogels; micelle; thermosensitive; biomedical; copolymer

1. Introduction

The word "hydrogel", according to Lee, Kwon and Park is due to an article published in 1894, but the first crosslinked network material that appeared in literature and that has been described by its typical hydrogel properties, was a polyhydroxyethylmethacrylate (HEMA) hydrogel developed much later, in 1960, by O. Wichterle and D. Lim, with the aim of using it in permanent contact applications with human tissues, i.e., as soft contact lenses [1].

Since then, hydrogels have been used as systems for drug controlled delivery, to facilitate the localized, sustained and prolonged release of a drug, thereby decreasing the number of administrations, avoiding side effects and following low doses [2].

The most widely studied environmentally responsive systems were temperature sensitive hydrogels, in which physical entanglements, hydrogen bonding, and hydrophobic interactions are the main features that constitute the crosslinks. Two different types of thermo-sensitive hydrogels exist that undergo gelation either by cooling below the upper critical gelation temperature (UCGT) or by heating above the lower critical gelation temperature (LCGT), respectively. Hydrogels with LCGT behavior and sol-to-gel transition at 37 °C have gained increasing attention in the biomedical field as carriers for cells, drugs, and biomolecules, since they allow encapsulation in mild conditions (temperature ≤ 37°C) [3].

Poloxamers and poloxamines are examples of these LCGT biocompatible thermoreversible hydrogels that were introduced in the 1950s by BASF (Iselin, NJ, USA) when they started being used for detergent development, but also in other areas, like agriculture, food, and paints [4].

Poloxamers or Pluronics® are a class of water-soluble nonionic triblock copolymers formed by polar (poly ethylene oxide) and non-polar (poly propylene oxide) blocks. which confer amphiphilic and surface active properties to the polymers. Their aqueous solutions undergo sol-to-gel transition with increasing the temperature above a LCGT; moreover, the coexistence of hydrophilic and hydrophobic monomers into block copolymers allows the formation of ordered structures in solution, the most common of these being the micelles. The formation of micelles in solution is a reversible and dynamic process useful for encapsulating hydrophobic drugs and delivering them into an aqueous environment.

They can be considered as smart polymers, for their stimuli-sensitive properties, due to the different behaviors of these polymers since they can modify their structure in function of pH, temperature and salt concentration [5]. For this reason, a variety of Pluronics is available on the market, differing for the molecular weight of the building blocks and for the hydrophobic–hydrophilic ratio, allowing the preparation of thermosensitive hydrogels with different properties, e.g., in terms of critical gelation concentration (CGC) and gelation time at physiological condition [3].

Thus, poloxamers represent a convenient choice in pharmaceutical technology and biomedical area due to their commercial availability, wide range of molecular weights, peculiar behavior and flexibility. Poloxamers are FDA approved and listed in the US and European Pharmacopoeia; they are non-toxic and non-irritant therefore they can be used as solubilizer, emulsifier, stabilizer, and administered through oral, parenteral, topical routes. As wetting agents, they are useful in ointments, suppository bases, and gels [6].

Poloxamer hydrogels use in drug release appeared at the beginning of the 1970s; they were a response in the search for new safer and faster treatments for the delivery of highly-effective therapeutic agents to a target cell, even if they have poor mechanical properties such as low tensile strength and low Young's modulus that limit their practical applications, sometimes even as medical device coatings [7].

Analysis of recent literature covering a range of treatment pathways and diseases, reveals a major emphasis on "smart" drug carriers developed with poloxamers. The different range of potential delivery methods is highlighted in this review by discussing how the poloxamer solution behavior enables multiple formulation processing routes, drug-encapsulating structures, and engagement with physiological barriers to drug passage.

The first research work concerned the treatment of thermal burns [8] followed by researches on the release of hormones [9], tetracycline [10], proteins [11], and more recently for norcantharidin delivery [12], heparin [13], and anti-HIV drugs [14]. In the last twenty years the numbers of papers related to poloxamer hydrogels for biomedical applications is exponentially increased (Figure 1).

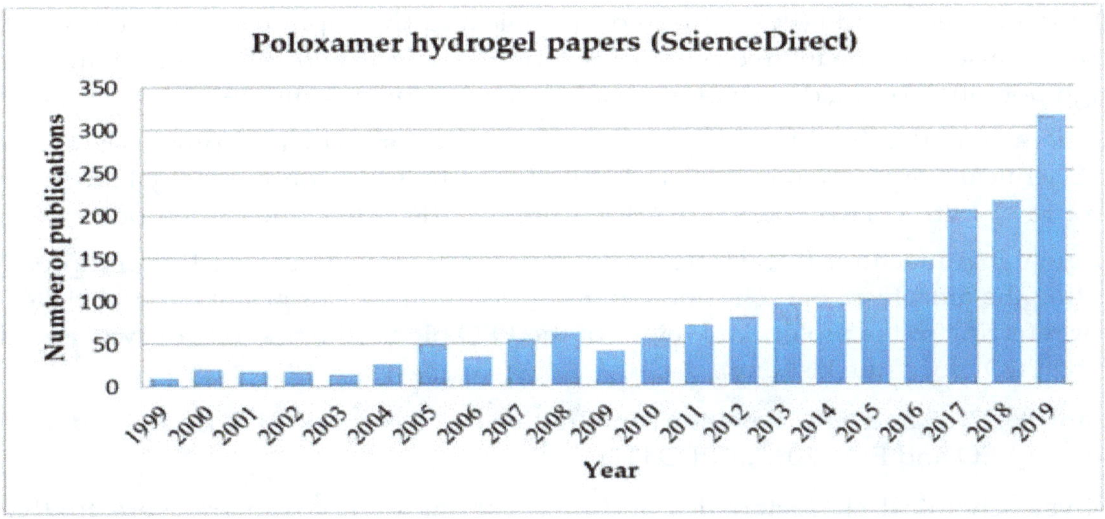

Figure 1. Histogram showing the increase in publications related to the keywords "poloxamer hydrogel" in Science Direct database during the past twenty years.

More recently such hydrogels have become especially attractive to the new field of "tissue engineering" as matrices for repairing and regenerating a wide variety of tissues and organs [15].

They have been successfully employed as scaffold-forming materials for cell printing technology, a computer-aided tissue engineering technology based on the layered deposition of cellularized hydrogels to form complex 3D constructs [16–18].

In this review the poloxamer hydrogels will be taken into consideration, giving an overview of their use as drug delivery systems (DDS) in different routes of administration, especially ophthalmic, transdermal, and vaginal ones. Finally, this paper focused on their potential in tissue and membrane regeneration, in the field of biomedical engineering and their application as micellar systems for gene delivery and cancer therapy.

2. Poloxamers

2.1. Poloxamers Properties

These polymers are synthetic triblock copolymers of poly(ethylene oxide)-b-poly(propylene oxide)-b-poly(ethylene oxide) (PEO-PPO-PEO) (Figure 2).

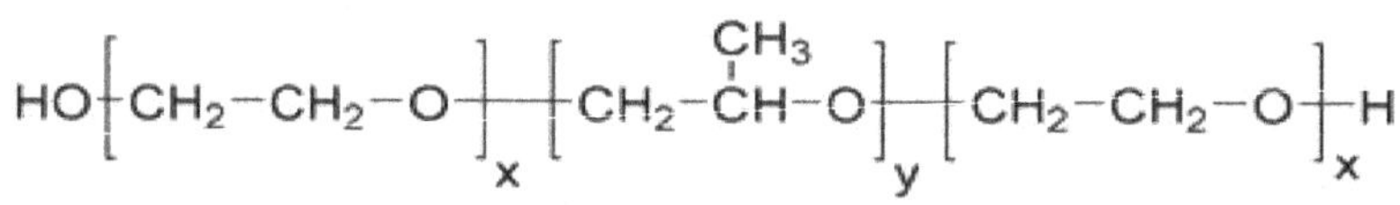

Figure 2. Chemical formula for poloxamers: x and y are the lengths of PEO and PPO: poly(ethylene oxide) and poly(propylene oxide) chains, respectively.

They are synthesized through the sequential addition of PO and EO monomers in the presence of an alkaline catalyst, such as sodium or potassium hydroxide, obtaining different copolymers with a different number of hydrophilic EO and hydrophobic PO units, which are also characterized by their distinct hydrophilic–lipophilic balance (HLB) value. Changes in the copolymer composition (PPO/PEO ratio) and molecular weight (PEO and PPO block length) during synthesis leads to macromolecular surface active agents with specific properties suitable in various technological areas.

Poloxamers appear in the form of liquids, pastes, and solids, depending on their molecular weights varying from 1100 to 14,000, offering a pool of more than 50 amphiphilic, water-soluble and polymorphic materials. Their water solubility is subjected by different ratio (1:9 to 8:2) between the chain of propylene oxide (PO) and ethylene oxide (EO) with hydrophobic and hydrophilic behavior, respectively [16]. These differences also alter the in vivo properties and interactions with cells and cell membranes, and provides high potential for the design of innovative nanomedicines and new biomaterials.

Poloxamers were the first block copolymers produced for industrial purposes, synthesized by Wyandotte Chemical Corporation in the late 1940s. Today they are commercially known by the trade names Pluronics®, Lutrol®, Kolliphor® (BASF), Antarox® (Rhodia), and Synperonics® (Croda).

The original manufacturer BASF introduced a specific nomenclature for Pluronics consisting of a letter indicating the morphism of each copolymer: L (for liquid), P (for paste) or F (for flakes) followed by a number referring to the molecular weight of the PPO block (the first one or two) and the weight fraction of the PEO block (the last one).

For example, P123 and F127 have the same molecular weight of PPO (in the order of 4000) but P123 has 30% of PEO and F127 70% of PEO [17].

The physicochemical characteristics and applications of Poloxamers were firstly reviewed extensively by Alexandridis and Hatton in 1995 [16]. In Figure 3, a 3D poloxamer modified pluronic grid showing the distribution of different copolymers, gathered according their physical state, is reported.

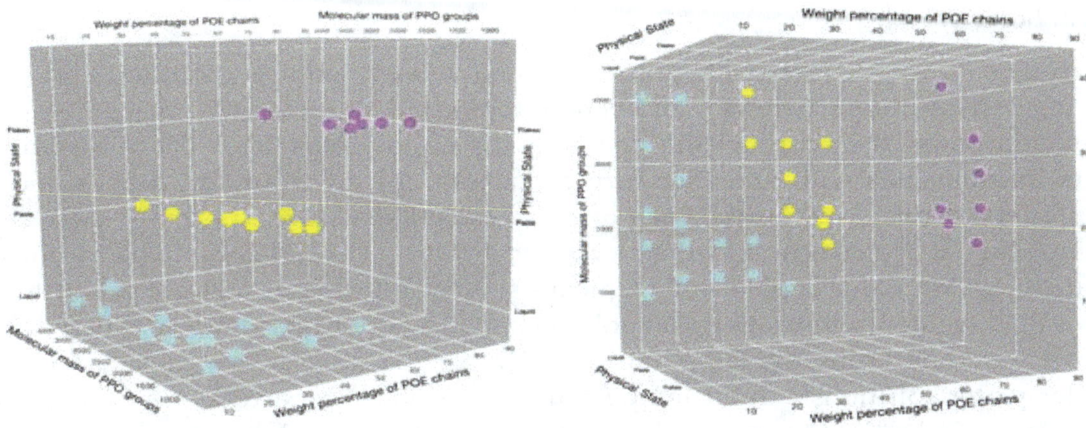

Figure 3. Poloxamers 3D distribution according to physical state (solid flakes = magenta; paste = yellow; liquid = blue), weight percentage of POE chains and molecular mass of the PPO groups (adapted from [16]).

The most significant physical properties of most common poloxamers, are reported in Table 1: average molecular weight, melting point expressed in °C, viscosity (Pa·s) measured at 25 °C, 60 °C, and 50 °C for pastes, liquids, and solids, respectively, surface tension at 0.1% at 25 °C (dyn cm^{-1}), hydrophilic–lipophilic balance (HLB) [4,17,19,20].

Table 1. Properties of the most common poloxamer poly(ethylene oxide)-b-poly(propylene oxide)-b-poly(ethylene oxide) (PEO-PPO-PEO) copolymers.

Poloxamer	Pluronic	PEO%	Average Molecular Weight	Melting Point (°C)	Viscosity (Pa·s)	Surface Tension (dyn cm^{-1})	HLB
P105	L35	50	1900	7	0.375	49	18–23
P108	F38	80	4700	48	0.260	52	>24
P122	L42	20	1630	−26	0.280	46	7–12
P123	L43	30	1850	−1	0.310	47	7–12
P124	L44	40	2200	16	0.440	45	12–18
P182	L62	20	2500	−4	0.450	43	1–7
P183	L63	30	2650	10	0.490	43	7–12
P184	L64	40	2900	16	0.850	43	12–18
P185	P65	50	3400	27	0.180	46	12–18
P188	F68	80	8400	52	1.000	50	>24
P212	L72	20	2750	−7	0.510	39	1–7
P215	P75	50	4150	27	0.250	43	12–18
P217	F77	70	6600	48	0.480	47	>24
P234	P84	40	4200	34	0.280	42	12–18
P235	P85	50	4600	34	0.310	42	12–18
P237	F87	70	7700	49	0.700	44	>24
P238	F88	80	11,400	54	2.300	48	>24
P288	F98	80	13,000	58	2.700	43	>24
P333	P103	30	4950	30	0.285	34	7–12
P334	P104	40	5900	32	0.390	33	12–18
P335	P105	50	6500	35	0.750	39	12–18
P338	F108	80	14,600	57	2.800	41	>24
P402	L122	20	5000	20	1.750	33	1–7
P403	P123	30	5750	31	0.350	34	7–12
P407	F127	70	12600	56	3.100	41	18–23

Commonly used poloxamers include P188 (F-68 grade), P237 (F-87 grade), P338 (F-108 grade), and P407 (F-127 grade) types, which are freely soluble in water.

2.2. Poloxamers Behavior

The aqueous solution properties of poloxamers have been intensely studied and thoroughly reviewed owing to their unique behavior and benefit to myriad applications.

In water solutions, the amphiphilic character of copolymers lead the macromolecule to self-aggregate into micelles with an inner core constituted by hydrophobic blocks and an outer shell constituted by hydrophilic units. They are nano-sized structures, normally between 10 and 200 nm that appears at the critical micellization concentration (CMC) and at critical micellization temperature (CMT). CMC value of poloxamer aqueous solutions decreases with increasing temperature and number of PEO segments, indicating that polymers with a larger hydrophobic (PPO) domain form micelles at lower concentrations and temperatures [21].

Poloxamer water solutions exhibit temperature sensitivity, in particular a "thermoreversible gelation" [21] for sufficiently concentrated samples; they show a sol-gel transition around 37 °C (physiological temperature) and gel-sol transition around 50 °C, being able to produce thermoreversible gels, some already approved by the Food and Drug Administration, which present great interest in food additives, drug delivery carriers in cosmetics, pharmaceutical ingredients, and tissue engineering [5,17]

Several mechanisms have been proposed for this behavior, the first one was related to the gel transition that was due to changes in micellar properties (Figure 4).

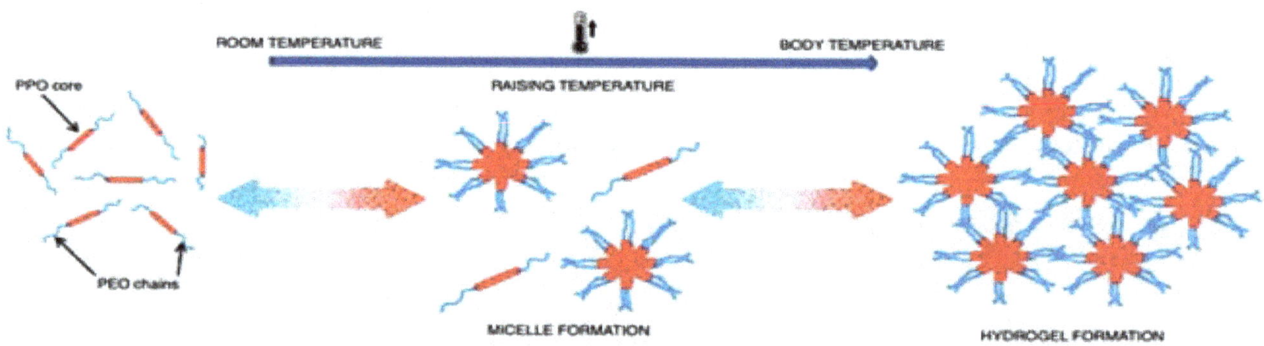

Figure 4. Schematic representation for hydrogel formation.

Thanks to their core–shell architecture, the hydrophobic core can act as a drug-loading site, creating a space for the encapsulation of hydrophobic drugs through the establishment of physical or chemical interactions. The properties of the outer shell and inner core have an influence in the drug release, that can promote an easier or sustained release of the drug. Due the properties above mentioned, polymeric micelles can transport several drugs, improving the circulation time, as well as the enhanced permeability and retention effect. Moreover, these systems exhibit low-risk of chronic toxicity since the polymeric micelles are disassembled in vivo, in single polymer chains that can be excreted by kidneys.

In order to prepare polymeric micelles for drug encapsulation, different methods can be used, however, the more common are the direct dissolution, dialysis, evaporation or film method, freeze-drying, microphase separation, and the oil-in-water emulsion [22].

The method depends, mostly, on the solubility of the copolymer and the drug in an aqueous medium. Some other aspects are also important to an efficient drug incorporation, such as copolymer characteristics, molecular weight and HLB. The structural and chemical characterization of polymeric micelles are important features to take into account in the development of these nanocarriers, since they have a direct influence on the efficiency of these drug release forms, in terms of size, polydispersion index, zeta potential, encapsulation efficiency (EE), and drug loading capacity (DL) [23].

Other researchers [24] discussed gelation as a function of thermodynamical parameters. The enthalpy of gelation depends on CMC and temperature, the value change in the case of poloxamers gelation is unfavorable unlike the gelatine gelation where a great enthalpy change occurred.

The useful concentration for gel formation is the same as for poloxamers with the same PPO/PEO ratio and it decreases with the increasing of polymer molecular weight, denoting the significance of this parameter. While the presence of electrolytes reduces gel transition temperature, enthalpy of gel formation is not significantly changed by the addition of other substances. This behavior suggests that entropy plays the major role in the gelation process.

For all these behaviors, the poloxamers were used for the study and for the development of innovative pharmaceutical forms in different administration routes.

3. Drug Delivery Systems (DDS)

Poloxamer sol-gel reversible hydrogels have attracted the attention for practical biomedical and pharmaceutical applications because of constituents solubility, biocompatibility with biological systems and easy administration of pharmaceutical formulations. The pharmaceutical and biomedical fields covered by the use of poloxamers including solubilization of hydrophobic drugs, controlled release, biomacromolecule delivery (e.g., proteins and genes) and tissue engineering.

Most applications involve the use of Poloxamer P407 and include delivery of protein/peptide drugs [25], such as insulin [26], interleukin-2 [27], epidermal growth factor [28], bone morphogenic protein [29], fibroblastic growth factor, and endothelial cell growth factor [30].

In recent years these hydrogels have been used as carriers for most routes of administration, the most interesting are discussed below.

3.1. *Poloxamers for Oftalmic Administration*

The thermoreversible gels have shown a growing interest at ocular level because they combine peculiar characteristics: i.e., the formulation when applied is sol (it performs like eye drops) and becomes gel with body temperature (it performs like ointment) increasing the in situ residence time.

The most well-known ocular drug delivery system is eye drops, but they have a short residence time because they are quickly drained through the nasolacrimal route resulting in frequent dosage regimen which leads to an increase in side effects and poor patient compliance.

Poloxamers P407 and P188 are among the most commonly used in this case for their good water solubility, solution clearness, optimal viscosity, and ocular tissue safety.

Recent works have focused on the best formulation to obtain a hydrogel with useful features for ocular administration and without toxicity. About this point Al Khateb et al. [31] studied two formulations containing poloxamers, i.e., P407 and P188, with different gelation properties depending on concentration solutions and the ratio of their mixtures. Transparent gels were obtained only in the case of 20% w/w P407 and P188 solutions. Furthermore, these preparations were non-toxic or irritating to the corneal mucosa and then suitable for application in ocular drug delivery.

Fathalla Z.M.A. et al. [32] studied the blend of the same two poloxamers for a controlled ocular delivery of ketorolac tromethamine (KT). The most promising gel formulations, loaded with KT, were those containing the mixtures of P407:P188 23:10 w/v% and 23:15 w/v% respectively. These gels do not present toxicity and do not irritate the conjunctiva and cornea.

In recent years other polymers have been added to poloxamers-based gels to obtain different drug release characteristics and to modify the rheological properties.

Among these works, Yu et al. [33] has to be remembered for the synthesis of a cross-linked hydrogel system containing carboxymethyl chitosan (CMC) and poloxamer P407, where the presence of CMC with biological properties could improve hydrogel biocompatibility. This formulation, containing nepafenac (NP) as a model drug, showed good rheological properties at gelation temperature (32–33 °C) and a sustained release of NP from hydrogel, so as to be considered a pH–temperature-responsive ophthalmic drug delivery system.

Another approach, with good results, involved the introduction of various colloidal carrier systems to easily load poorly soluble drugs into poloxamers hydrogels.

Lou et al. [34] incorporated curcumin-loaded albumin nanoparticles into a hydrogel based on a mixture of P407/P188 for local ocular administration, to treat diabetic retinopathy. This formulation, which became a gel when exposed to eye temperature, may be applied as eye drops. Nanoparticles provided the sustained drug release while the presence of hydrogel prolonged the in situ residence time.

Finally, Almeda et al. [35] reported the combination of lipid nanoparticles and a thermoresponsive polymer with mucomimetic properties (poloxamer P407). The incorporated nanoparticles showed an average size below 200 nm, a good positive zeta potential and an efficiency of ibuprofen encapsulation of about 90%. The optimal poloxamer concentration in thermoreversible gel was 15% (w/w) Pluronic® F-127. The formulation did not present a relevant cytotoxicity and showed a sustained release of ibuprofen over several hours. The strategy proposed in this work can be successfully applied to increase bioavailability and therapeutic efficacy of conventional eyedrops.

3.2. Poloxamers for Transdermal Administration

Transdermal drug delivery is a valid alternative to the oral and parenteral route because it offers several advantages: Avoidance the hepatic first pass, good compliance by the patient, and easy access. The most studied formulations for this route contained poloxamer P407, as a polymer, and as drugs those with anti-inflammatory [36,37], analgesic [38], local anesthetic [39], and cardiac [40,41] activity, rarely are present preparations containing big molecules such as arginine, vasopressin, and insulin [42,43].

Generally in these topical preparations it is necessary to introduce an enhancer substance which is able to facilitate the passage through the stratum corneum (thickness of 10 to 15 μm) which is the main barrier to drug penetration.

In the last decade the penetration enhancers have been replaced by the microneedles (MNs) that have the capacity to permeate the stratum corneum and infuse the active ingredient in the deep areas of the skin.

Microneedles are needles similar to the ones useful for hypodermic injections but they present different sizes: from 1–100 microns in length and 1 micron in diameter (Figure 5). They are manufactured with silicon [44,45], metals such as stainless steel, palladium, nickel and titanium [46–48], carbohydrates including galactose, maltose, and polysaccharide [49–51], glass [52], ceramics [53], and various other polymers [54,55]. MNs are fabricated in backing that can be applied to the substrate like a patch carrying different drugs by penetrating through the skin, mucosal tissue and sclera [56–59]. Their dissolution has to be taken into consideration because it can influence drug delivery [60,61].

One of the most recent researches regards sol-gel transition property of poloxamers to obtain in situ forming hydrogel microneedles, for the delivery of methotrexate to treat solid tumors [62]. The use of this drug by transdermal route is generally limited by its relatively high molecular weight and hydrophilicity. For this purpose four formulations were prepared with two different methotrexate concentrations (0.2% and 0.4% w/w) with poloxamer P407 (20% w/w) and without, using the last one as a control, replacing the polymer with deionized water. In this study, it was confirmed the sol-gel transition of the formulations at skin temperature (32 °C), maintaining skin barrier function and skin viscoelastic properties after administration of the formulations. In vitro drug diffusion studies, using a Franz cell, showed that the formulations containing methotrexate (0.2% and 0.4%) without P407 released overall drug after 22 and 35 h respectively, while the one with P407 after 72 h. For this reason it is possible to conclude that the poloxamer-based formulations provided a steady and sustained delivery.

In an even more recent work, the formation of depots of thermoreversible poloxamers in skin micropores using MNs to transdermal drug delivery has been reported for the first time [63]. Sodium fluorescein (FS) was used as model drug to study in vitro permeation at different concentrations. In order to crate pores into the skin and to overcome the stratum corneum MNs have been used, then the drug loaded poloxamer solution was applied to fill pores, subsequently an in situ gelation at skin temperature of 32 °C occurred.

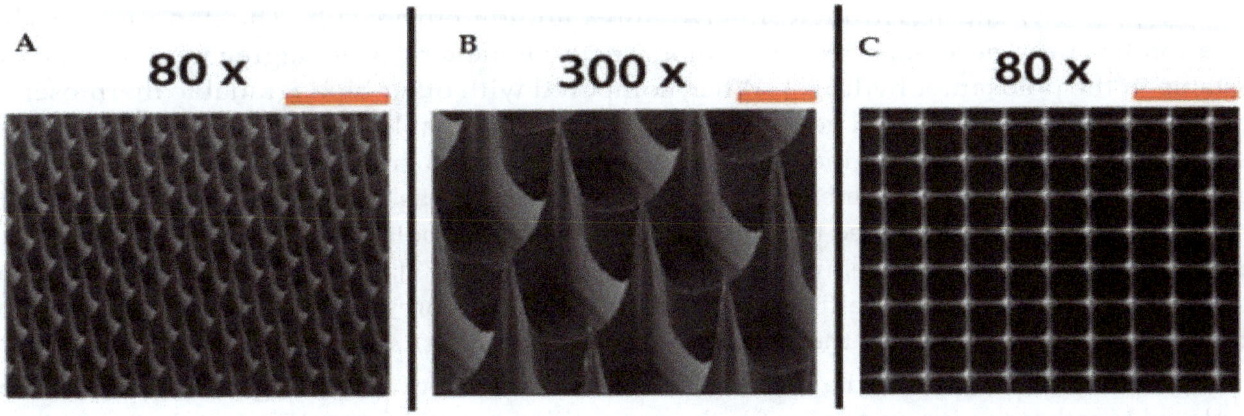

Figure 5. Scanning electron microscopy images of microneedle arrays imaged from a lateral view (**A**,**B**) and from the top side (**C**). Scale bars represent 500 μm (80×) (**A**,**C**) and 100 μm (300×) (**B**) (adapted from [64]).

For this goal poloxamers P407, P237, and P338 were used at different concentrations (from 15 to 30% w/w in water) loading different amounts of fluorescein.

The formulations were characterized for their rheological properties and in situ gel formation. The distribution of FS in skin tissue was tracked by confocal laser microscopic analysis with higher intensity of FS in MN-treated skin tissues. The in vitro fluorescein release studies were carried out using vertical Franz diffusion cells. The release profiles indicated that the concentration of fluorescein (0.1%, 0.3%, and 0.5% w/w) was a variable parameter that significantly affects drug release as well as the type of poloxamer used. In particular P338 and P237 0.1–0.3% FS-loaded formulations provided a total drug release during 16 h while 0.5% FS-loaded provided a release for 20 h. Moreover, for a longer time (about 24 h), the release from P407 formulations was comparable. All the poloxamers depots started dissolving according to the dominant hydrophilic interactions and gels did not remain intact. It was concluded that P407 provided the best release for a longer duration and it was selected as the best drug delivery for in vitro permeation assays. These studies confirmed that drug loading is not a limitation and permeation of FS after MN treatment was found in more controlled manner and for a long time when compared to a permeation across untreated skin sample.

3.3. *Poloxamers for Vaginal Administration*

Another interesting pathway exploited in drug delivery systems is the vaginal route, allowing both the systemic and local absorption of drugs poorly absorbed after oral administration [65–67]. The vagina has a vast network of blood vessels that make easy the systemic absorption, avoiding deactivation at gastrointestinal level and hepatic first pass. Mucoadhesive pharmaceutical forms have been studied for this district due to the presence of mucus which increases permeability. The thermoreversible systems, appropriately modified with polymers that promote mucoadhesion, allow to obtain a sustained drug release and a good bioavailability without altering the vaginal physiology [68].

After application of poloxamers for vaginal administration occurring gelation favored a long permanence of drugs on the administration site to promote a drug controlled release [69]. Vaginal drug delivery is based on the exploitation of polymers which are able not only to gelify at physiological temperature but also to adhere to the vaginal mucosa improving the in situ residence time.

A brief description of recent reports in the literature, based on poloxamer formulations by vaginal route, is given below.

In the first work [70] the authors investigated a novel amphotericin B (AmB) release system in the form of nanosuspension loaded into a poloxamer P407/P188 hydrogel. P407 (20% w/w) and P188 (5% w/w) were dissolved in AmB nanosuspension, the AmB NPs thermogel were characterized regarding nanoparticle features (particle size, zeta potential, morphology) and gel behavior (rheology, stability, in vitro drug release, and in vitro and in vivo anti-Candida efficiency). The nanosuspension-gel combination has been necessary because nanoparticles alone tended to aggregate while they were more stable in the poloxamer hydrogel. When compared with other biodegradable thermosensitive hydrogel, such as polyester-based gels, poloxamer were not capable of an in vivo degradation. This property is really suitable for vaginal delivery because it means grater safety in use. Another very important element in the development of vaginal formulations was mucoadhesion; poloxamers have lower adhesion properties compared to compounds such as Carbopol, the addition of some bioadhesive materials into P407/P188 thermogel would be a feasible path [71–73]. Finally, the in vivo anti-Candida assay showed a better antifungal efficiency of AmB in the thermoreversible gel when compared with commercial effervescent tablets at the same drug dose (2.5 mg/Kg).

A second paper [74] described a novel vaginal delivery strategy consisting of two pharmaceutical forms placed together to give an expansible thermal gelling aerosol foam (ETGFA) that combined the advantages of foam and gel penetration and carrier retention in vaginal canal, respectively.

ETGA was prepared adding an optimized amount of P407 (18–22% w/w) and P188 (0–5% w/w), achieved by evaluating the gelation temperature, the adhesive agents (arabic gum, sodium carboxymethyl cellulose, sodium alginate, and xanthan gum) and silver nanoparticles to obtain a drug concentration of 1% w/w. To study a better performance in foam expansion and duration, propane/butane 80/20 v/v and dimethyl ether were compared as propellants. The formulation was characterized in regards of rheology, foam expansion, adhesiveness and drug release. ETGA showed a better extended drug release (over 4 h) dose –dependent antimicrobial effects on the vaginal flora and no tissue irritation when compared to a commercial antimicrobial gel. These results indicated that ETGA could be a suitable formulation for vaginal drug delivery.

4. Tissue Regeneration Scaffolders

Tissue engineering, in this last decade, has emerged in the biomedical field because it allows researchers to create specific devices that represent in vivo tissues that can be replaced or increased to address current therapeutic challenges [75].

Poloxamers have received special attention for tissue regeneration based on their biocompatibility, low cytotoxicity, and good rheological properties [76].

In particular, the area the most explored deals with regeneration of bone tissue. The use of growth factors such as bone morphogenetic protein-2 (BMP-2) for bone repair has been reported [77,78] but it is very expensive and easily loose its integrity. Recently, other compounds that have received interest were statins because they altered bone metabolism through different mechanisms [79–81]. Their bioavailability after oral administration was low and a real bone healing cannot be expected. For this reason different delivery systems for local delivery of statins have been evaluated. The study of incorporation of rosuvastatin (RSV)-loaded chitosan/chondroitin sulfate nanoparticles into a thermosensitive hydrogel is reported below [82]. At first this research considered nanoparticles preparation and optimization, thereafter it dealt with the characterization of thermosensible hydrogels.

Gel formulation consisted of poloxamer P407 (18–20% w/v), hyaluronic acid (HA) 1–3% w/v and hydroxypropyl methylcellulose (2% w/v) to stabilize the formulation itself.

HA [83] and P407 had also positive effects on articular cartilage, simulating the regenerative process within the joint. The study showed that gel provided a low viscosity at 4 °C and gelification at 35 °C; drug release from nanoparticles, inserted into the hydrogel, was around 60% after 48 h, while it was completely released from nanoparticles alone within 12 h. This behavior indicated that the drug release was controlled and sustained.

Moreover, the hydrogel formulation showed an improvement in osteoblast viability and proliferation due to the used polymer and the biological properties of the nanoparticle delivery system.

Another paper [84] reported the design of a cryogel scaffold for the regeneration of an intervertebral disc tissue (nucleus pulposus NP). NP is located inside the vertebral discs and has the function of absorbing the pressure exerted on the spine and keeping the vertebrae separated. The symptoms of NP degeneration are pain and limited mobility of the extremities. It is composed of up to 90% water, type II collagen and proteoglycans [85]. This study focused on the preparation of a novel gelatin-P407 cryogel (in different ratio: 1:1,2:1, 4:1,5:1, 7:1, or 10:1 respectively) as an alternative to the spinal fusion procedure. The composite hydrogel was tested by the following assays: Pore analysis, swelling potential, stability, mechanical integrity and cellular infiltration. The inclusion of P407 in the cryogel was designed to increase swelling ratio, due its hydrophilic nature, since in the NP degradation there is a rapid water loss. All sample presented a high swelling ratio after 24 h, mechanical durability and stability for 28 days in a body-like environment. The 7:1 and 10:1 gel scaffolds showed the most ideal pore diameters and a profuse cell infiltration after only 14 days.

In recent years, 3D printing technology has become important in the biomedical field and in particular the use of thermoreversible gels that with their sol-gel characteristics can be very useful in tissue regeneration [86].

The principle on which the 3D printer is based is to lay a filament of polymeric material which is deposited layer upon layer until the desired system is obtained in 3 dimensions.

Bioprinting systems can be classified into three types: Laser based, jetting based, and extrusion based; recent techniques such as magnetic bioprinting and electrohydrodynamic jetting have been used in tissue engineering.

Hydrogels requirements for 3D bioprinting of ideal engineered tissues should be the following [87]: High porosity, rapid gelation, shape retention, and immunological issue avoidance.

Thermoreversible hydrogels have been successfully applied thanks to their gelation characteristics as they quickly pass from sol-gel state and are also easily extruded from 3D printers [88].

P407 showed good printability [86] but it was not suitable for long-term cell viability. As reported by the recent work [89] it is used, combined with gelatin to create a biocompatible hydrogel for vascular channels, for molds, exploiting its excellent rheological behavior, under shear stress, and its elasticity.

In addition to bioprintability, biological properties of hydrogels played a crucial role in successful tissues regeneration [90]. One of the major disadvantages of available hydrogel materials was that they do not facilitate differentiation of cells into multiple linkages. Despite this, thermoresponsive hydrogels may be very useful for tissue engineering applications and they will become part of the advancement in bio printing technology.

5. Poloxamer as Micellar Systems

Polymeric micelles generated by poloxamers with peculiar characteristics and under specific conditions are exploited as nanometric drug carriers [91]. They have taken hold in recent years as they are able to solubilize poorly water-soluble drugs [36] and decrease undesirable cellular interactions [92,93]. In this review chapter, two recent applications (gene delivery and cancer therapy) of poloxamer micelles have been taken into account.

The development of gene delivery carriers has emerged as a promising technology in transporting genes directly to the target site as therapeutic factors [94]. Current gene transfer vectors used in regenerative medicine approaches included no viral [95] and viral vehicles [96]. The complexation of DNA with cationic polymers (polyplexes) or lipids (lipoplexes) protected DNA against degradation by nucleases and serum components creating a less negative surface charge. They can be designed to target specific cell types through receptor–ligand interactions [97], but these systems exhibited aggregation tendency, a low transfection efficiency and short time transgene expression levels [98]. The use of poloxamers has been described as a tool to increase efficiency of viral gene transfer, obtaining a localized delivery into targets or protecting the vectors.

In the last decade many works that focused the attention on gene delivery were published; the most recent and significant studies are here summarized.

Many researchers have studied the recombinant adeno-associated viral (rAAV) carriers as adapted gene transfer vectors to direct human cartilagine in regenerative medicine [99–101]. However, their use is limited cause their rapid neutralization by the presence of antibodies or heparin which prevent their binding to the viral receptor, present on the cell surface. In this regard, based on the use of polymeric biocompatible materials the combining of direct rAAV-mediated gene transfer with tissue engineering approaches, may offer efficient alternatives.

In this study [102] the possibility of providing rAAV to cartilage regenerative cells via self-assembled poloxamers was evaluated. The formulations consisted of P188 and P407 (2% w/v i.e., above CMC)/rAAV or poloxamine/rAAV were directly incubated within monolayer cultures of hMSCs, cartilagine regenerative cells. At thisoptimized concentration the two poloxamers were more efficient in increasing gene expression over time than a treatment lacking them.

The highest rAAV gene transfer occurred when the PEO/PPO ratio was shifted to hydrophilicity (HLB > 24) using a concentration above CMC (2%) (89.5–94.6% efficiencies with up to 2.7-fold increase in transgene expression for at least 21 days, suggesting that micelles may be better carriers than unimers).

In another paper [103], lentiviral vectors (LV) used for the transduction of human and nonhuman cells were taken into consideration. The optimal transduction conditions for efficient LV gene delivery into target cells depended on a number of factors, including cell density, purity of lentiviral preparation, virus transduction units (TU), multiplicity of infection (MOI) and presence of adjuvants that facilitate transduction [104–106]. These researches identified and validated novel adjuvants for improving transduction efficiency, in particular five representatives poloxamers (P402, P235, P188, P407, and P338). P338 proved to be the best choice since it produced low toxicity and effective viral transduction, especially in difficult-to-transduce cells of T-cell origin.

Further application strategies with poloxamer regard cancer therapy [4]. Poloxamers have gained interest in the field of oncology because of their ability to developed stable systems with the capability of efficient drugs encapsulation and deliver. They usually present small sizes and self-assembling behavior in micellar systems in an aqueous medium, good stability in physiological medium and they avoid the deactivation by RES organs improving consequently drug bioavailability [22,107].

In this biomedical and pharmaceutical area the most recent works in the literature are reported. The first one concerned the use of poloxamer micelles containing a dye (CyFaP) as photo-acoustic imaging (PAI) contrast for mammary neoplastic tissue [108]. In this formulation, dye was inserted in P407 (10% w/v) micelle dropwise under constant stirring. Serum stability studies, cell viability assays, deep tissue penetration and in vivo biodistribution studies were performed. This work has shown that poloxamer micelles are effective for PAI as they penetrate more deeply into breast cancer tissue and are also useful for lymphatic mapping.

The second work [109] explored the anticancer activity of Salinomycin (SAL), an antibiotic isolated from Streptomyces albus [110], that has recently been reported as being effective against tumor cells and mainly to inhibit growth of a specific cancer cell sub-population: CSC. The main goal of the research was the encapsulation of SAL into an innovative poloxamer micelles (PM) system and a further evaluation of in vitro PM-SAL delivery in bacterial and in eukaryotic tumor cells. PM formulations containing P407 and SAL in different amounts were defined with a two multivariate experimental design (DoE) to get the best preparation conditions. Micelles were characterized for size by dynamic light scattering, for their zeta potential and for the encapsulation efficiency. Their in vitro activity was conducted in bacterial cell culture and A549 (adenocarcinoma cell line) cell culture. In conclusion, these micelles seem to be able to deliver SAL into human cancer cells promoting a high drug intracellular accumulation, greatly decreasing toxicity on healthy cells.

Finally, a combined study between radiation therapy and systemic chemotherapeutics to provide both local radiosensitization and systemic control of tumor disease has been reported [111,112]. This study showed the development of a single micelles formulation consisting of multiple poloxamers (MPMs) containing PARP (poly ADP- ribose polymerase) inhibitor talazoparib (Tal) and PI3K (phosphoinositol-3-kinase) inhibitor buparlisib (Bup). When administered during a radiotherapy cycle, that would increase the therapeutic activity of the two drugs in a preclinical model [113]. The performed formulation was made of poloxamer mixture (P103 and P407) obtaining micelles (MPMs) via a modified nanoprecipitation method [114]. MPMs were characterized by dynamic light scattering, to determine size, zeta potential and polydispersity, and by transmission electron microscopy (TEM).

It was also observed that MPMs modulate drug release depending on pH; this behavior is a very useful tool, as the change in pH at tumor level (pH 6.8) would result in a faster release than what occurs when they are circulating in the blood stream (pH 7.4). Furthermore, metabolic assays confirmed that the use of both Tal and Bup synergistically enhanced in vitro cytotoxicity. The in vitro therapeutic activity of the two drugs was studied by a colony-forming assay and a DNA damage assay.

In vivo experiments have shown that the administration of this new MPMs formulation during the course of radiotherapy gave promising results into the enhanced tumor control. The results of this study confirmed that it is important to carry on the development and advancement of combination therapies, especially with the aim of enhancing the outcomes of patients in late-stage and metastatic disease.

6. Summary

Poloxamers are peculiar synthetic tri-block copolymers composed of two poly(ethylene oxide) units and a poly(propylene oxide) one with amphiphilic properties. The dual character, confers to the copolymers interesting properties that can be controlled and changed by different PPO/PEO ratios. These polymers exhibit thermogelling behavior at strategical physiological temperatures.

The most used and studied poloxamer P407, at a concentration of 20% w/w in water, is able to convert the solution to a clear gel by warming the system from room (25 °C) to body temperature (near 37 °C). This thermoresponsive feature has made it attractive for several applications including injectable and topical pharmaceutical formulations, where the material may flow through an applicator or syringe before forming a gel upon contact with the body (35–37 °C).

Because of their biocompatibility and nontoxicity poloxamers have been widely utilized in biomedical applications. In this review their usefulness as thermoreversible hydrogels in the most significant routes of administration (i.e., ocular, transdermic and vaginal route) was reported. Moreover, the latest frontiers have been highlighted for what concerns poloxamers employed in tissue engineering and in gene and cancer therapy.

References

1. Wichterle, O.; Lim, D. Hydrophilic Gels for Biological Use. *Nature* **1960**, *185*, 117–118. [CrossRef]
2. Buwalda, S.J.; Boere, K.W.; Dijkstra, P.J.; Feijen, J.; Vermonden, T.; Hennink, W.E. Hydrogels in a historical perspective: From simple networks to smart materials. *J. Control. Release* **2014**, *190*, 254–273. [CrossRef] [PubMed]
3. Gioffredi, E.; Boffito, M.; Calzone, S.; Giannitelli, S.M.; Rainer, A.; Trombetta, M.; Mozetic, P.; Chiono, V. Pluronic F127 hydrogel characterization and biofabrication in cellularized constructs for tissue engineering applications. *Procedia Cirp* **2016**, *49*, 125–132. [CrossRef]
4. Almeida, M.; Magalhães, M.; Veiga, F.; Figueiras, A. Poloxamers, poloxamines and polymeric micelles: Definition, structure and therapeutic applications in cancer. *J. Polym. Res.* **2018**, *25*, 31. [CrossRef]
5. Aguilar, M.R.; Elvira, C.; Gallardo, A.; Vázquez, B.; Román, J.S. Smart Polymers and Their Applications as Biomaterials. In *Topics in Tissue Engineering*; Ashammakhi, N., Reis, R.L., Chiellini, E., Eds.; Biomaterials and Tissue Engineering Group: Oulu, Finland, 2007; Volume 3.
6. Johnston, T.P.; Palmer, W.K. Mechanism of poloxamer 407-induced hypertriglyceridemia in the rat. *Biochem. Pharm.* **1993**, *46*, 1037–1042. [CrossRef]
7. Li, J.; Stachowski, M.; Zhang, Z. Application of responsive polymers in implantable medical devices and biosensors. In *Switchable and Responsive Surfaces and Materials for Biomedical Applications*; Woodhead Publishing: Sawston, UK; Cambridge, UK, 2015.
8. Nalbandian, R.M.; Henry, R.L.; Wilks, H.S. Artificial skin. II. Pluronic F-127 Silver nitrate or silver lactate gel in the treatment of thermal burns. *J. Biomed. Mater. Res.* **1972**, *6*, 583–590. [CrossRef] [PubMed]

9. Law, T.; Florence, A.T.; Whateley, T.L. Some chemically modified poloxamer hydrogels-controlled release of prostaglandin-e2 and testosterone. *Int. J. Pharm.* **1986**, *33*, 65–69. [CrossRef]
10. Esposito, E.; Carotta, V.; Scabbia, A.; Trombelli, L.; D'Antona, P.; Menegatti, E.; Nastruzzi, C. Comparative analysis of tetracycline-containing dental gels: Poloxamer- and monoglyceride-based formulations. *Int. J. Pharm.* **1996**, *142*, 9–23. [CrossRef]
11. Stratton, L.P.; Dong, A.; Manning, M.C.; Carpenter, J.F. Drug delivery matrix containing native protein precipitates suspended in a poloxamer gel. *J. Pharm. Sci.* **1997**, *86*, 1006–1010. [CrossRef]
12. Xie, M.H.; Ge, M.; Peng, J.B.; Jiang, X.R.; Wang, D.S.; Ji, L.Q.; Ying, Y.; Wang, Z. In-vivo anti-tumor activity of a novel poloxamer-based thermosensitive in situ gel for sustained delivery of norcantharidin. *Pharm. Dev. Technol.* **2019**, *24*, 623–629. [CrossRef]
13. He, C.; Ji, H.; Qian, Y.; Wang, Q.; Liu, X.; Zhao, W.; Zhao, C. Heparin-based and heparin-inspired hydrogels: Size-effect, gelation and biomedical applications. *J. Mater. Chem. B* **2019**, *7*, 1186–1208. [CrossRef]
14. Tian, W.; Han, S.; Huang, X.; Han, M.; Cao, J.; Liang, Y.; Sun, Y. LDH hybrid thermosensitive hydrogel for intravaginal delivery of anti-HIV drugs. *Artif. Cells Nanomed. Biotechnol.* **2019**, *47*, 1234–1240. [CrossRef] [PubMed]
15. Hoffman, A.S. Hydrogels for biomedical applications. *Adv. Drug Deliv. Rev.* **2012**, *64*, 18–23. [CrossRef]
16. Alexandridis, P.; Hatton, T.A. Poly(ethylene oxide)-poly(propylene oxide)-poly (ethylene oxide) block copolymer surfactants in aqueous solutions and at interfaces: Thermodynamics, structure, dynamics, and modeling. *Colloids Surf. A Physicochem. Eng. Asp.* **1995**, *96*, 1–46. [CrossRef]
17. Singh-Joy, S.D.; McLain, V.C. Safety Assessment of Poloxamers 101, 105, 108, 122, 123, 124, 181, 182, 183, 184, 185, 188, 212, 215, 217, 231, 234, 235, 237, 238, 282, 284, 288, 331, 333, 334, 335, 338, 401, 402, 403, and 407, Poloxamer 105 Benzoate, and Poloxamer 182 Dibenzoate as Used in Cosmetics. *Int. J. Toxicol.* **2008**, *27*, 93–128.
18. Pitto-Barry, A.; Barry, N.P. Pluronic®block-copolymers in medicine: From chemical and biological versatility to rationalization and clinical advances. *Polym. Chem.* **2014**, *5*, 3281–3496. [CrossRef]
19. Jeong, B.; Kim, S.W.; Bae, Y.H. Thermosensitive sol–gel reversible hydrogels. *Adv. Drug Deliv. Rev.* **2012**, *64*, 154–162. [CrossRef]
20. Devi, D.R.; Sandhya, P.; Hari, B.V. Poloxamer: A novel functional molecule for drug delivery and gene therapy. *J. Pharm. Sci. Res.* **2013**, *5*, 159–165.
21. Alexandridis, P.; Holzwarth, J.F.; Hatton, T.A. Micellization of Poly(Ethylene Oxide)-Poly(Propylene Oxide)-Poly(Ethylene Oxide) Triblock Copolymers in Aqueous-Solutions-Thermodynamics of Copolymer Association. *Macromolecules* **1994**, *27*, 2414–2425. [CrossRef]
22. Simões, S.M.; Figueiras, A.R.; Veiga, F.; Concheiro, A.; Alvarez-Lorenzo, C. Polymeric micelles for oral drug administration enabling loco regional and systemic treatments. *Expert Opin. Drug Deliv.* **2015**, *12*, 297–318. [CrossRef]
23. Ahmad, Z.; Shah, A.; Siddiq, M.; Kraatz, H.B. Polymeric micelles as drug delivery vehicles. *RSC Adv.* **2014**, *4*, 17028–17038. [CrossRef]
24. Vadnere, M.; Amidon, G.L.; Lindenbaum, S.; Haslam, J.L. Thermodynamic studies on the gel-sol transition of some pluronic polyols. *Int. J. Pharm.* **1984**, *22*, 207. [CrossRef]
25. Cho, C.W.; Cho, Y.S.; Lee, H.K.; Yeom, Y.I.; Park, S.N.; Yoon, D.Y. Improvement of receptor-mediated gene delivery to HepG2 cells using an amphiphilic gelling agent. *Biotechnol. Appl. Biochem.* **2000**, *32*, 21–26. [CrossRef] [PubMed]
26. Morishita, M.; Barichello, J.M.; Takayama, K.; Chiba, Y.; Tokwa, S.; Nagai, T. Pluronic F-127 gels incorporating highly purified unsaturated fatty acids for buccal delivery of insulin. *Int. J. Pharm.* **2001**, *212*, 289–293. [CrossRef]
27. Johnston, T.P.; Punjabi, M.A.; Froelich, C.J. Sustained delivery of interleukin-2 from a Poloxamer 407 gel matrix following intraperitoneal injection in mice. *Pharm. Res.* **1992**, *9*, 425–434. [CrossRef]
28. DiBiase, M.D.; Rhodes, C.T. Investigations of epidermal growth factor in semisolid formulations. *Pharm. Acta Helv.* **1991**, *66*, 165–169.
29. Clokie, C.M.; Urist, M.R. Bone morphogenic protein excipients: Comparative observations on poloxamer. *Plast. Reconstr. Surg.* **2000**, *105*, 628–637. [CrossRef]
30. Hom, D.B.; Medhi, K.; Assefa, G.; Juhn, S.K.; Johnston, T.P. Vascular effects of sustained-release fibroblast growth factors. *Ann. Otol. Rhinol. Laryngol.* **1996**, *105*, 109–116. [CrossRef]

31. Al Khateb, K.; Ozhmukhametova, E.K.; Mussin, M.N.; Seilkhanov, S.K.; Rakhypbekov, T.K.; Lau, W.M.; Khutoryanskiy, V.V. In situ gelling systems based on Pluronic F127/Pluronic F68 formulations for ocular drug delivery. *Int. J. Pharm.* **2016**, *502*, 70–79. [CrossRef]
32. Fathalla, Z.M.; Vangala, A.; Longman, M.; Khaled, K.A.; Hussein, A.K.; El-Garhy, O.H.; Alany, R.G. Poloxamer-based thermoresponsive ketorolac tromethamine in situ gel preparations: Design, characterisation, toxicity and transcorneal permeation studies. *Eur. J. Pharm. Biopharm.* **2017**, *114*, 119–134. [CrossRef]
33. Yu, S.; Zhang, X.; Tan, G.; Tian, L.; Liu, D.; Liu, Y.; Yang, X.; Pan, W. A novel pH-induced thermosensitive hydrogel composed of carboxymethyl chitosan and poloxamer cross-linked by glutaraldehyde for ophthalmic drug delivery. *Carbohydr. Polym.* **2017**, *155*, 208–217. [CrossRef] [PubMed]
34. Lou, J.; Hu, W.; Tian, R.; Zhang, H.; Jia, Y.; Zhang, J.; Zhang, L. Optimization and evaluation of a thermoresponsive ophthalmic in situ gel containing curcumin-loaded albumin nanoparticles. *Int. J. Nanomed.* **2014**, *9*, 2517–2525.
35. Almeida, H.; Lobão, P.; Frigerio, C.; Fonseca, J.; Silva, R.; Sousa Lobo, J.M.; Amaral, M.H. Preparation, characterization and biocompatibility studies of thermoresponsive eyedrops based on the combination of nanostructured lipid carriers (NLC) and the polymer Pluronic F-127 for controlled delivery of ibuprofen. *Pharm. Dev. Technol.* **2017**, *22*, 336–349. [CrossRef] [PubMed]
36. Cafaggi, S.; Russo, E.; Caviglioli, G.; Parodi, B.; Stefani, R.; Sillo, G.; Leardi, R.; Bignardi, G. Poloxamer 407 as a solubilising agent for tolfenamic acid and as a base for a gel formulation. *Eur. J. Pharm. Sci.* **2008**, *35*, 19–29. [CrossRef] [PubMed]
37. Ur-Rehman, T.; Tavelin, S.; Gröbner, G. Effect of DMSO on micellization, gelation and drugrelease profile of Poloxamer 407. *Int. J. Pharm.* **2010**, *394*, 92–98. [CrossRef] [PubMed]
38. Liaw, J.; Lin, Y.C. Evaluation of poly(ethylene oxide)–poly(propylene oxide)–poly(ethylene oxide) (PEO–PPO–PEO) gels as a release vehicle for percutaneous fentanyl. *J. Control. Release* **2000**, *68*, 273–282. [CrossRef]
39. Shin, S.C.; Cho, C.W.; Yang, K.H. Development of lidocaine gels for enhanced local anesthetic action. *Int. J. Pharm.* **2004**, *287*, 73–78. [CrossRef]
40. Suedee, R.; Bodhibukkana, C.; Tangthong, N.; Amnuaikit, C.; Kaewnopparat, S.; Srichana, T. Development of a reservoir-type transdermal enantioselective-controlled delivery system for racemic propranolol using a molecularly imprinted polymer composite membrane. *J. Control. Release* **2008**, *129*, 170–178. [CrossRef]
41. Stamatialis, D.F.; Rolevink, H.H.M.; Koops, G.H. Transdermal timolol delivery from a Pluronic gel. *J. Control. Release* **2006**, *116*, 53–65. [CrossRef]
42. Nair, V.; Panchagnula, R. Poloxamer gel as vehicle for transdermal iontophoretic delivery of arginine vasopressin: Evaluation of in vivo performance in rats. *Pharm. Res.* **2003**, *47*, 555–562. [CrossRef]
43. Pillai, O.; Panchagnula, R. Transdermal delivery of insulin from poloxamer gel: Ex vivo and in vivo skin permeation studies in rat using iontophoresis and chemical enhancers. *J. Control. Release* **2003**, *89*, 127–140. [CrossRef]
44. Donnelly, R.F.; Morrow, D.I.; McCarron, P.A.; Woolfson, A.D.; Morrissey, A.; Juzenas, P.; Juzeniene, A.; Iani, V.; McCarthy, H.O.; Moan, J. Microneedle-mediated intradermal delivery of 5-aminolevulinic acid: Potential for enhanced topical photodynamic therapy. *J. Control. Release* **2008**, *129*, 154–162. [CrossRef] [PubMed]
45. Khanna, P.; Flam, B.R.; Osborn, B.; Strom, J.A.; Bhansali, S. Skin penetration and fracture strength testing of silicon dioxide microneedles. *Sens. Actuators A* **2011**, *170*, 180–186. [CrossRef]
46. Chandrasekaran, S.; Brazzle, J.D.; Frazier, A.B. Surface micromachined metallic microneedles. *J. Microelectromech. Syst.* **2003**, *12*, 281–288. [CrossRef]
47. Gill, H.S.; Prausnitz, M.R. Coating formulations for microneedles. *Pharm. Res.* **2007**, *24*, 1369–1380. [CrossRef] [PubMed]
48. Parker, E.R.; Rao, M.P.; Turner, K.L.; Meinhart, C.D.; MacDonald, N.C. Bulk micromachined titanium microneedles. *J. Microelectromech. Syst.* **2007**, *16*, 289–295. [CrossRef]
49. Donnelly, R.F.; Morrow, D.I.; Singh, T.R.; Migalska, K.; McCarron, P.A. Processing difficulties and instability of carbohydrate microneedle arrays. *Drug Deliv. Ind. Pharm.* **2009**, *35*, 1242–1254. [CrossRef]
50. Lee, K.; Lee, C.Y.; Jung, H. Dissolving microneedles for transdermal drug administration prepared by stepwise controlled drawing of maltose. *Biomaterials* **2011**, *32*, 3134–3140. [CrossRef]
51. Li, G.; Badkar, A.; Nema, S.; Kolli, C.S.; Banga, A.K. In vitro transdermal delivery of therapeutic antibodies using maltose microneedles. *Int. J. Pharm.* **2009**, *368*, 109–115. [CrossRef]

52. Wang, P.M.; Cornwell, M.; Hill, J.; Prausnitz, M.R. Precise microinjection into skin using hollow microneedles. *J. Investig. Derm.* **2006**, *126*, 1080–1087. [CrossRef]
53. Bystrova, S.; Luttge, R. Micromolding for ceramic microneedle arrays. *Microelectron. Eng.* **2011**, *88*, 1681–1684. [CrossRef]
54. Ito, Y.; Murano, H.; Hamasaki, N.; Fukushima, K.; Takada, K. Incidence of low bioavailability of leuprolide acetate after percutaneous administration to rats by dissolving microneedles. *Int. J. Pharm.* **2011**, *407*, 126–131. [CrossRef]
55. Noh, Y.W.; Kim, T.H.; Baek, J.S.; Park, H.H.; Lee, S.S.; Han, M.; Shin, S.C.; Cho, C.W. In vitro characterization of the invasiveness of polymer microneedle against skin. *Int. J. Pharm.* **2010**, *397*, 201–205. [CrossRef]
56. Sachdeva, V.; Banga, A.K. Microneedles and their applications. *Recent Pat. Drug Deliv. Formul.* **2011**, *5*, 95–132. [CrossRef]
57. Thakur, R.R.S.; Fallows, S.J.; McMillan, H.L.; Donnelly, R.F.; Jones, D.S. Microneedle-mediated intrascleral delivery of in situ forming thermoresponsive implants for sustained ocular drug delivery. *J. Pharm Pharm. Pharmacol.* **2014**, *66*, 584–595. [CrossRef]
58. Gilger, B.C.; Abarca, E.M.; Salmon, J.H.; Patel, S. Treatment of acute posterior uveitis in a porcine model by injection of triamcinolone acetonide into the suprachoroidal space using microneedles. *Investig. Ophthalmol. Vis. Sci.* **2013**, *54*, 2483–2492. [CrossRef]
59. Patel, S.R.; Lin, A.S.; Edelhauser, H.F.; Prausnitz, M.R. Suprachoroidal drug delivery to the back of the eye using hollow microneedles. *Pharm. Res.* **2011**, *28*, 166–176. [CrossRef]
60. Roxhed, N.; Griss, P.; Stemme, G. Membrane-sealed hollow microneedles and related administration schemes for transdermal drug delivery. *Biomed. Microdevices* **2008**, *10*, 271–279. [CrossRef]
61. Ovsianikov, A.; Chichkov, B.; Mente, P.; Monteiro-Riviere, N.A.; Doraiswamy, A.; Narayan, R.J. Two photon polymerization of polymer–ceramic hybrid materials for transdermal drug delivery. *Int. J. Appl. Ceram Technol.* **2007**, *4*, 22–29. [CrossRef]
62. Sivaraman, A.; Banga, A.K. Novel in situ forming hydrogel microneedles for transdermal drug delivery. *Drug Deliv. Transl. Res.* **2017**, *7*, 16–26. [CrossRef]
63. Khan, S.; Minhas, M.U.; Tekko, I.A.; Donnelly, R.F.; Thakur, R.R.S. Evaluation of microneedles-assisted in situ depot forming poloxamer gels for sustained transdermal drug delivery. *Drug Deliv. Transl. Res.* **2019**, *9*, 764–782. [CrossRef] [PubMed]
64. Leone, M.; van Oorschot, B.H.; Nejadnik, M.R.; Bocchino, A.; Rosato, M.; Kersten, G.; O'Mahony, C.; Bouwstra, J.; van der Maaden, K. Universal applicator for digitally-controlled pressing force and impact velocity insertion of microneedles into skin. *Pharmaceutics* **2018**, *10*, 211. [CrossRef] [PubMed]
65. Sahoo, C.K.; Nayak, P.K.; Sarangi, D.K.; Sahoo, T.K. Intra vaginal drug delivery system: An overview. *Am. J. Adv. Drug Deliv.* **2013**, *1*, 43–55.
66. Ndesendo, V.M.; Pillay, V.; Choonara, Y.E.; Buchmann, E.; Bayever, D.N.; Meyer, L.C. A review of current intravaginal drug delivery approaches employed for the prophylaxis of HIV/AIDS and prevention of sexually transmitted infections. *AAPS Pharmscitech* **2008**, *9*, 505–520. [CrossRef] [PubMed]
67. Hussain, A.; Ahsan, F. The vagina as a route for systemic drug delivery. *J. Control. Release* **2005**, *103*, 301–313. [CrossRef] [PubMed]
68. Taurin, S.; Almomen, A.A.; Pollak, T.; Kim, S.J.; Maxwell, J.; Peterson, C.M.; Owen, S.C.; Janát-Amsbury, M.M. Thermosensitive hydrogels a versatile concept adapted to vaginal drug delivery. *J. Drug Target.* **2018**, *26*, 533–550. [CrossRef] [PubMed]
69. Caramella, C.M.; Rossi, S.; Ferrari, F.; Bonferoni, M.C.; Sandri, G. Mucoadhesive and thermogelling systems for vaginal drug delivery. *Adv. Drug Deliv. Rev.* **2015**, *92*, 39–52. [CrossRef]
70. Ci, T.; Yuan, L.; Bao, X.; Hou, Y.; Wu, H.; Sun, H.; Cao, D.; Ke, X. Development and anti-Candida evaluation of the vaginal delivery system of amphotericin B nanosuspension-loaded thermogel. *J. Drug Target.* **2018**, *26*, 829–839. [CrossRef]
71. Ibrahim, E.S.; Ismail, S.; Fetih, G.; Shaaban, O.; Hassanein, K.; Abdellah, N. Development and characterization of thermosensitive pluronic-based metronidazole in situ gelling formulations for vaginal application. *Acta Pharma.* **2012**, *62*, 59–70. [CrossRef]
72. Xuan, J.-J.; Yan, Y.D.; Oh, D.H.; Choi, Y.K.; Yong, C.S.; Choi, H.G. Development of thermosensitive injectable hydrogel with sustained release of doxorubicin: Rheological characterization and in vivo evaluation in rats. *Drug Deliv.* **2011**, *18*, 305–311. [CrossRef]

73. Hani, U.; Shivakamuar, H.G. Development of miconazole nitrate thermosensitive bioadhesive vaginal gel for vaginal candidiasis. *Am. J. Adv. Drug Deliv.* **2013**, *3*, 358–368.
74. Mei, L.; Chen, J.; Yu, S.; Huang, Y.; Xie, Y.; Wang, H.; Pan, X.; Wu, C. Expansible thermal gelling foam aerosol for vaginal drug delivery. *Drug Deliv.* **2017**, *24*, 1325–1337. [CrossRef] [PubMed]
75. Holland, I.; Logan, J.; Shi, J.; McCormick, C.; Liu, D.; Shu, W. 3D biofabrication for tubular tissue engineering. *Bio-Des. Manuf.* **2018**, *1*, 89–100. [CrossRef] [PubMed]
76. Doğan, A.; Yalvaç, M.E.; Şahin, F.; Kabanov, A.V.; Palotás, A.; Rizvanov, A.A. Differentiation of human stem cells is promoted by amphiphilic pluronic block copolymers. *Int. J. Nanomed.* **2012**, *7*, 4849–4860.
77. Bessa, P.C.; Casal, M.; Reis, R.L. Bone morphogenetic proteins in tissue engineering: The road from laboratory to clinic, part II (BMP delivery). *J. Tissue Eng. Regen. Med.* **2008**, *2*, 81–96. [CrossRef]
78. Gittens, S.A.; Uludag, H. Growth factor delivery for bone tissue engineering. *J. Drug Target.* **2001**, *9*, 407–429. [CrossRef]
79. Han, Q.Q.; Du, Y.; Yang, P.S. The role of small molecules in bone regeneration. *Future Med. Chem.* **2013**, *5*, 1671–1684. [CrossRef]
80. Laurencin, C.T.; Ashe, K.M.; Henry, N.; Kan, H.M.; Lo, K.W.-H. Delivery of small molecules for bone regenerative engineering: Preclinical studies and potential clinical applications. *Drug Discov. Today* **2014**, *19*, 794–800. [CrossRef]
81. Zhang, Y.; Bradley, A.D.; Wang, D.; Reinhardt, R.A. Statins, bone metabolism and treatment of bone catabolic diseases. *Pharm. Res.* **2014**, *88*, 53–61. [CrossRef]
82. Rezazadeh, M.; Parandeh, M.; Akbari, V.; Ebrahimi, Z.; Taheri, A. Incorporation of rosuvastatin-loaded chitosan/ chondroitin sulfate nanoparticles into a thermosensitive hydrogel for bone tissue engineering: Preparation, characterization, and cellular behavior. *Pharm. Dev. Technol.* **2019**, *24*, 357–367. [CrossRef]
83. Muzzarelli, R.A.; Greco, F.; Busilacchi, A.; Sollazzo, V.; Gigante, A. Chitosan, hyaluronan and chondroitin sulfate in tissue engineering for cartilage regeneration: A review. *Carbohydr. Polym.* **2012**, *89*, 723–739. [CrossRef] [PubMed]
84. Temofeew, A.; Hixon, K.R.; McBride-Gagyi, S.H.; Scott, A. Sell The fabrication of cryogel scaffolds incorporated with poloxamer 407 for potential use in the regeneration of the nucleus pulposus. *J. Mater. Sci. Mater. Med.* **2017**, *28*, 36–47. [CrossRef] [PubMed]
85. Pattappa, G.; Li, Z.; Peroglio, M.; Wismer, N.; Alini, M.; Grad, S. Diversity of intervertebral disc cells: Phenoztype and function. *J. Anat.* **2012**, *221*, 480–496. [CrossRef] [PubMed]
86. Suntornnond, R.; An, J.; Chua, C.K. Bioprinting of Thermoresponsive Hydrogels for Next Generation Tissue Engineering: A Review. *Macromol. Mater. Eng.* **2017**, *302*, 1600266. [CrossRef]
87. Chung, J.H.; Naficy, S.; Yue, Z.; Kapsa, R.; Quigley, A.; Moulton, S.E.; Wallace, G.G. Bio-ink properties and printability for extrusion printing living cells. *Biomater. Sci.* **2013**, *1*, 763. [CrossRef]
88. Nicmodeus, G.D.; Bryant, S.J. Cell encapsulation in biodegradable hydrogels for tissue engineering applications. *Tissue Eng Part B Rev.* **2008**, *14*, 149–165.
89. Kolesky, D.B.; Truby, R.L.; Gladman, A.S.; Busbee, T.A.; Homan, K.A.; Lewis, J.A. 3D Bioprinting of Vascularized, Heterogeneous Cell-Laden Tissue Constructs. *Adv. Mater.* **2013**, *25*, 3124–3130. [CrossRef]
90. Hospodiuk, M.; Dey, M.; Sosnoski, D.; Ozbolat, I.T. The bioink: A comprehensive review on bioprintable materials. *Biotechnol. Adv.* **2017**, *35*, 217–239. [CrossRef]
91. Aliabadi, H.M.; Lavasanifar, A. Polymeric micelles for drug delivery. *Expert Opin. Drug Deliv.* **2006**, *3*, 139–162. [CrossRef]
92. Kabanov, A.V.; Lemieux, P.; Vinogradov, S.; Alakhov, V. Pluronic block copolymers: Novel functional molecules for gene therapy. *Adv. Drug Deliv. Rev.* **2002**, *54*, 223–233. [CrossRef]
93. Anderson, R.A. Micelle formation by oxyethylene-oxypropylene polymers. *Pharm. Acta Helv.* **1972**, *47*, 304–308. [PubMed]
94. Rey-Rico, A.; Cucchiarini, M. Controlled release strategies for raav-mediated gene delivery. *Acta Biomater.* **2016**, *29*, 1–10. [CrossRef] [PubMed]
95. Niidome, T.; Huang, L. Gene therapy progress and prospects: Nonviral vectors. *Gene Ther.* **2002**, *9*, 1647–1652. [CrossRef] [PubMed]
96. Rey-Rico, A.; Cucchiarini, M. Recent tissue engineering-based advances for effective rAAV-mediated gene transfer in the musculoskeletal system. *Bioengineered* **2016**, *7*, 175–188. [CrossRef]

97. De Laporte, L.; Cruz Rea, J.; Shea, L.D. Design of modular non-viral gene therapy vectors. *Biomaterials* **2006**, *27*, 947–954. [CrossRef]
98. Wang, W.; Li, W.; Ma, N.; Steinhoff, G. Non-viral gene delivery methods. *Curr. Pharm. Biotechnol.* **2013**, *14*, 46–60.
99. Cucchiarini, M.; Madry, H. Gene therapy for cartilage defects. *J. Gene Med.* **2005**, *7*, 1495–1509. [CrossRef]
100. Madry, H.; Cucchiarini, M. Advances and challenges in gene-based approaches for osteoarthritis. *J. Gene Med.* **2013**, *15*, 343–355. [CrossRef]
101. Johnstone, B.; Alini, M.; Cucchiarini, M.; Dodge, G.R.; Eglin, D.; Guilak, F.; Madry, H.; Mata, A.; Mauck, R.L.; Semino, C.E.; et al. Tissue engineering for articular cartilage repair—The state of the art. *Eur. Cell Mater.* **2013**, *25*, 248–267. [CrossRef]
102. Rey-Rico, A.; Venkatesan, J.K.; Frisch, J.; Rial-Hermida, I.; Schmitt, G.; Concheiro, A.; Madry, H.; Alvarez-Lorenzo, C.; Cucchiarini, M. PEO–PPO–PEO micelles as effective rAAV-mediated gene delivery systems to target human mesenchymal stem cells without altering their differentiation potency. *Acta Biomater.* **2015**, *27*, 42–52. [CrossRef]
103. Höfig, I.; Atkinson, M.J.; Mall, S.; Krackhardt, A.M.; Thirion, C.; Anastasov, N. Poloxamer synperonic F108 improves cellular transduction with lentiviral vectors. *J. Gene Med.* **2012**, *14*, 549–560. [CrossRef] [PubMed]
104. Millington, M.; Aendt, A.; Boyd, M.; Applegate, T.; Shen, S. Towards a clinically relevant lentiviral transduction protocol for primary human CD34 haematopoietic stem/progenitor cells. *PLoS ONE* **2009**, *4*, 6461. [CrossRef] [PubMed]
105. Birmingham, A.; Anderson, E.; Sullivan, K.; Reynolds, A.; Boese, Q.; Leake, D.; Karpilow, J.; Khvorova, A. A protocol for designing siRNAs with high functionality and specificity. *Nat. Protoc.* **2007**, *9*, 2068–2078. [CrossRef] [PubMed]
106. Takahashi, K.; Tanabe, K.; Ohnuki, M.; Narita, M.; Ichisaka, T.; Tomoda, K.; Yamanaka, S. Induction of pluripotent stem cells from adult human fibroblasts by defined factors. *Cell* **2007**, *131*, 861–872. [CrossRef] [PubMed]
107. Alvarez-Lorenzo, C.; Rey-Rico, A.; Sosnik, A.; Taboada, P.; Concheiro, A. Poloxamine-based nanomaterials for drug delivery. *Front. Biosci.* **2012**, *337*, 303–305. [CrossRef] [PubMed]
108. Chitgupi, U.; Nyayapathi, N.; Kim, J.; Wang, D.; Sun, B.; Li, C.; Carter, K.; Huang, W.C.; Kim, C.; Xia, J.; et al. Surfactant-Stripped Micelles for NIR-II Photoacoustic Imaging through 12 cm of Breast Tissue and Whole Human Breasts. *Adv. Mater.* **2019**, *31*, 1–10. [CrossRef]
109. Sousa, C.; Gouveia, L.F.; Kreutzer, B.; Silva-Lima, B.; Maphasa, R.E.; Dube, A.; Videira, M. Polymeric Micellar Formulation Enhances Antimicrobial and Anticancer Properties of Salinomycin. *Pharm. Res.* **2019**, *36*, 83. [CrossRef]
110. Naujokat, C.; Steinhart, R. Salinomycin as a drug for targeting human cancer stem cells. *J. Biomed. Biotechnol.* **2012**, *20*, 44–46. [CrossRef]
111. Steel, G.G.; Peckham, M.J. Exploitable Mechanisms in Combined Radiotherapy-Chemotherapy: The Concept of Additivity. *Int. J. Radiat. Oncol. Biol. Phys.* **1979**, *5*, 85–91. [CrossRef]
112. Seiwert, T.Y.; Salama, J.K.; Vokes, E.E. The Concurrent Chemoradiation Paradigm—General Principles. *Nat. Rew. Clin. Oncol.* **2007**, *4*, 86–100. [CrossRef]
113. DuRoss, A.N.; Neufeld, M.J.; Landry, M.R.; Rosch, J.G.; Eaton, C.T.; Sahay, G.; Thomas, C.R., Jr.; Sun, C. Micellar Formulation of Talazoparib and Buparlisib for Enhanced DNA Damage in Breast Cancer Chemoradiotherapy. *ACS Appl. Mater. Interfaces* **2019**, *11*, 12342–12356. [CrossRef] [PubMed]
114. Fessi, H.; Puisieux, F.; Devissaguet, J.P.; Ammoury, N.; Benita, S. Nanocapsule Formation by Interfacial Polymer Deposition Following Solvent Displacement. *Int. J. Pharm.* **1989**, *55*, R1–R4. [CrossRef]

8

Mechanistic Studies on the Absorption-Enhancing Effects of Gemini Surfactant on the Intestinal Absorption of Poorly Absorbed Hydrophilic Drugs in Rats

Tammam Alama [1], Kosuke Kusamori [2], Masaki Morishita [1], Hidemasa Katsumi [1], Toshiyasu Sakane [3] and Akira Yamamoto [1,*]

1 Department of Biopharmaceutics, Kyoto Pharmaceutical University, Misasagi, Yamashina-Ku, Kyoto 607-8414, Japan; abowaleed87@gmail.com (T.A.); morishita@mb.kyoto-phu.ac.jp (M.M.); hkatsumi@mb.kyoto-phu.ac.jp (H.K.)

2 Laboratory of Biopharmaceutics, Faculty of Pharmaceutical Sciences, Tokyo University of Science, 2641 Yamazaki, Noda, Chiba 278-8510, Japan; kusamori@rs.tus.ac.jp

3 Department of Pharmaceutical Technology, Kobe Pharmaceutical University, Higashinada-ku, Kobe 658-8558, Japan; sakane@kobepharma-u.ac.jp

* Correspondence: yamamoto@mb.kyoto-phu.ac.jp

Abstract: Generally, the use of absorption enhancers might be the most effective approaches to ameliorate the enteric absorption of poorly absorbed substances. Among numerous absorption enhancers, we already reported that a gemini surfactant, sodium dilauramidoglutamide lysine (SLG-30) with two hydrophobic and two hydrophilic moieties, is a novel and promising adjuvant with a high potency in improving the absorption safely. Here, we examined and elucidated the absorption-improving mechanisms of SLG-30 in the enteric absorption of substances. SLG-30 increased the intestinal absorption of 5(6)-carboxyfluorescein (CF) to a greater level than the typical absorption enhancers, including sodium glycocholate and sodium laurate, as evaluated by an *in situ* closed-loop method. Furthermore, SLG-30 significantly lowered the fluorescence anisotropy of dansyl chloride (DNS-Cl), suggesting that it might increase the fluidity of protein sections in the intestinal cell membranes. Moreover, SLG-30 significantly lowered the transepithelial-electrical resistance (TEER) values of Caco-2 cells, suggesting that it might open the tight junctions (TJs) between the enteric epithelial cells. Additionally, the levels of claudin-1 and claudin-4 expression decreased in the presence of SLG-30. These outcomes propose that SLG-30 might improve the enteric transport of poorly absorbed substances through both transcellular and paracellular routes.

Keywords: absorption enhancer; gemini surfactant; intestinal absorption; poorly absorbed drug; Caco-2 cells

---

1. Introduction

The enteric epithelium represents a physical barrier for the intestinal absorption of most substances to the systemic-circulation. It is well-established that the enteric epithelium acts as an impervious barrier against many pathogens and toxins through its complicated structure, although it can permit the intestinal absorption of nutrients [1]. The most important barrier against the permeability of drugs is the brush-border membranes of the enteric epithelial cells, which can restrict the passage of drugs through cells into the systemic circulation. The other important barrier is the tight junction between the adjacent cells, which is an aqueous route for compounds of molecular weight less than 500 Da [2–4]. These two barriers are considered great hurdles when some drugs are transported across the intestinal epithelial cells, assuming that drugs could survive the harsh environment and the decomposition in the gastrointestinal tract [5,6]. Therefore, the major routes for drugs to be absorbed by the intestinal cells are the transcellular and paracellular routes [7–9]. This could be a serious problem for a wide range of newly discovered and synthesized drugs, especially peptide and protein drugs, which also suffer from enzymatic deterioration [10] in the gastrointestinal tract before reaching the enteric cell membrane.

A variety of systems have been tested to improve the enteric absorption of poorly absorbed substances [1]. Of all these approaches, the use of absorption enhancers is a promising way to improve the enteric absorption of poorly absorbed substances [11–20]. It was reported that typical absorption enhancers involving medium chain fatty acids (e.g., sodium laurate, sodium caprate, and sodium caprylate) could improve the absorption of poorly absorbed substances such as antibiotics, peptide and protein drugs, and bisphosphonates [11–20]. However, most of the typical absorption-enhancers usually prompt irritation along with damage to enteric membranes.

Gemini surfactants are a new type of absorption enhancers with a rather different structure than the typical ones [21]. The structure is composed of two hydrophilic heads connected with a linker and two hydrophobic tails. This structure makes the CMC values of gemini-type surfactants lower than the CMC values of typical surfactants with an equal chain length [21]. However, the effects of gemini surfactants on the enteric absorption of substances and how they improve absorption are seldom studied.

We previously reported SLG-30, a gemini surfactant, increased the enteric absorption of hydrophilic poorly absorbed substances [22]. As shown in Figure 1, the hydrophilic heads of SLG-30 have two amino acid derivatives, i.e., two glutamic acid moieties, linked through a lysine spacer, and two hydrophobic chains of twelve carbons each [23]. We showed that SLG-30 might be safe *in vitro* and *in vivo* and may be a very efficient absorption enhancer, which can possibly be used as an adjuvant in oral formulations for increasing the enteric absorption of poorly absorbed hydrophilic substances. However, we did not compare the effectiveness of SLG-30 with that of typical absorption enhancers regarding the enteric absorption of substances. Moreover, the absorption-enhancing mechanisms of SLG-30 in improving the enteric absorption of poorly absorbed substances were not clearly understood.

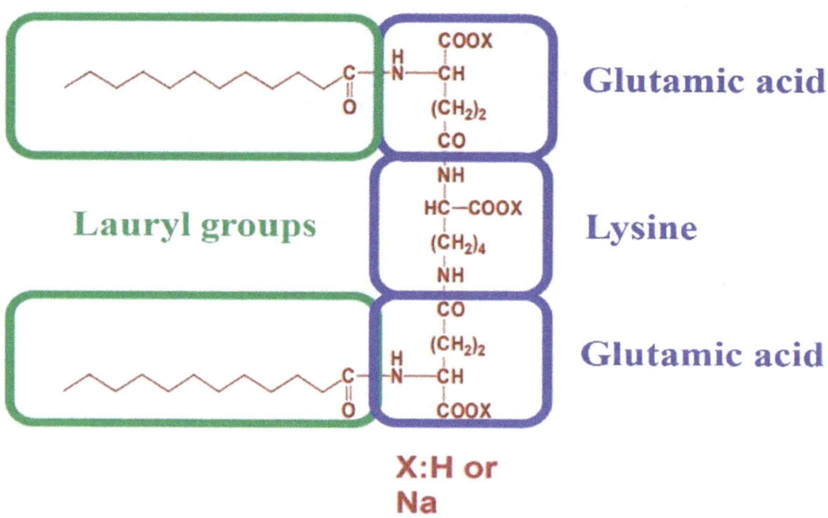

Figure 1. The chemical structure of a gemini surfactant, SLG-30. The hydrophilic moiety of this surfactant has two derivatives of amino acid, i.e., two glutamic acid moieties, linked through a lysine spacer, while the hydrophobic moieties are lauric acid.

The purpose of this study was to study the difference between SLG-30, a gemini surfactant, with typical absorption enhancers, including sodium glycocholate and sodium laurate, regarding absorption-enhancing performance. Furthermore, we also examined and clarified the possible absorption-enhancing mechanisms of SLG-30 on the enteric absorption of substances.

2. Materials and Methods

2.1. Materials

Male Wistar rats, weighing 250–300 g, were purchased from SLC, Inc. (Hamamatsu, Shizuoka, Japan). SLG-30 was kindly supplied by Asahi Kasei Chemicals Co. (Tokyo, Japan). CF was obtained from Eastman Kodak Co. (Rochester, NY, USA). LDH-Cytotoxicity Test Wako, sodium glycocholate (NaGC), sodium laurate, and tma-DPH (1-(4-(trimethylamino)phenyl)-6-phenylhexa-1,3,5-hexatriene-p-toluenesulfonate) were purchased from Wako Pure Chemical Industries, Ltd. (Osaka, Japan). DPH (1,6-diphenyl-1,3,5-hexatriene) and Hank's balanced salt solution (HBSS) were purchased from Sigma-Aldrich Chemical Co. (St. Louis, MO, USA). Dansyl chloride (DNS-Cl) was purchased from Santa Cruz Biotechnology, Inc. (Dallas, Texas, USA). Anti-claudin-1, anti-β-actin (rabbit monoclonal antibodies), and goat anti-rabbit IgG HRP-linked antibodies were purchased from Cell Signaling Technology® (Danvers, MA, USA). Anti-claudin-4 (mouse monoclonal antibodies) and rabbit anti-mouse IgG HRP-linked antibodies were purchased from Invitrogen™ (Carlsbad, CA, USA). Chemi-Lumi One Ultra kit, Dulbecco's modified Eagle medium (DMEM) with 4500 mg/L glucose, nonessential amino acids (MEM–NEAA), antibiotic–antimycotic mixture stock (10,000 U/mL penicillin, 10,000 μg/mL streptomycin, and 25 μg/mL amphotericin B in 0.85% sodium chloride), and 0.25% trypsin-1 mM EDTA solution were purchased from Nacalai Tesque Inc. (Kyoto, Japan). Human colon adenocarcinoma-derived Caco-2 cell line was purchased from Dainippon Sumitomo Pharma Co., Ltd. (Osaka, Japan). Fetal bovine serum (FBS) was purchased from Gibco® Life Technologies (Grand Island, NE, USA). All other reagents used in the experiments were of analytical grade.

2.2. *In Vivo Enteric Absorption Studies*

The enteric absorption of CF was examined by an *in situ* closed-loop method, as reported previously [22,24]. The experiments were carried out in accordance with the guidelines of the Animal Ethics Committee at Kyoto Pharmaceutical University. The protocols were approved by this Committee (permit number: 16-12-069, permit date: 14 April 2016). The rats were starved overnight for approx. 16 h pre-dosing, but water was freely available. After inducing anesthesia with sodium pentobarbital which was administered intraperitoneally at a dose of 32 mg/kg body weight, the rats were placed under a heat lamp to maintain a body temperature at around 37 °C, and the intestines were exposed using a midline-abdominal incision. After the bile duct was ligated, the intestines were washed with phosphate buffered saline (PBS, pH 7.4), and the remaining buffer solution was expelled with air. Enteric cannulation was performed at both ends using polyethylene tubing, and the distal parts of the small intestines were clipped by forceps. The dosing solutions (3 mL) with or without absorption enhancers kept at 37 °C, were directly introduced into the lumen of the enteric loop through a cannulated opening in the proximal part of the small enteric loop, which was then closed by clipping with another forceps. The jugular vein was exposed, and approx. 0.3 mL of blood was collected via a direct puncture into heparinized syringes at predetermined time intervals up to 240 min. The samples were immediately centrifuged at 12,000 rpm (15,000× *g*) for a period of 5 min to obtain the plasma fraction, which was stored on ice for further analysis. CF fluorescence signals in these plasma samples were detected after the treatment with the same volume of acetonitrile using a fluorescence spectrophotometer, Powerscan1 HT supplied by BioTek Instruments (Winooski, VT, USA) at an excitation wavelength of 485 nm and an emission wavelength of 535 nm. There was no significant background fluorescence in the plasma when the fluorescence intensities of CF were determined in this study. The peak drug concentrations (C_{max}) and the time to reach the peak drug concentrations (T_{max}) in the plasma were directly determined from the plasma concentration–time profiles. The area under the curve (AUC) was calculated by the trapezoidal method from pre-dose (time zero) till the administration of the final sample. The absorption enhancement ratios of CF, with or without absorption enhancers, were calculated as follows:

$$\text{Absorption enhancement ratio} = \text{AUC}_{\text{with enhancer}} / \text{AUC}_{\text{control without enhancer}}$$

2.3. *Preparation of Brush Border Membrane Vesicles (BBMVs)*

To prepare BBMVs, we followed the methods as reported previously [25–27] with a slight modification. Briefly, an *in situ* small intestinal loop was prepared in each rat, as mentioned above, and then, PBS (pH 7.4) was administered into the loop. The fat was trimmed off from the small intestine and mesentery. Then, the whole small intestine was soaked in ice-cold PBS (pH 7.4). The small intestine was divided into 10 cm segments. Mucosa was scraped out with a slide glass from each of these segments and used for subsequent studies. BBMVs were prepared by the divalent cation precipitation method using $MgCl_2$ in the presence of ethylenebis (oxyethylenenitrilo) tetraacetic acid (EGTA) [25–27]. Briefly, the collected mucosa was homogenized in a buffer containing mannitol (300 mM), EGTA (5 mM), and Tris (pH 7.4) (12 mM) by using a tissue homogenizer. An aqueous solution of 10 mM magnesium chloride was added to the homogenate. The homogenate was centrifuged at 3000× *g* for 15 min. The supernatant was then centrifuged at 32,000× *g* for 30 min. The pellet was resuspended in a buffer containing mannitol (300 mM), EGTA (5 mM), and Tris (pH 7.4) (12 mM) by using a 26-G needle. The protein concentration was determined by the BCA method using bovine serum albumin as a standard, and the final concentration was adjusted to 1 mg/ml in each Eppendorf tube. The samples were frozen by liquid nitrogen and kept at −80 °C for further studies.

2.4. *Measurement of Membrane Fluidity by Fluorescence Polarization*

The BBMVs (100 μg protein) were incubated with 1 μM DPH, with 0.5 μM tma-DPH or with 5 μM DNS-Cl in HEPES-Tris buffer (25 mM HEPES, 5.4 mM KCl, 1.8 mM $CaCl_2$, 0.8 mM $MgSO_4$, 140 mM NaCl, 5 mM glucose, pH 7.4 adjusted by 1 M Tris) in the dark at 37 °C for 30 min [25,28]. Then, various concentrations (0.1% *v*/*v*, 0.25% *v*/*v*, 0.5% *v*/*v*, and 1.0% *v*/*v*) of SLG-30 were added. Then, the samples were incubated in the dark for 1 min at 37 °C. For the control group, the same procedure was carried out by adding the HEPES-Tris buffer only. The fluorescence intensities and the steady-state polarization of fluorescence expressed as the fluorescence anisotropy, r, of the labeled membrane vesicles were measured at 37 °C. The excitation and emission wavelengths were λ_{ex} = 360 nm, and λ_{em} = 430 nm for DPH and tma-DPH and λ_{ex} = 380 nm and λ_{em} = 480 nm for DNS-Cl. The measurements were carried out by using a Hitachi Spectrofluorometer (F-2000 Spectrofluorometer, Hitachi Seisakusho Corp, Yokohama, Japan) equipped with a polarizer set.

The fluorescence anisotropy (r) was calculated using the following equation:

$$\mathrm{r} = \frac{I_V - I_H}{I_V + 2I_H}$$

where I_V and I_H respectively represent the perpendicular and parallel fluorescence intensities to the polarized excitation plane [29].

2.5. *Measurement of Transepithelial Electrical Resistance (TEER) and the Transport of CF Using Caco-2 cell Monolayers*

Caco-2 cells (passage 45) were cultured in 175-cm^2 culture flask (Thermo Fisher Scientific™, Waltham, MA, USA). The culture medium consisted of DMEM containing 10% FBS, 0.1 mM MEM–NEAA, 2 mM glutamine, 100 U/mL penicillin, and 100 μg/mL streptomycin [30]. Cells were cultured in a humidified atmosphere of 5% CO_2 at 37 °C. The culture medium was changed every two days. When the cultured Caco-2 cells became sub-confluent, they were seeded onto 12-mm Transwell® with 0.4-μm pore polycarbonate membrane inserts (Corning Inc., New York, NY, USA) at a density of 1×10^5 cells/insert. The transepithelial transport studies were performed when the transepithelial electrical resistance (TEER) values were more than 500 Ω·cm^2 (i.e., after 21 days) [17,18].

Briefly, after removing the incubation medium by aspiration, the apical and basal sides were washed thrice by Hank's Balanced Salt (HBSS) solution (pH 7.4). The cells were incubated in HBSS (pH 6.0) for the apical side and HBSS (pH 7.4) for the basal side for 20 min at 37 °C. HBSS supplemented with 1 mg/mL glucose was used in all cell culture experiments. After removing the washing solution by aspiration, 500 μL of 10 μM CF in a HBSS (pH 6.0) solution with or without various concentrations (0.001% *v/v*, 0.01% *v/v*, 0.025% *v/v*, 0.05% *v/v*, and 0.1% *v/v*) of SLG-30, 0.1% (*w/v*) and 1% (*w/v*) NaGC or 0.05% (*w/v*) sodium laurate were added to the apical side at zero time, whereas precisely 1500 μL of HBSS (pH 7.4) was added to the basal side at 37 °C. The cells were kept at 37 °C and 5% CO_2 and were continuously agitated on a shaker during the transport experiments.

The TEER values were measured by Millicell® (ERS-2 Volt-Ohm Meter, Billerica, MA, USA) at the predetermined times up to 24 h, and the initial values were considered as 100%. The samples from the basal side were withdrawn at predetermined time points up to 24 h. The samples were replaced with an equal volume of HBSS (pH 7.4). CF was determined as previously mentioned. The apparent permeability coefficients P_{app} (cm/s) for the transported CF was determined by the following equation:

$$P_{app} = \frac{dX_R}{dt} \times \frac{1}{A} \times \frac{1}{C_0}$$

where P_{app} is the apparent permeability coefficient in centimeters per second, X_R is the amount of CF in moles in the receptor side, $\frac{dX_R}{dt}$ is the flux across the monolayer, A is the diffusion area (i.e., in square centimeters), and C_0 is the initial concentration of CF in the donor side in moles per milliliter.

2.6. Assessment of Caco-2 Cell Damage

After the transport studies were over, the solution on the apical side of each well was collected. Cell injury caused by SLG-30 was determined by tracking the LDH release [31,32]. The cell precipitate and the monolayers left on the filters were solubilized with 1% (*v/v*) Triton X-100. The solutions from apical sides and the lysates were centrifuged for 7 min at 200× *g* at a temperature of 4 °C. The activities of LDH in the supernatant were measured. ($LDH_{release}$) stands for the activity of the LDH released into the apical side in the existence of SLG-30. (LDH_{cell}) stands for the activity of the LDH obtained from the cell lysate. $LDH_{released}\%$ was calculated by the following equation:

$$LDH_{release}\% = LDH_{release} \times 100/(LDH_{release} + LDH_{cells})$$

2.7. Western Blotting

Western blotting was performed by the method described previously with slight modifications [33,34]. Three male Wistar rats weighing 250 g were prepared to perform an *in situ* closed-loop method on the small intestine, as mentioned above. A control study, a treatment study, and a pretreatment study were conducted on the first, second, and third rat, respectively. For the control study, only PBS solution (pH 7.4) was administered into the small intestine, and then, the rat was sacrificed, while for the treatment study, SLG-30 was administered for 1 h, and then, the rat was sacrificed without washing the SLG-30 out. The pretreatment study was performed by administrating SLG-30 for 1 h then washing it out with PBS solution (pH 7.4), followed by sacrificing the rat after 4 h. The small intestine (60 cm) of three rats was taken and treated, as mentioned above, for extracting the BBMVs. The total protein amount of each sample was adjusted to 30 μg.

The expression levels of proteins from the claudin family, in the homogenate of the small intestine membrane, were evaluated by western blotting. Briefly, equal amounts of protein samples (30 μg protein) were mixed with an SDS buffer solution and electrophoretically separated on SDS-polyacrylamide (15%) gels. The separated proteins were transferred to a polyvinylidene difluoride (PVDF) membrane. After blocking in 5% skim milk in Tris-buffered saline (pH 7.4) for 1 h at room temperature, the PVDF membrane was incubated overnight in a blocking buffer with diluted (1:1000) monoclonal antibodies for claudin-1, claudin-4, and β-actin at 4 °C. Subsequently, the PVDF membrane was washed three times using Tris-buffered saline containing 0.05% Tween 20 (TTBS), followed by incubation with peroxidase-conjugated anti-rabbit IgG antibody for claudin-1 and β-actin, and with peroxidase-conjugated anti-rabbit IgG antibody for claudin-4 for 1 h at room temperature. The signals were visualized by luminescence imaging (Fujifilm Luminescent Image Analyzer LAS4000 System, Tokyo, Japan). The intensity of each signal was corrected using the values obtained from the β-actin bands, and the relative protein intensity was expressed as the fold change compared to the relative protein intensity in the normal group.

2.8. Statistical Analysis

The results are expressed as the mean ± S.E. of at least three experiments. The statistical significance between groups was analyzed using Dunnett's test; $p < 0.05$ was regarded to be significant. Significance levels are denoted (**) $p < 0.01$, (*) $p < 0.05$, and (n.s.) not significantly different. The number of experiments is indicated by n.

3. Results

3.1. *In Vivo* Comparative Study between SLG-30 and Typical Surfactants Including Sodium Glycocholate and Sodium Laurate

First, the effects of 0.5% (v/v) SLG-30 and 1% (w/v) sodium glycocholate (NaGC) on the enteric absorption of CF were examined by an *in situ* closed-loop method, and the effectiveness of SLG-30 was compared with that of NaGC (a typical absorption enhancer). As Figure 2 shows, the enteric absorption of CF was significantly improved in the existence of 0.5% (v/v) SLG-30, and the $AUC_{0\rightarrow240}$ of CF was 16 times higher than that of the control group, as opposed to 4.5 times in the presence of 1% (w/v) NaGC. The absorption improvement of CF in the existence of 0.5% (v/v) SLG-30 was about 3.5 times higher than that in the existence of 1% (w/v) NaGC (Table 1). As shown in Figure 1, SLG-30 contains two moieties of fatty acid (lauric acid). Therefore, in order to clarify whether SLG-30 is effective as a whole compound or whether the effectiveness is related to lauric acid, a degradation product of SLG-30, we also studied the absorption improvement effect of 0.5% (w/v) sodium laurate in the small intestines by the *in situ* closed-loop method. We found that the T_{max} of CF in the case of sodium laurate-treated samples is approximately 15 min. Thereafter, the concentrations of CF decreased quickly and continuously until the end of the experiment. Contrarily, SLG-30 greatly increased the concentrations of CF until T_{max} (180 min), followed by a decrease, as revealed in Figure 2 and Table 1. The absorption improvement ratio of CF for SLG-30 was approximately 6 times higher than that of sodium laurate.

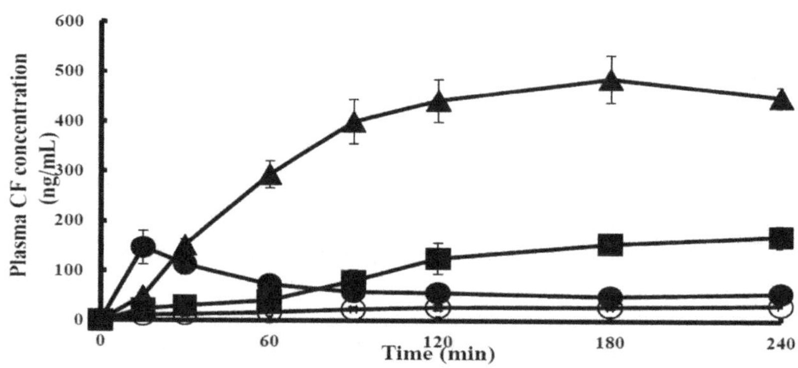

Figure 2. The profile of concentration vs. time course of 5(6)-carboxyfluorescein (CF) in the plasma after an enteric administration with SLG-30, a gemini surfactant, or typical absorption enhancers including sodium glycocholate and sodium laurate by an *in situ* closed-loop method. The results are expressed as the mean ± S.E. (n = 3). Keys: (○) Control, (▲) 0.5% (v/v) SLG-30, (•) 0.5% (w/v) sodium laurate, and (■) 1% (w/v) sodium glycocholate.

Table 1. A summary of the pharmacokinetic parameters of CF (0.5 mg/kg) after its administration with 0.5% (*v*/*v*) SLG-30, 0.5% (*w*/*v*) sodium laurate, and 1% (*w*/*v*) sodium glycocholate into rat small intestines by an in situ closed-loop method.

Absorption Enhancer	Conc.	C_{max} (ng/mL)	T_{max} (min)	$AUC_{0\rightarrow240}$ (ng·min/mL)	Enhancement Ratio
Control		-	-	5450 ± 700	-
SLG-30	0.5% (*v*/*v*)	487 ± 4	180 ± 0	87,200 ± 6000 **	16.0
Sodium laurate	0.5% (*w*/*v*)	375 ± 2	15 ± 0	14,700 ± 1950	2.7
Sodium glycocholate	1% (*w*/*v*)	172 ± 2	180 ± 0	24,500 ± 3700 *	4.5

The results are expressed as the mean ± S.E. (n = 3). ** $p < 0.01$, * $p < 0.05$, when compared with the control group.

3.2. *Effects of SLG-30 on the Membrane Fluidity of Small Intestines in Rats*

One of the important absorption-enhancing mechanisms of absorption enhancers is that they increase the membrane fluidity of the enteric membrane, thereby increasing the enteric absorption of poorly absorbed substances through a transcellular route. To examine the effect of SLG-30 on the enteric membrane fluidity, DPH, tma-DPH, and DNS-Cl, which can bind to different portions of the lipid bilayers (i.e., inner, outer, and protein portion, severally) were used as fluorescence probes in this study. Any decrease in the fluorescence anisotropy of these markers represents an increase in the membrane fluidity of BBMVs. Figure 3A–C shows that cholesterol, used as a positive control, increased the fluorescence anisotropy, which indicates a decrement in the membrane fluidity of BBMVs. Figure 3A shows that SLG-30 slightly decreased the fluorescence anisotropy of DPH compared to that of the control group. However, as Figure 3B shows, SLG-30 did not decrease, but significantly increased the tma-DPH fluorescence anisotropy. However, SLG-30 significantly reduced the fluorescence anisotropy of DNS-Cl in a dose dependent pattern (** $p < 0.01$ vs. control group) (Figure 3C). These findings propose that the membrane fluidity in the protein section of the enteric membranes could be significantly augmented by SLG-30, while it also slightly augmented the membrane fluidity in the inner section of the lipid bilayers.

(A)

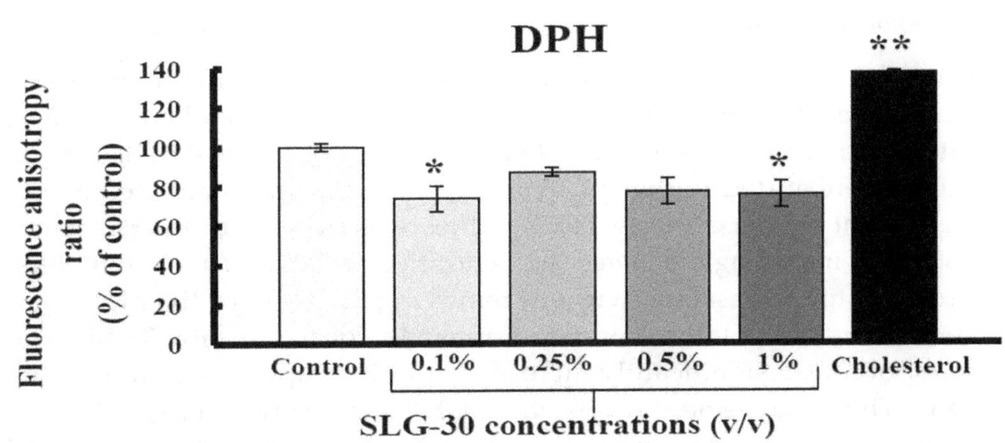

Figure 3. *Cont.*

(B)

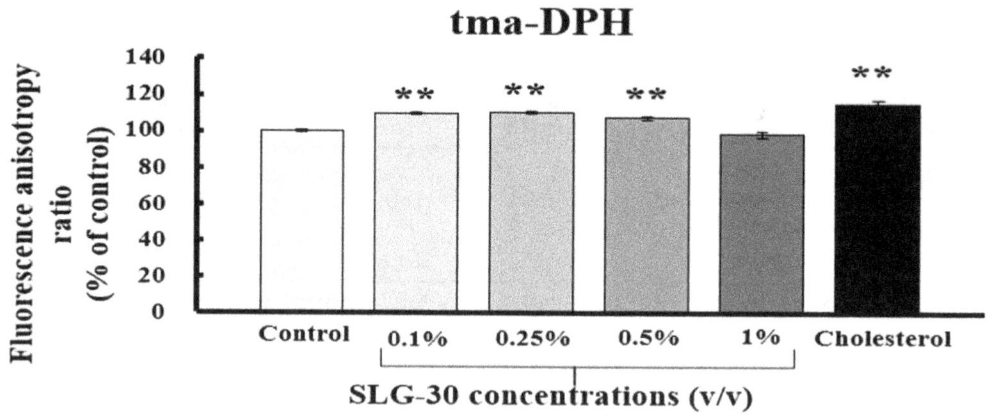

(C)

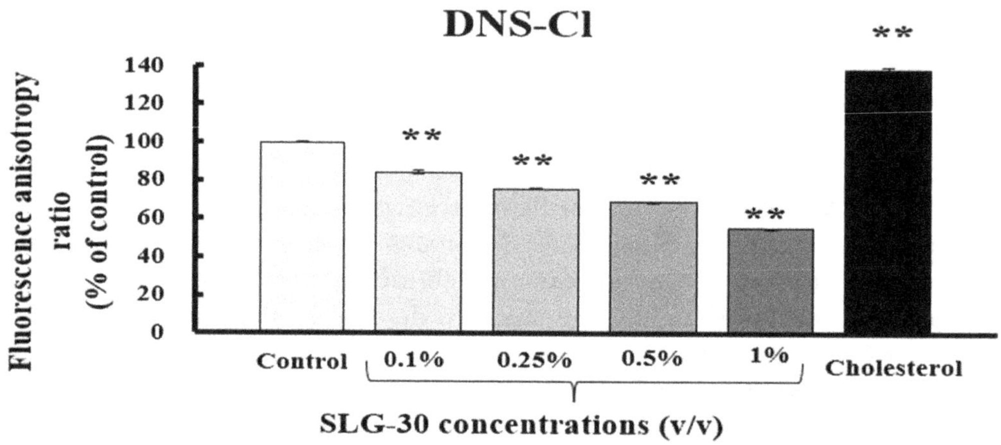

Figure 3. The effect of SLG-30 on the membrane fluidity of brush-border membrane vesicles (BBMVs). DPH (**A**), tma-DPH (**B**), and DNS-Cl (**C**) were used as fluorescein probes of inner lipid bilayers, outer lipid bilayers, and the protein portion of the enteric membranes. The absolute concentrations of DPH, tma-DPH, and DNS-Cl were 1 μM, 0.5 μM, and 5 μM, respectively. The results are expressed as the mean ± S.E. ($n = 4$). ** $p < 0.01$, n.s. not significantly different when compared with the control.

3.3. Effect of SLG-30 on TEER and Transport of CF in Caco-2 Cell Monolayers

We also estimated the effects of SLG-30 on the TEER values and the transport of poorly absorbed substances through the paracellular route by using Caco-2 cell monolayers. CF solutions in HBSS with or without various concentrations of SLG-30 (i.e., 0.001% *v*/*v*, 0.01% *v*/*v*, 0.025% *v*/*v*, 0.05% *v*/*v*, and 0.1% *v*/*v*) were added to the apical side of the cells and incubated at 37 °C. As shown in Figure 4A, a significant decrease in the TEER values was noticed in the presence of SLG-30 at all concentrations studied, including the lowest concentration of 0.001% (*v*/*v*), in the first hour. The TEER values did not recover to the baseline (without removing SLG-30) for the higher concentrations, but they started to recover for the lower concentrations. In contrast to the TEER results, as shown in Figure 5, the transport of CF significantly increased after 24 h upon coadministration with SLG-30 at all concentrations. The enhancement ratios of the CF transport were 6, 7, 9, 11, and 12 times higher than the control group for SLG-30 concentrations of 0.001% (*v*/*v*), 0.01% (*v*/*v*), 0.025% (*v*/*v*), 0.05% (*v*/*v*), and 0.1% (*v*/*v*), respectively.

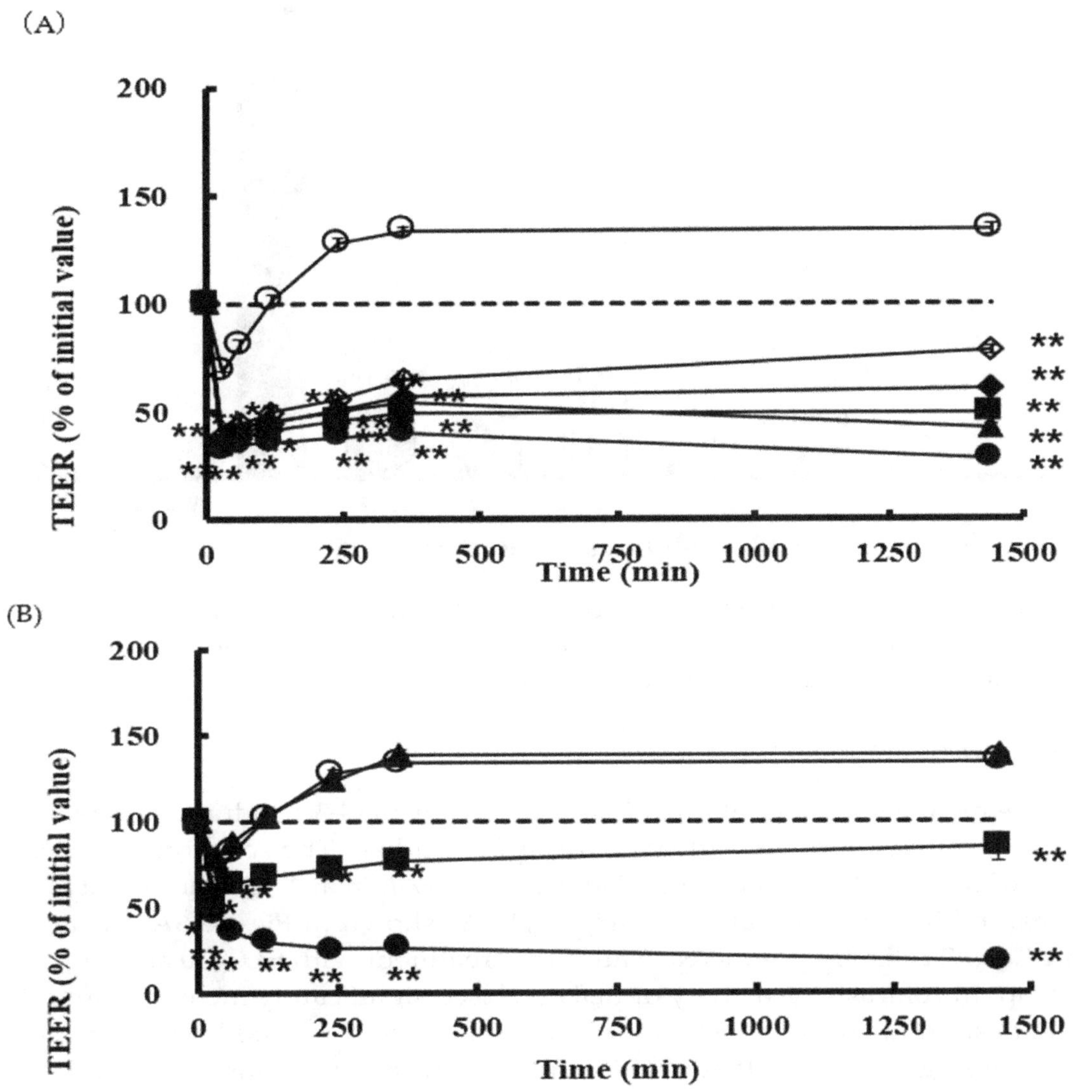

Figure 4. The TEER values in the existence of (**A**) SLG-30 and (**B**) sodium glycocholate and sodium laurate in Caco-2 cell monolayers. The results are expressed as the mean ± S.E. (n = 3). ** $p < 0.01$, n.s. not significantly different when compared with the control. Keys for Figure 4A: (○) Control, (◇) 0.001% (v/v) SLG-30, (◆) 0.01% (v/v) SLG-30, (■) 0.025% (v/v) SLG-30, (▲) 0.05% (v/v) SLG-30, and (•) 0.1% (v/v) SLG-30. Keys for Figure 4B: (○) Control, (▲) 0.1% (w/v) sodium glycocholate, (■) 1% (w/v) sodium glycocholate, and (•) 0.05% (w/v) sodium laurate.

Parallel studies were performed with 0.1% (w/v) and 1% (w/v) NaGC and with 0.05% (w/v) sodium laurate. Figure 4B shows that TEER values were significantly reduced in the presence of 0.05% (w/v) sodium laurate without recovering to the baseline within the period of the experiment. In the case of 1% (w/v) NaGC, the TEER values significantly decreased then recovered to the baseline at the end of the experiment. Almost no effect was seen with 0.1% (w/v) NaGC on the TEER values. As shown in Figure 5, 0.05% (w/v) sodium laurate significantly increased (94 times) the transport of CF as compared to that observed in the control group; 1% (w/v) NaGC also significantly increased the transport of CF to a lesser extent than SLG-30 (i.e., 5 times higher than the control group). Further, 0.1% (w/v) NaGC had an insignificant effect on the transport of CF through Caco-2 cells (Figure 5).

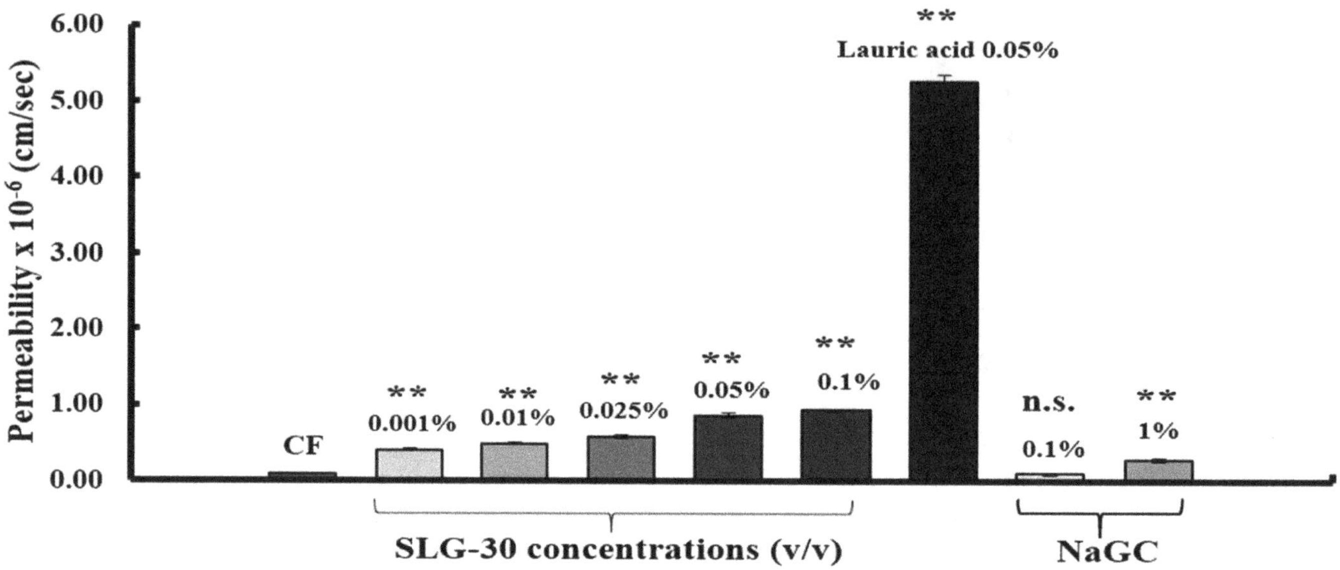

Figure 5. The permeability of CF in the presence of SLG-30, sodium glycocholate, and sodium laurate across Caco-2 cell monolayers: The results are expressed as the mean ± S.E. (n = 3). ** $p < 0.01$, n.s. not significantly different when compared with the control.

3.4. Assessment of Caco-2 Cells Injury

To assess the membrane injury of Caco-2 cells caused by SLG-30, sodium laurate, and NaGC, the LDH activities were measured right after the transport studies. The solutions were collected from the apical sides of wells and then centrifuged at 200× g for 7 min at 4 °C. The activity of the released LDH was measured in the supernatant ($LDH_{release}$). As shown in Figure 6A, the activity of LDH released from Caco-2 cells did not increase after the treatment with SLG-30 as compared to that in the control group. In contrast, the activity of LDH released significantly increased after the treatment with 0.05% (*w*/*v*) sodium laurate. Neither 0.1% (*w*/*v*) nor 1% (*w*/*v*) of NaGC increased the release of LDH. These findings proposed that SLG-30 did not cause serious injury to the cell membranes. Figure 6B shows the relationship between the effects of SLG-30 and typical absorption enhancers on the CF permeability across Caco-2 cells on one side and their toxic effects on the other side. While the absorption-improving effect of SLG-30 is concentration-dependent, we found no serious injury to enteric membrane irrespective of SLG-30 concentrations.

3.5. Estimation of Claudin Proteins by Western Blotting

As described above, SLG-30 might open the tight junctions of the intestinal epithelium, thus increasing the movement of substances through the paracellular route. However, the mechanism by which SLG-30 might open the tight junctions was not elucidated. Therefore, we finally evaluated the expression levels of claudin-1 and claudin-4 by western blotting. Figure 7A shows the bands of western blotting for claudin-1 and claudin-4 after a treatment with 0.5% (*v*/*v*) SLG-30. The treatment with 0.5% (*v*/*v*) SLG-30 decreased the intensity of the claudin-1 and claudin-4 bands by 57% and 64%, respectively, as shown in Figure 7B,C. The expression levels of claudin-1 and claudin-4 were about 64% and 45% less than the control, respectively, after the pretreatment study.

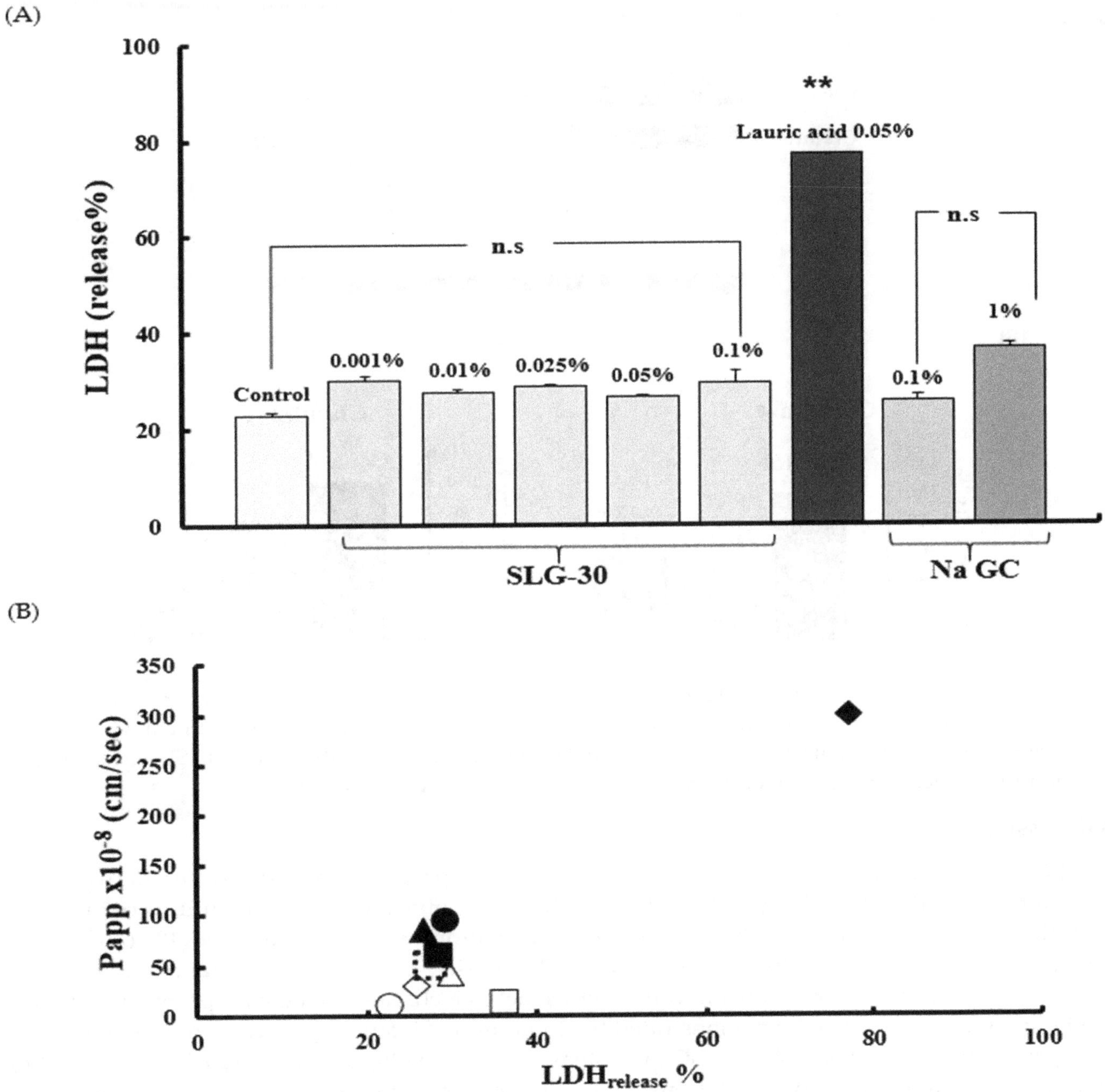

Figure 6. (**A**) The evaluation of the membrane toxicity of Caco-2 cells monolayers in the existence of SLG-30, sodium glycocholate, and sodium laurate and (**B**) the relationship between the effects of SLG-30 and typical absorption enhancers on the CF permeability across Caco-2 cells and their toxic effects: The results are expressed as the mean ± S.E. ($n = 6$). ** $p < 0.01$, n.s. not significantly different when compared with the control. Keys for Figure 6B: (○) Control, (Δ) 0.001% (v/v) SLG-30, (◘) 0.01% (v/v) SLG-30, (■) 0.025% (v/v) SLG-30, (▲) 0.05% (v/v) SLG-30, (•) 0.1% (v/v) SLG-30. (◇) 0.1% (w/v) sodium glycocholate, (□) 1% (w/v) sodium glycocholate, and (◆) 0.05% (w/v) sodium laurate.

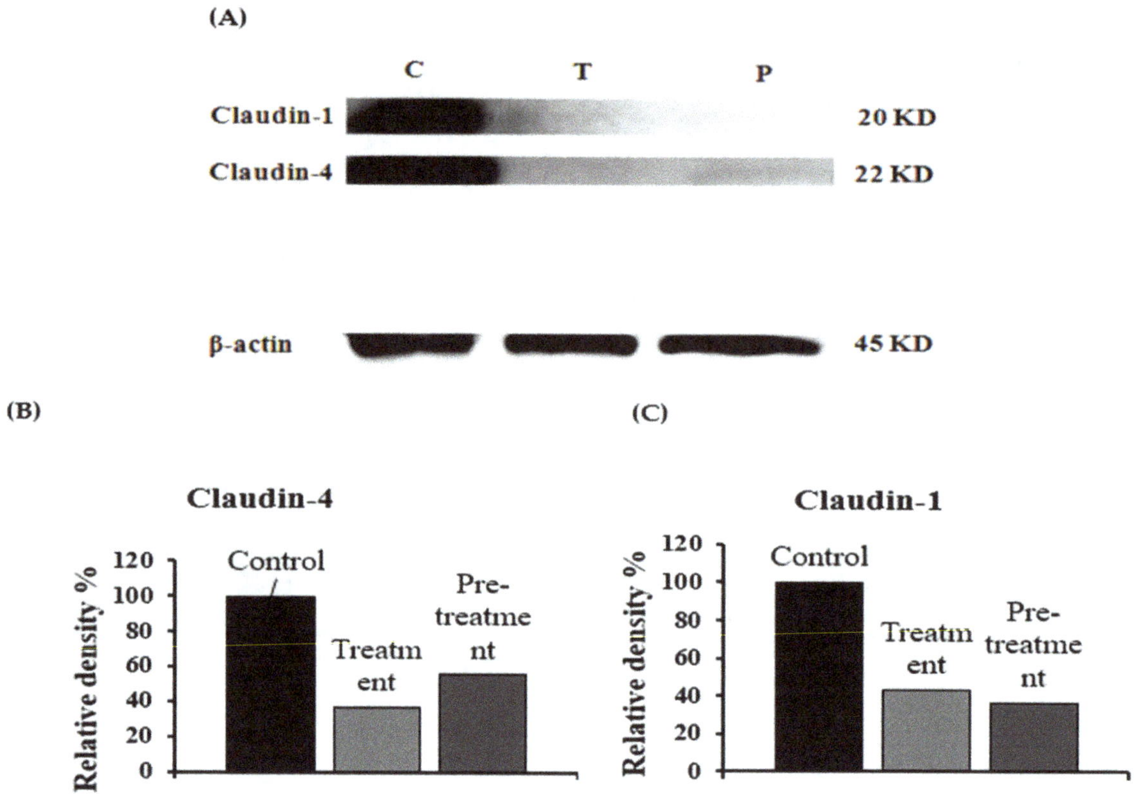

Figure 7. Western blot images of claudin-1 and claudin-4 (**A**): The expression levels of claudin-1 (**B**) and claudin-4 (**C**) in the rat small intestine were quantitatively calculated after a treatment with 0.5% (*v*/*v*) SLG-30 for 1 h. Control, without treatment; treatment, treatment with 0.5% (*v*/*v*) SLG-30 for 1 h; and pretreatment, pretreatment for 1 h. The proteins were extracted after 4 h.

4. Discussion

SLG-30 is a gemini surfactant with good surface-active properties and it is different from typical surfactants of similar chain lengths [21]. In this study, the efficacy of SLG-30 in improving enteric absorption was compared with that of a typical absorption enhancer. We used 1% (*w*/*v*) NaGC, a typical bile salt, as a typical absorption enhancer. Previously, it was proposed that bile acids interact with cell membranes to form reverse micelles, which act as a channel to increase permeation [35]. On the other hand, previous reports demonstrated the inhibition of insulin hydrolysis in different mucosal homogenates of rats by 1% (*w*/*v*) NaGC (a protease inhibitor) [36]. As shown in Figure 2, 1% (*w*/*v*) NaGC improved the absorption of CF from the small intestine to a much lower range than SLG-30. As shown in Table 1, the $AUC_{0\rightarrow240}$ value of CF in the presence of 0.5% *v*/*v* SLG-30 is 3.5 times greater than that in the presence of 1% (*w*/*v*) NaGC. These findings suggested that the absorption-enhancing effect of SLG-30, a gemini surfactant, is more potential than typical absorption enhancers.

We also studied the absorption-improving effect of sodium laurate, as a typical absorption enhancer and a major component of SLG-30 molecule. From Figure 2, we conclude that the effect of sodium laurate on the enteric absorption of CF was quite low and rapid, probably because sodium laurate itself was absorbed into the bloodstream due to its low molecular weight (approximately 288 Da), leading to a decrease in the concentration of sodium laurate at the site of absorption. This could explain the lower T_{max} observed for sodium laurate than for SLG-30. Table 1 also shows the difference between the $AUC_{0\rightarrow240}$ values of CF in the presence of SLG-30 and sodium laurate. Therefore, SLG-30 by itself, rather than sodium laurate, a degradation product of SLG-30, could improve the enteric absorption of poorly absorbable substances. These results provided three outcomes: firstly, the superiority of the enteric absorption-enhancing effects SLG-30 over typical absorption enhancers. Secondly, SLG-30 was effective as a whole compound and not because of lauric acid moieties present in the SLG-30 molecule. Finally, SLG-30 was stable in the intestines and was not degraded to its basic components.

In this study, we examined and elucidated the absorption-enhancing mechanisms of SLG-30 in improving the enteric absorption of poorly absorbed substances. Of all the absorption-enhancing mechanisms, an increase in the membrane fluidity is one of the most important mechanisms of action of many absorption enhancers. Labeling the cell membrane with fluorescent compounds allows the tracking of membrane fluidity changes by fluorescence polarization techniques [25,28]. Enteric BBMVs were used to study the membrane lipid fluidity in the presence of SLG-30. This was done by measuring the fluorescence intensities and calculating the fluorescence anisotropies of DPH, tma-DPH, and DNS-Cl [37,38]. As shown in Figure 3A, SLG-30 slightly decreased the anisotropy of DPH; meanwhile, it decreased the anisotropy of DNS-Cl in a dose-dependent pattern, as shown in Figure 3C. These results suggested that SLG-30 has a great effect on the protein portion of the cell membrane with a mild effect on the inner portion between the phospholipids bilayers. However, it did not have an effect on the outer portion of the phospholipid bilayers, as indicated in Figure 3B.

Caco-2 cell monolayers were used in this study to understand the mechanism by which SLG-30 could improve the absorption of chemical compounds and peptides. Caco-2 monolayers are more susceptible to the cytotoxic influences of permeation enhancers than whole enteric tissue [39,40]. For this reason, we used low concentrations of SLG-30, i.e., 0.0001% (*v*/*v*), 0.001% (*v*/*v*), 0.025% (*v*/*v*), 0.05% (*v*/*v*), and 0.1% (*v*/*v*), and a low concentration of CF (10 μM). When SLG-30 was added at concentrations used in *in vivo* studies, the cells were detached and severely injured. The TEER values usually decreased when the tight junctions between the adjacent cells were opened. In the present study, SLG-30 at all concentrations, significantly decreased the TEER values, suggesting that this enhancer might open the tight junctions, even at low concentrations, thereby increasing the transport of CF. The TEER values did not recover to the baseline when high concentrations of SLG-30 were used, while in the *in vivo* absorption studies, we noticed that the concentrations of CF in the plasma decreased [22]. This distinction might be explained by the nature of Caco-2 cells, which are more sensitive than the enteric cells and have a lower ability to remove any substance away from the cell surface than in vivo enteric cells [12,40].

In the present work, we also compared the effects of typical absorption enhancers and SLG-30 on Caco-2 cells. As shown in Figure 5B, the effects of NaGC were consistent with the results of previous report [24] and with the *in vivo* studies. NaGC at a concentration of 1% (*w*/*v*) might also open the tight junctions to an extent lower than SLG-30. The cumulative amounts of CF (Figure 7) after using 1% (*w*/*v*) NaGC was also less than that obtained after using 0.001% (*v*/*v*) of SLG-30, thus confirming the superiority of SLG-30 over NaGC. Figure 4B also indicates that sodium laurate significantly decreased the TEER values without recovering and, with a significant cumulative amount of CF (Figure 5), even more than that of 0.1% (*v*/*v*) SLG-30, while in the in vivo studies, the absorption enhancement ratio for SLG-30 was better than that of sodium laurate. This discrepancy can be partially explained by the highly toxicity effects of sodium laurate on Caco-2 cells. As Figure 6A shows, the amount of LDH released from Caco-2 cells was significant, and sodium laurate might cause a disintegration of Caco-2 cell monolayers and a rupture of cell membranes which led to a high permeability of CF to the basal side.

We previously reported the *in vivo* safety of SLG-30, as an absorption enhancer for the enteric epithelium [22]. The results of toxicity studies on Caco-2 cells (Figure 6A) also confirm the safety of SLG-30 on the intestinal epithelium. Apparently, SLG-30 might loosen the tight junctions to an extent enough for drug permeability but not enough to cause cell detachment, as in the case of sodium laurate, or to cause damage to the cell membrane, as suggested by the normal release of LDH.

Many previous studies have suggested the importance of claudin family proteins (molecular masses of approx. 23 kDa) to tight junctions to function properly [41,42]. Occludin family proteins are also important tight junction components. However, the deletion of occludin did not cause a disturbance of the TJs barrier function [43], and whether occludin is a major part of TJs remains unclear.

Claudins, which have molecular weight of approx. 23 kDa, comprise a multigene family consisting of more than 20 members. In our experiment, we studied the levels of claudin-1 and claudin-4 after treatment with 0.5% (*v*/*v*) SLG-30. The expression levels of both claudin-1 and claudin-4 were impaired (Figure 7A), suggesting that the loosening of TJs might be connected to the decrease in the levels of these proteins and that SLG-30 increased enteric transport of substances through the paracellular route. The pretreatment studies indicated that these proteins levels recovered, although at different rates, which could explain the partially reversible effects of SLG-30 [22]. It seems that the tight junctions might need more than 4 h for recovery. However, other proteins involved in TJs should be tested, including occludin and ZO-1, and further studies are required to understand the underlying mechanism of the decrease in these protein levels.

These findings also suggested that SLG-30 might enhance the enteric absorption of substances through a paracellular route in addition to a transcellular route.

5. Conclusions

Comparative studies conducted *in vivo* and *in vitro* showed that SLG-30, a gemini surfactant, had a greater absorption-improving effect than typical absorption enhancers, including NaGC and sodium laurate. Furthermore, the study also suggested that SLG-30 was stable in the intestines and acted as a whole compound to ameliorate the enteric absorption of poorly absorbed substances. The *in vitro* evaluation of membrane damage results confirmed the safety of SLG-30 on the enteric membrane. SLG-30 might also improve absorption through the transcellular route by changing the membrane fluidity. In addition, *in vitro* mechanistic studies suggested that SLG-30 might affect tight junctions by decreasing the levels of claudin-1 and claudin-4; thus, SLG-30 might open TJs and enhance the permeability through the paracellular route.

Author Contributions: Conceptualization, A.Y.; methodology, T.A. and A.Y.; software, T.A.; validation, T.A. and H.K.; formal analysis, T.A.; investigation, T.A., K.K., and M.M.; resources, A.Y.; data curation, T.A. and H.K..; writing—original draft preparation, T.A.; writing—review and editing, H.K., T.S., and A.Y.; visualization, T.A.; supervision, A.Y.; project administration, A.Y.; funding acquisition, A.Y.

References

1. Beg, S.; Swain, S.; Rizwan, M.; Irfanuddin, M.; Malini, D.S. Bioavailability enhancement strategies: Basics, formulation approaches and regulatory considerations. *Curr. Drug Deliv.* **2011**, *8*, 691–702. [CrossRef]
2. Adson, A.; Raub, T.J.; Burton, P.S.; Barsuhn, C.L.; Hilgers, A.R.; Audus, K.L.; Ho, N.F. Quantitative approaches to delineate paracellular diffusion in cultured epithelial cell monolayers. *J. Pharm. Sci.* **1994**, *83*, 1529–1536. [CrossRef]
3. Antosova, Z.; Mackova, M.; Kral, V.; Macek, T. Therapeutic application of peptides and proteins: Parenteral forever? *Trends Biotechnol.* **2009**, *27*, 628–635. [CrossRef]
4. Mitic, L.L.; Anderson, J.M. Molecular architecture of tight junctions. *Annu. Rev. Physiol.* **1998**, *60*, 121–142. [CrossRef] [PubMed]
5. Fricker, G.; Drewe, J. Current concepts in intestinal peptide absorption. *J. Pept. Sci.* **1996**, *2*, 195–211. [CrossRef] [PubMed]
6. Salamat-Miller, N.; Johnston, T.P. Current strategies used to enhance the paracellular transport of therapeutic polypeptides across the intestinal epithelium. *Int. J. Pharm.* **2005**, *294*, 201–216. [CrossRef] [PubMed]
7. Fix, J.A.; Engle, K.; Porter, P.A.; Leppert, P.S.; Selk, S.J.; Gardner, C.R.; Alexander, J. Acylcarnitines: Drug absorption-enhancing agents in the gastrointestinal tract. *Am. J. Physiol.* **1986**, *251*, G332–G340. [CrossRef]
8. Lee, V.H.L.; Yamamoto, A. Penetration and enzymatic barriers to peptide and protein absorption. *Adv. Drug Deliv. Rev.* **1989**, *4*, 171–207. [CrossRef]
9. Nellans, H.N. (B) Mechanisms of peptide and protein absorption. *Adv. Drug Deliv. Rev.* **1991**, *7*, 339–364. [CrossRef]
10. Pauletti, G.M.; Okumu, F.W.; Borchardt, R.T. Effect of size and charge on the passive diffusion of peptides across Caco-2 cell monolayers via the paracellular pathway. *Pharm. Res.* **1997**, *14*, 164–168. [CrossRef]

11. Aungst, B.J. Absorption enhancers: Applications and advances. *AAPS J.* **2012**, *14*, 10–18. [CrossRef] [PubMed]
12. Yamamoto, A.; Uchiyama, T.; Nishikawa, R.; Fujita, T.; Muranishi, S. Effectiveness and toxicity screening of various absorption enhancers in the rat small intestine: Effects of absorption enhancers on the intestinal absorption of phenol red and the release of protein and phospholipids from the intestinal membrane. *J. Pharm. Pharmacol.* **1996**, *48*, 1285–1289. [CrossRef] [PubMed]
13. Yamamoto, A.; Tatsumi, H.; Maruyama, M.; Uchiyama, T.; Okada, N.; Fujita, T. Modulation of intestinal permeability by nitric oxide donors: Implications in intestinal delivery of poorly absorbable drugs. *J. Pharmacol. Exp. Ther.* **2001**, *296*, 84–90. [PubMed]
14. Gao, Y.; He, L.; Katsumi, H.; Sakane, T.; Fujita, T.; Yamamoto, A. Improvement of intestinal absorption of water-soluble macromolecules by various polyamines: Intestinal mucosal toxicity and absorption-enhancing mechanism of spermine. *Int. J. Pharm.* **2008**, *354*, 126–134. [CrossRef]
15. Gao, Y.; He, L.; Katsumi, H.; Sakane, T.; Fujita, T.; Yamamoto, A. Improvement of intestinal absorption of insulin and water-soluble macromolecular compounds by chitosan oligomers in rats. *Int. J. Pharm.* **2008**, *359*, 70–78. [CrossRef] [PubMed]
16. Lin, Y.; Fujimori, T.; Kawaguchi, N.; Tsujimoto, Y.; Nishimi, M.; Dong, Z.; Katsumi, H.; Sakane, T.; Yamamoto, A. Polyamidoamine dendrimers as novel potential absorption enhancers for improving the small intestinal absorption of poorly absorbable drugs in rats. *J. Control. Release* **2011**, *149*, 21–28. [CrossRef]
17. Nakaya, Y.; Takaya, M.; Hinatsu, Y.; Alama, T.; Kusamori, K.; Katsumi, H.; Sakane, T.; Yamamoto, A. Enhanced oral delivery of bisphosphonate by novel absorption enhancers: Improvement of intestinal absorption of alendronate by *N*-acyl amino acid and *N*-acyl taurates and their absorption-enhancing mechanisms. *J. Pharm. Sci.* **2016**, *105*, 3680–3690. [CrossRef]
18. Alama, T.; Katayama, H.; Hirai, S.; Ono, S.; Kajiyama, A.; Kusamori, K.; Katsumi, H.; Sakane, T.; Yamamoto, A. Enhanced oral delivery of alendronate by sucrose fatty acids esters in rats and their absorption-enhancing mechanisms. *Int. J. Pharm.* **2016**, *515*, 476–489. [CrossRef]
19. Dahlgren, D.; Roos, C.; Johansson, P.; Tannergren, C.; Lundqvist, A.; Langguth, P.; Sjöblom, M.; Sjögren, E.; Lennernas, H. The effects of three absorption-modifying critical excipients on the *in vivo* intestinal absorption of six model compounds in rats and dogs. *Int. J. Pharm.* **2018**, *547*, 158–168. [CrossRef]
20. Maher, S.; Mrsny, R.J.; Braydenc, D.J. Intestinal permeation enhancers for oral peptide delivery. *Adv. Drug Deliv. Rev.* **2016**, *106*, 277–319. [CrossRef]
21. Hait, S.K.; Moulik, S.P. Gemini surfactants: A distinct class of self- assembling molecules. *Curr. Sci. Gemini Surfactants* **2002**, *82*, 1101–1111.
22. Alama, T.; Kusamori, K.; Katsumi, H.; Sakane, T.; Yamamoto, A. Absorption-enhancing effects of gemini surfactant on the intestinal absorption of poorly absorbed hydrophilic drugs including peptide and protein drugs in rats. *Int. J. Pharm.* **2016**, *499*, 58–66. [CrossRef]
23. Kaneko, D.; Olsson, U.; Sakamoto, K. Self-assembly in some *N*-lauroyl-L-glutamate/water Systems. *Langmuir* **2002**, *18*, 4699–4703. [CrossRef]
24. Yamamoto, A.; Taniguchi, T.; Rikyuu, K.; Tsuji, T.; Fujita, T.; Murakami, M.; Muranishi, S. Effects of various protease inhibitors on the intestinal absorption and degradation of insulin in rats. *Pharm. Res.* **1994**, *11*, 1496–1500. [CrossRef]
25. Bhor, V.M.; Sivakami, S. Regional variations in intestinal brush border membrane fluidity and function during diabetes and the role of oxidative stress and non-enzymatic glycation. *Mol. Cell. Biochem.* **2003**, *252*, 125–132. [CrossRef]
26. Ganapathy, V.; Mendicino, J.F.; Leibach, F.H. Transport of glycyl-L-proline into intestinal and renal brush border vesicles from rabbit. *J. Biol. Chem.* **1981**, *256*, 118–124.
27. Prabhu, R.; Balasubramanian, K.A. A novel method of preparation of small intestinal brush border membrane vesicles by polyethylene glycol precipitation. *Anal. Biochem.* **2001**, *289*, 157–161. [CrossRef]
28. Koga, K.; Kusawake, Y.; Ito, Y.; Sugioka, N.; Shibata, N.; Takada, K. Enhancing mechanism of Labrasol on intestinal membrane permeability of the hydrophilic drug gentamicin sulfate. *Eur. J. Pharm. Biopharm.* **2006**, *64*, 82–91. [CrossRef]
29. Ohyashiki, T.; Sakata, N.; Matsui, K. A decrease of lipid fluidity of the porcine intestinal brush-border membranes by treatment with malondialdehyde. *J. Biochem.* **1992**, *111*, 419–423. [CrossRef]

30. Hidalgo, I.J.; Raub, T.J.; Borchardt, R.T. Characterization of the human colon carcinoma cell line (Caco-2) as a model system for intestinal epithelial permeability. *Gastroenterology* **1989**, *96*, 736–749. [CrossRef]
31. Choksakulnimitr, S.; Masuda, S.; Tokuda, H.; Takakura, Y.; Hashida, M. *In vitro* cytotoxicity of macromolecules in different cell culture systems. *J. Control. Release* **1995**, *34*, 233–241. [CrossRef]
32. Quan, Y.S.; Hattori, K.; Lundborg, E.; Fujita, T.; Murakami, M.; Muranishi, S.; Yamamoto, A. Effectiveness and toxicity screening of various absorption enhancers using Caco-2 cell monolayers. *Biol. Pharm. Bull.* **1998**, *21*, 615–620. [CrossRef]
33. Sugibayashi, K.; Onuki, Y.; Takayama, K. Displacement of tight junction proteins from detergent-resistant membrane domains by treatment with sodium caprate. *Eur. J. Pharm. Sci.* **2009**, *36*, 246–253. [CrossRef]
34. Takizawa, Y.; Kishimoto, H.; Kitazato, T.; Tomita, M.; Hayashi, M. Changes in protein and mRNA expression levels of claudin family after mucosal lesion by intestinal ischemia/reperfusion. *Int. J. Pharm.* **2012**, *426*, 82–89. [CrossRef]
35. Gordon, G.S.; Moses, A.C.; Silver, R.D.; Flier, J.S.; Carey, M.C. Nasal absorption of insulin: Enhancement by hydrophobic bile salts. *Proc. Natl. Acad. Sci. USA* **1985**, *82*, 7419–7423. [CrossRef]
36. Yamamoto, A.; Hayakawa, E.; Lee, V.H. Insulin and proinsulin proteolysis in mucosal homogenates of the albino rabbit: Implications in peptide delivery from nonoral routes. *Life Sci.* **1990**, *47*, 2465–2474. [CrossRef]
37. Rinken, A.; Harro, J.; Engström, L.; Oreland, L. Role of fluidity of membranes on the guanyl nucleotide-dependent binding of cholecystokinin-8S to rat brain cortical membranes. *Biochem. Pharmacol.* **1998**, *55*, 423–431. [CrossRef]
38. Schedl, H.P.; Christensen, K.K.; Clark, E.D.; Buettner, G.R. Surface charge, fluidity, and calcium uptake by rat intestinal brush-border vesicles. *Biochim. Biophys. Acta Biomembr.* **1995**, *1234*, 81–89. [CrossRef]
39. Aungst, B.J. Intestinal permeation enhancers. *J. Pharm. Sci* **2000**, *89*, 429–442. [CrossRef]
40. Chao, A.C.; Nguyen, J.V.; Broughall, M.; Griffin, A.; Fix, J.A.; Daddona, P.E. *In vitro* and *in vivo* evaluation of effects of sodium caprate on enteral peptide absorption and on mucosal morphology. *Int. J. Pharm.* **1999**, *191*, 15–24. [CrossRef]
41. Morita, K.; Furuse, M.; Fujimoto, K.; Tsukita, S. Claudin multigene family encoding four-transmembrane domain protein components of tight junction strands. *Proc. Natl. Acad. Sci. USA* **1999**, *96*, 511–516. [CrossRef] [PubMed]
42. Sonoda, N.; Furuse, M.; Sasaki, H.; Yonemura, S.; Katahira, J.; Horiguchi, Y.; Tsukita, S. Clostridium perfringens enterotoxin fragment removes specific claudins from tight junction strands: Evidence for direct involvement of claudins in tight junction barrier. *J. Cell Biol.* **1999**, *147*, 195–204. [CrossRef] [PubMed]
43. Balda, M.S.; Whitney, J.A.; Flores, C.; González, S.; Cereijido, M.; Matter, K. Functional dissociation of paracellular permeability and transepithelial electrical resistance and disruption of the apical-basolateral intramembrane diffusion barrier by expression of a mutant tight junction membrane protein. *J. Cell Biol.* **1996**, *134*, 1031–1034. [CrossRef] [PubMed]

9

Trimethyl Chitosan Hydrogel Nanoparticles for Progesterone Delivery in Neurodegenerative Disorders

Maria Cristina Cardia [1], Anna Rosa Carta [2], Pierluigi Caboni [1], Anna Maria Maccioni [1], Sara Erbì [1], Laura Boi [2], Maria Cristina Meloni [1], Francesco Lai [1,*] and Chiara Sinico [1]

1 Department of Life and Environmental Sciences, Unit of Drug Sciences, University of Cagliari, 09124 Cagliari, Italy; cardiamr@unica.it (M.C.C.); caboni@unica.it (P.C.); maccion@unica.it (A.M.M.); erbisara@gmail.com (S.E.); mariacristina.meloni@unica.it (M.C.M.); sinico@unica.it (C.S.)

2 Department of Biomedical Sciences, University of Cagliari, 09124 Cagliari, Italy; acarta@unica.it (A.R.C.); laurettaboi@hotmail.it (L.B.)

* Correspondence: frlai@unica.it

† This work is dedicated to the memory of Prof. Sandro Fenu and Prof. Sandra Dessì.

Abstract: Progesterone is a sex hormone which shows neuroprotective effects in different neurodegenerative disorders, including Parkinson's disease, stroke, and Alzheimer's disease. However, the pharmacokinetic limitations associated with the peripheral administration of this molecule highlight the need for more efficient delivery approaches to increase brain progesterone levels. Since the nose-to-brain administration of mucoadhesive hydrogel nanoparticles is a non-invasive and convenient strategy for the delivery of therapeutics to the central nervous system, in this work, progesterone-loaded hydrogel nanoparticle formulations have been prepared, characterized, and tested in vivo. Nanoparticles, loaded with different progesterone concentrations, have been obtained by polyelectrolyte complex formation between trimethyl chitosan and sodium alginate, followed by ionotropic gelation with sodium tripolyphosphate as a cross-linking agent. All formulations showed a mean diameter ranging from 200 nm to 236 nm, a polydispersity index smaller than 0.23, and a high progesterone encapsulation efficiency (83–95%). The zeta potential values were all positive and greater than 28 mV, thus ensuring nanoparticles stability against aggregation phenomena as well as interaction with negative sialic residues of the nasal mucosa. Finally, in vivo studies on Sprague–Dawley male rats demonstrated a 5-fold increase in brain progesterone concentrations compared to basal progesterone level after 30 min of hydrogel nanoparticle inhalation.

Keywords: trimethyl chitosan; progesterone; brain; hydrogel nanoparticles

1. Introduction

In recent years, research has focused on the potential repurposing of sex hormones, particularly progesterone (PG), for the treatment of neurodegenerative disorders, including Parkinson's disease (PD), stroke, and Alzheimer's disease [1,2]. Use of PG in PD initially raised interest following evidence of the higher incidence in men than in women [3,4]. PD is a complex pathology comprising multiple pathological events; therefore, molecules with several mechanisms of action, such as PG, are valuable options as neuroprotective agents [5]. Preclinical studies have suggested a neuroprotective effect of low doses of PG administered in several models of PD [6,7]. Similarly, the neuroprotective action of PG was also found in models of traumatic brain injury in both human and experimental animals [8–10] and is under investigation for cognitive impairment in Alzheimer's disease [11]. Therefore, while current evidence points to PG as a valid and promising therapeutic approach for several CNS disorders, the pharmacokinetic limitations associated with the peripheral administration of this molecule highlight a need for more efficient delivery approaches to increase its brain levels.

In particular, oral administration of PG is characterized by low bioavailability. Indeed, its rapid absorption is associated with an elevated clearance rate due to intestine and first-pass metabolism [12,13]. Moreover, PG absorption is influenced by food intake, formulation excipients, and drug crystal diameter [14]. Several PG derivatives with a higher stability have been synthetized, but their use often relates to different undesirable effects, such as a decrease in total high-density lipoprotein cholesterol and an increased risk of fetal malformations [12,14]. For these reasons, in order to overcome low oral bioavailability, parenteral PG administration routes have been explored. Intravenous and intramuscular administrations determine high serum PG concentrations [12,13]; however, in the case of chronic therapy, daily injections can be uncomfortable and are characterized by low patient compliance.

Therefore, as several high-molecular-weight drugs have shown promising results in the treatment of CNS disorders, alternative routes for brain delivery are steadily investigated [15,16]. Nose-to-brain administration is a non-invasive and convenient strategy for the delivery of therapeutics to the CNS, bypassing the blood-brain barrier (BBB). Indeed, the nasal cavity can be employed not only for local administration, but also for the systemic delivery of different therapeutic agents (e.g., peptides, proteins, stem cells, etc.) due to its large surface area and high degree of vascularization. Drug administered by this route can enter the brain principally using olfactory or trigeminal nerve pathways. Moreover, other pathways involving vasculature, cerebrospinal fluid, and the lymphatic system have been individuated [17,18].

Even though it is often not easy to identify the exact pathways that an intranasally administered molecule follows to penetrate the CNS, it has been observed that different experimental factors can influence the amount and rate of brain accumulation. Usually, an increase in the drug contact time (residence time) with the nasal mucosa enhances the overall nose-to-brain drug delivery. In particular, it has been demonstrated that the use of mucoadhesive hydrogel nanoparticles (NPs) can increase the residence time and, consequently, the brain bioavailability of loaded drugs [19,20].

N,N,N-Trimethyl chitosan (TMC) is a hydrophilic polymer obtained by chitosan methylation which is able to form a stable gel in presence of sodium alginate (SA), an anionic water-soluble polysaccharide composed of alternating blocks of a-L-guluronic and b-D-mannuronic acid (b 1–4 linked) [21]. Similarly to chitosan, it is characterized by low toxicity, good biodegradability, and biocompatibility. However, compared to chitosan, TMC shows a higher positive charge and consequently, good solubility at all physiological pH values. Moreover, TMC shows excellent mucoadhesive properties as well as the ability to improve the paracellular permeation of hydrophilic compounds by means of interactions with the tight junctions [22,23].

With the aim of both identifying a more effective route for PG administration and clarifying whether the mucoadhesive properties of TMC can affect its brain accumulation, in this work we prepared PG-loaded TMC hydrogel NPs for PG brain delivery.

PG-loaded hydrogel NPs were prepared by polyelectrolyte complex formation between TMC and SA followed by ionotropic gelation with sodium tripolyphosphate (TPP) as a cross-linking agent. NPs were characterized in terms of size, size distribution, surface charge, and encapsulation efficiency. Moreover, NP stability and in vitro PG release were assessed. Finally, brain PG accumulation was evaluated in vivo on Sprague–Dawley male rats after PG hydrogel NP inhalation.

2. Materials and Methods

2.1. Materials

Low-molecular-weight chitosan, sodium iodide, *N*-methyl-pyrrolidinone, methyl iodide, sodium chloride, sodium hydroxide, sodium alginate, sodium tripolyphosphate, and deuterated PG (D9-PG) were purchased from Sigma Aldrich. PG was purchased from Galeno (Carmignano, Italy). For the in vivo experiments Sprague–Dawley rats were purchased from Envigo (Huntingdon, England, UK).

2.2. TMC Synthesis and Characterization

The synthesis of TMC was performed starting with low-molecular-weight chitosan, slightly revising already reported procedures [21]. Chitosan (2 g) and sodium iodide (4.8 g) were dispersed in *N*-methylpyrrolidinone (80 mL) into a three empty flasks immersed in a water bath. The suspension was stirred vigorously with a paddle stirrer at a controlled temperature (60 °C) for 20 min. After stabilization of the temperature, an NaOH solution (11 mL, 15% *w/w*) and methyl iodide (12 mL) were added to the mixture, keeping the temperature at 60 °C (± 5 °C) for 60 min. Then, methyl iodide (5 mL) and NaOH solution (10 mL, 15% *w/w*) were added again to the mixture, and the suspension was stirred at 60 °C for 6 h. The mixture was allowed to reach room temperature under stirring overnight, and the resulting brown colored suspension was concentrated under vacuum and dialyzed against bidistilled water. To replace the I^- counterions with Cl^- counterions, the obtained polymer was treated with an NaCl solution (10% *w/w*, room temperature, overnight) and lyophilized. The dried polymer is stable at room temperature until the time of use and no further purification is needed. TMC was characterized by Proton Magnetic Resonance (^{1}H-NMR) spectroscopy to assess the degree of quaternization. TMC samples were prepared solubilizing freeze-dried TMC in D_2O (5 mg/1 mL). Spectra were determined on a Varian INOVA500 (Palo Alto, CA, USA) spectrometer at 27 °C and were recorded with the water suppression technique. Chemical shifts are expressed as δ value.

2.3. NP Preparation and Characterization

A water dispersion of SA (1 mg/mL) was added to a TMC dispersion (2 mg/mL) containing D9-PG or PG at different concentrations to obtain six different formulations (PGNP0, PGNP0.1, PGNP0.5, PGNP0.7, PGNP1, PGNP1D) as reported in Table 1. The mixture was kept under constant magnetic stirring (~1000 rpm) at room temperature for one hour and then sodium tripolyphosphate (TPP, 1 mg/mL) was added as cross-linking agent (~1000 rpm for 30 min). The volumetric ratio between TMC/SA/TPP was fixed to 6:1:2. A light opalescence revealed NP formation. PG concentrations in the final formulations were (0, 0.1, 0.5, 0.7, and 1 mg/mL).

The average diameter (nm ± SD) and polydispersity index (PDI) of all the formulations were determined by Photon Correlation Spectroscopy (PCS), using a Zetasizer nano-ZS (Malvern Instruments, Worcestershire, UK) Then, 0.2 mL of each formulation were diluted with bidistilled water up to 10 mL and backscattered by a helium-neon laser (633 nm) at an angle of 173° and a constant temperature of 25 °C.

ζ potential (ZP) was determined using the same instrument by means of the M3-PALS (Mixed Mode Measurement-Phase Analysis Light Scattering) technique, which measures the particle electrophoretic mobility. All the measurements were made in triplicate.

Morphology of freeze-dried nanoparticles was examined by scanning electron microscope (SEM). The samples were fixed on a brass stub using carbon double-sided tape. Pictures were then taken at an excitation voltage of 20 kV using a Dual-beam Fei Nova Nano Lab 600 (Hillsboro, OR, USA), equipped with a high-brightness FEG source reaching resolutions up to 5 nm.

2.4. Stability Studies

Stability studies were carried out for 28 days on NP dispersions stored at 4 °C. At preselected time intervals, the refrigerated formulations were allowed to warm to room temperature under magnetic stirrer for 30 min and then the average diameter, polydispersity index, and ζ potential were determined as previously described. All the measurements were taken in triplicate.

2.5. Evaluation of Encapsulation Efficiency

The encapsulation efficiency of the PG containing NPs was estimated by means of an indirect method. NP dispersions were centrifuged at 15,000 rpm for 15 min at 4 °C (Scilogex mod. D3024R,

Rocky Hill, CT, USA) and the PG amount in the supernatant was determined by High Performance Liquid Chromatography (HPLC).

The encapsulation efficiency (EE%) was calculated using the following equation:

$$EE\% = \frac{PG_{TOT} - PG_{SURN}}{PG_{TOT}} \times 100 \quad (1)$$

In the calculation of EE% (Equation (1)), PG_{TOT} corresponds to the total amount of PG used in each sample preparation and PG_{SURN} is the amount of PG in the supernatant after centrifugation. All the measurements were made in triplicate.

PG content was quantified at 254 nm using a Flexar–Perkin Elmer HPLC equipped with a UV detector and a computer-integrating apparatus. The column was a C18 reversed-phase and the mobile phase was a mixture of acetic acid solution (0.5% *v/v*) and methanol (10:90 *v/v* and pH = 3.92) at a flow rate of 1.2 mL/min. The retention time was 3.75 min ± 0.01 s. A standard calibration curve was built up by using working standard solutions. Calibration graphs were plotted according to the linear regression analysis, which gave a correlation coefficient value (R^2) of 0.999.

2.6. *In Vitro Drug Release Studies*

In vitro PG release studies were performed using Franz cells. A dialysis membrane (Spectra/Por® Dialysis Membrane MWCO: 12–14 kD) was previously hydrated with bidistilled water for 24 h and then fixed between the two compartments of Franz cells. The receiving compartment was filled with a water/ethanol solution (40:60 *v/v*) maintained under constant agitation and at controlled temperature (37 °C). In the donor compartment, 500 µL of the samples (PGNP0.1, PGNP0.5, PGNP0.7, PGNP1) were deposited. At preselected intervals (15, 30, 45, 60, 120, 180, 240, and 300 min), the total content of the receiving compartment (~6.5 mL) was withdrawn, replaced with pre-thermostated, fresh water/ethanol solution, and analyzed by HPLC for PG content. All the analyses were performed in triplicate.

2.7. *In Vitro Biocompatibility*

The RPMI 2650 human nasal septum carcinoma cell line (Sigma Aldrich, Milan, Italy) was grown as a monolayer in 75 cm^2 flasks, and incubated in 100% humidity and 5% CO_2 at 37 °C, using RPMI1640 supplemented with fetal bovine serum, penicillin/streptomycin, and fungizone as culture medium. For toxicity studies, cells were seeded into 96-well plates (7.5 × 103 cells/well) and, after 24 h, were treated for 24 h with PGNP1D-deuterated PG-loaded nanoparticles and related unloaded formulations at different dilutions corresponding to 0.5, 5, 15, and 40 µg/mL of PG. After incubation, cells were washed three times with fresh medium and their viability was determined by the (3(4,5-dimethylthiazolyl-2)-2,5-diphenyltetrazolium bromide) colorimetric assay (MTT), adding 200 µL of MTT reagent (0.5 mg/mL in PBS) to each well. After 2–3 h, the formed formazan crystals were dissolved in DMSO and their concentration was spectrophotometrically quantified at 570 nm with a microplate reader (Synergy 4, Reader BioTek Instruments, AHSI S.P.A, Bernareggio, Monza and Brianza, Italy). All experiments were repeated at least three times. Results are shown as percent of cell viability in comparison with non-treated control cells (100% viability).

2.8. *In Vivo Studies*

PGNP1D nanoparticle formulation, containing 1 mg/mL of D9-PG (Table 1), was tested on male Sprague–Dawley rats ($n = 16$, weight range 270–300 g). Rats were immobilized in a plexiglass restrainer and exposed to PGNP1D or empty NPs by inhalation via an aerosol apparatus (Nebula M2000, Air Liquide Medical Systems, Bovezzo, Italy).

The rate of flow of the aerosol apparatus was about 0.3 mL/min. The administered dose was approximatively 1 mg/kg per minute or 0.3 mg per animal per minute, since the PG concentration of the PGNP1D nanoparticle formulation is 1 mg/mL. At 15 min, 30 min, 1 h, and 2 h after continuous inhalation, rats were deeply anesthetized and sacrificed by decapitation. Brains and blood were rapidly collected and processed to determine the amount of D9-PG.

All experimental procedures met the guidelines and protocols approved by the European Community (2010/63 UE L 276 20/10/2010) and by the Ethical Commission for Animal Care and Use at the University of Cagliari and Italian Ministry of Health (pr. # 1293/2015-PR, 18/12/2015).

2.9. *Progesterone and Deuterated Progesterone (D9-PG) in Plasma and Brain GC-MS Analysis*

Quantities of D9-PG in plasma and brain tissue was determined by GC-MS analysis. Plasma samples were initially thawed on ice, and then 200 µL of plasma were withdrawn and extracted with 250 µL of an ice-cold mixture of methanol/water (3:1 *v/v*). Samples were then loaded on C18 columns (Agilent Technologies, Palo Alto, CA, USA), which were previously activated with 2 mL of methanol and 2 mL of bidistilled water. One mL of methanol was added to each SPE column and recovered. The purified extract was then evaporated to dryness using a gentle nitrogen stream.

Brain samples were initially weighed and thawed on ice. Then, 2 mL of a methanol/acetic acid (99:1 *v/v*) solution were added to each sample, which was homogenated with a Potter-Elvehjem PTFE pestle and glass tube homogenizer and left overnight. Samples were then centrifugated for 15 min at 4000 rpm and recovered. The pellet was dissolved and extracted again using 0.5 mL of the methanol/acetic acid solution. After centrifugation of the latter obtained solution, the two extracts were combined and evaporated to dryness. Brain and plasma samples were finally derivatized using 100 µL heptafluorobutyric acid (HFBA) and 200 µL acetone. After 30 min at 35 °C, 600 µL hexane were added before GC-MS analysis.

The derivatized samples were analyzed with a Hewlett Packard 6850 Gas Chromatograph, 5973 mass selective detector, and 7683B series injector (Agilent Technologies, Palo Alto, CA, USA), using helium as the carrier gas at 1.0 mL min^{-1} flow. One µL of samples was injected in the split-less mode and resolved on a 30 m × 0.25 mm × 0.25 µm DB-5MS column (Agilent Technologies, Palo Alto, CA, USA). Inlet, interface, and ion source temperatures were 250, 250, and 230 °C, respectively. Oven starting temperature was set to 50 °C, and the final temperature to 230 °C with a heating rate of 5 °C/min for 36 min and then for 2 min at constant temperature. GC-MS mass spectra were recorded in the selected ion monitoring mode (SIM) recording the 510, 495, 425 *m/z* ions for PG and deuterated PG.

2.10. *Statistical Analysis of Data*

Results are expressed as the mean ± standard deviation and significance was tested at the 0.01 or 0.05 level of probability (*p*). For size, zeta potential, drug accumulation, and cytotoxicity, analysis of variance (one way-ANOVA) followed by post-hoc Bonferroni correction were used to substantiate statistical differences between groups using XLSTAT for Excel.

3. Results and Discussion

3.1. *TMC Synthesis*

In this study PG-loaded hydrogel NPs were prepared by ionotropic gelation technique, using a mixture of TMC/SA and TPP as cross-linker. TMC was synthesized as already reported [21]. The procedure was reproducible and allowed us to obtain TMC with a high degree of quaternization (DQ = 70%), simply extending the reaction time up to seven hours. By means of this procedure, we were able to reduce the methylating agent (CH_3I) amount and, as demonstrated by ^{1}H-NMR data, avoid the formation of undesirable side products (such as TMC with a high degree of methoxylation in position 3 and 6 of the glucosamine ring), which decrease the polymer water solubility. Besides, we avoided the use of organic solvents in purification steps.

3.2. Preparation and Characterization of Nanoparticles

The NP composition was selected based on results obtained in an our previous preformulation study in which the effect of both polymers (TMC and SA) and cross-linker (TPP) ratio was deeply investigated [21]. In particular, in this work the volumetric ratio of TMC, SA, and TPP solution was kept constant (6:1:2). Moreover, the amount of TMC was kept higher than that of SA in order to obtain NPs with positive surface charge, useful to promote the interaction with negative sialic residues of the nasal mucosa. Starting from the above reported composition, we prepared five PG NP formulations (PGNP 0, PGNP0.1, PGNP0.5, PGNP0.7, and PGNP1) loaded with different drug concentrations (0, 0.1, 0.5, 0.7, and 1 mg/mL, respectively). Moreover, a D9-PG-loaded NP dispersion was also prepared (PGNP1D, 1 mg/mL). Deuterated drug-loaded NPs have been used for in vivo studies in order to distinguish endogenous and administered PG after the inhalation experiment. Empty (PGNP0) and PG or D9-PG-containing NPs (PGNP0.1, PGNP0.5, PGNP0.7, PGNP1, PGNP1D) were fully characterized by average diameter (nm ± SD), polydispersity index (PDI), ζ potential (ZP), and encapsulation efficiency (EE%) (Table 1). As shown in Table 1, the incorporation of PG or D9-PG led only to a slight variation of the NP mean diameter, PDI, and ζ potential values when compared to the unloaded NP. Indeed, all formulations (unloaded and loaded) showed a mean diameter ranging from 200 nm and 236 nm and a polydispersity index always smaller than 0.23, thus indicating a fairly narrow size distribution.

The zeta potential values, all positive and greater than 28 mV, should ensure NP stability against aggregation phenomena. In general, all loaded formulations showed a high EE%. The amount of PG used for the preparation of the different formulations seems to have only a small influence on the drug encapsulation efficiency (EE%). Indeed, PGNP0.1, prepared with the smallest PG concentration (0.1 mg/mL), showed the highest EE% (95%), but PGNP1, with the highest PG concentration (1 mg/mL) can also incorporate a very high amount of drug (EE% 83).

NP morphology was evaluated via scanning electron microscopy. In Figure 1 an SEM image of freeze-dried PGNP1D nanoparticles is reported. As can be seen, freeze-dried PG-loaded NPs have a regular and rounded shape. Moreover, SEM analyses confirmed the fact that nanoparticles with a mean diameter comparable with that measured by photon correlation spectroscopy are still present in the lyophilized samples.

Table 1. Composition mean diameter (nm), polydispersity index (PDI), and zeta potential (ZP, mV) of freshly prepared progesterone (PG)-loaded nanoparticles. Results are expressed as means of three independent measurements ± standard deviations. EE%: encapsulation efficiency. PGNP0, PGNP0.1, PGNP0.5, PGNP0.7, and PGNP1: PG NP formulations loaded with drug concentrations of 0, 0.1, 0.5, 0.7, and 1 mg/mL, respectively. NP: nanoparticle.

Sample	PG Concentration (mg/mL)	D9-PG Conccentration (mg/mL)	Mean Diameter (nm ± SD)	PDI (±SD)	ZP (mV ± SD)	EE%
PGNP0	-	-	208 ± 5	0.19 ± 0.01	+28 ± 2	/
PGNP0.1	0.1	-	222 ± 9	0.23 ± 0.08	+28 ± 1	95 ± 3
PGNP0.5	0.5	-	227 ± 6	0.23 ± 0.04	+30 ± 1	88 ± 5
PGNP0.7	0.7	-	236 ± 6	0.25 ± 0.03	+31 ± 2	85 ± 5
PGNP1	1	-	198 ± 4	0.22 ± 0.02	+29 ± 1	83 ± 2
PGNP1D	-	1	204 ± 5	0.25 ± 0.03	+27 ± 1	80 ± 1

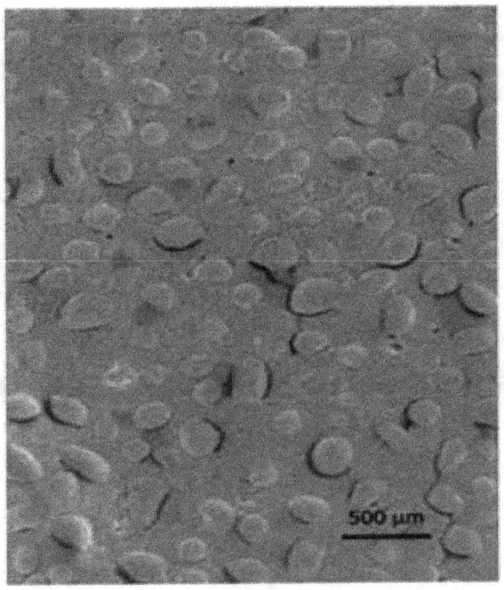

Figure 1. Scanning electron microscopy image of freeze-dried PGNP1D nanoparticles.

3.3. Stability of NPs

Stability studies were performed for 4 weeks, monitoring the variations in size, PDI, and ζ potential of NPs stored at 4 °C (Figures 2 and 3). As shown in Figure 2, the NP mean diameter growth over the studied period was moderate (ranging around 30%). Indeed, all formulations showed a mean diameter of approximately 300 nm after 28 days of storage at 4 °C and, in particular, the smallest size (~290 nm) was measured for PGNP1. Also, polydispersity index values increased after 28 days, thus confirming the fact that NP weak aggregation phenomena occur during storage. Once again, the formulation PGNP1 showed the smallest PDI (nearby 0.30). As expected, zeta potential remains positive for all NP, and almost stable in a narrow range (26–35 mV) over the monitored period (Figure 3).

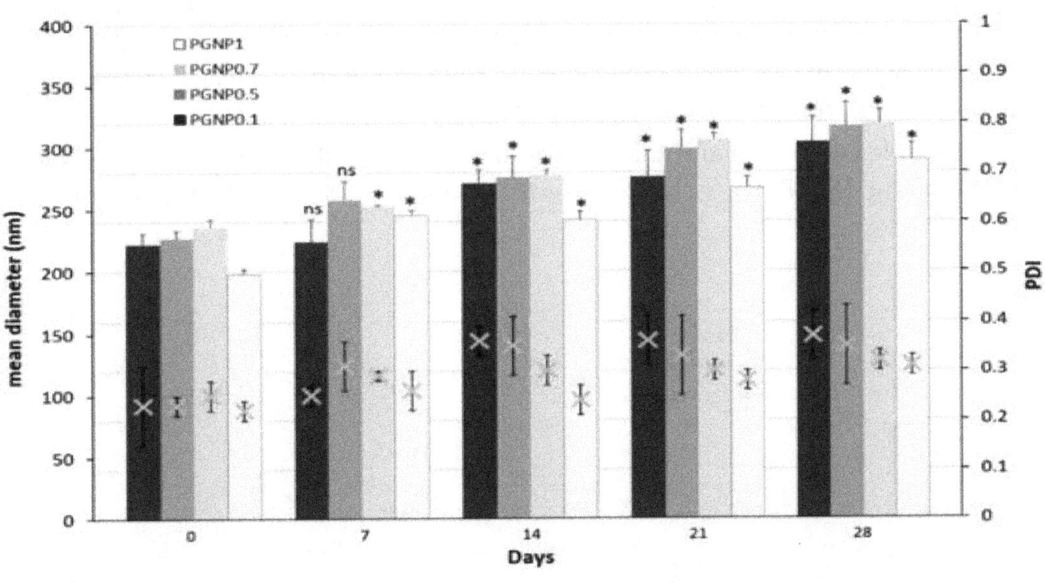

Figure 2. Variation of mean diameter and polydispersity index (PDI) of PG-loaded nanoparticles during 28 days of storage at 4 °C. Results are expressed as means of three independent measurements ± standard deviations. For each formulation, statistical analysis was performed comparing the mean diameter value at each time point with respect to that at time zero. * = different from day 0 ($p \leq 0.05$), ns indicates not significant data ($p > 0.05$).

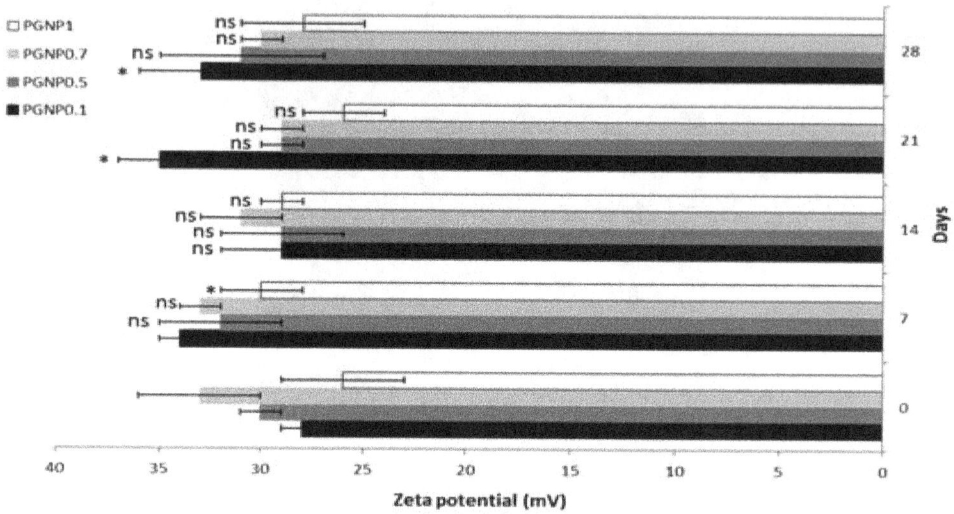

Figure 3. Zeta potential of PG-loaded nanoparticles during 28 days of storage at 4 °C. Results are expressed as means of three independent measurements ± standard deviations. For each formulation, statistical analysis was performed comparing the zeta potential value at each time point with respect to that at time zero. * = different from day 0 ($p \leq 0.05$), ns indicates not significant data ($p > 0.05$).

3.4. *PG Release from NPs*

The PG release from hydrogel NPs was studied over a period of 5 h in a water/ethanol (40:60 *v/v*) solution to ensure sink conditions. To this aim, 500 μL of each samples (PGNP0.1, PGNP0.5, PGNP0.7, PGNP1) were deposited in the Franz cell donor compartment while the receiving compartment was filled with a water/ethanol solution (40:60 *v/v*) maintained at 37 °C and under constant agitation. Results reported in Figure 4 show no burst release for all formulations, thus demonstrating that PG is effectively incorporated into the hydrogel nanoparticles matrix. The PG release profile from formulations PGNP1, PGNP0.7, and PGNP0.5 showed a similar trend, with the release rate directly related to the loaded drug concentration. As for PG release from NPs with the lowest PG concentration, namely PGNP0.1, the rate is significantly the lowest (50.52%). This behavior suggested that the main mechanism by which PG is released from NPs should be a concentration-dependent diffusion process rather than a consequence of matrix hydrogel erosion.

Starting from the release results and taking also into account stability data, we decided to perform the in vivo studies using PGNP1 but loaded with deuterated PG (D9-PG), namely the PGNP1D formulation (Table 1).

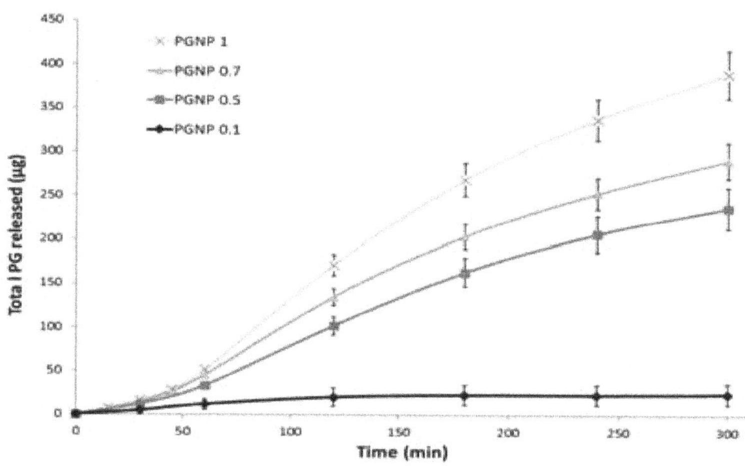

Figure 4. In vitro PG release in water/ethanol (40:60 *v/v*) solution from PG-loaded nanoparticles.

3.5. *In Vitro Biocompatibility*

To evaluate the biocompatibility of both PGNP1D-unloaded and deuterated PG-loaded nanoparticles, an in vitro cytotoxicity study was performed using the human nasal septum carcinoma cell line treated with different PG concentrations (0.5, 5, 15, and 40 μg/mL) for 24 h. As can be seen in Figure 5, the unloaded formulation did not induce any toxic effect on RPMI 2650 cells exposed for 24 h up to the highest tested dose. However, the presence of PG reduces the cell viability in an apparently dose-dependent manner. Indeed, at the dose of 40 μg/mL, a 61% cell viability, when compared to non-treated control cells, was observed. These results confirmed data already reported in the literature concerning the apoptosis effect produced by PG at high doses and prolonged exposition times on cells [24].

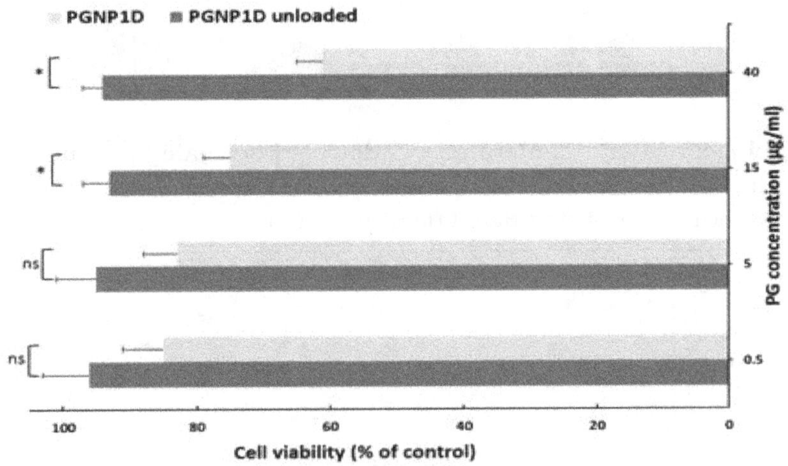

Figure 5. In vitro cytotoxicity studies of PGNP1D and relative unloaded formulations at different dilutions on the human nasal cell line RPMI 2650. The cell viability is recorded as percentage cell viability in comparison with non-treated control cells (100% viability). Results are represented as mean ± SD from three independent experiments. The asterisks indicate statistically significant data (* = $p \leq 0.05$), ns indicates not significant data ($p > 0.05$).

3.6. *In Vivo Studies*

In vivo studies have been carried out on male rats in order to have an animal model with levels of PG as constant as possible. Indeed, the level of endogenous PG in female rats depends on the estrus phase, and thus it is much more variable than in males [25]. To discriminate endogenous PG from exogenous PG, we administered the PGNP1D or empty nanoparticles via aerosol, and we measured plasma and brain levels of both D-9-progesterone and endogenous progesterone at progressive time points (Figures 6 and 7). Results showed that deuterated PG reached a plasma concentration six-fold higher than endogenous PG as soon as 15 min after nanoparticles inhalation, which lasted for 30 min. Plasma levels of deuterated PG decreased to values close to that of endogenous PG 60 min after inhalation (Figure 6). Analysis of brain tissue showed that deuterated PG increased to a concentration significantly higher than endogenous PG when measured 30 min and 60 min after inhalation, and it returned to endogenous PG level 120 min after inhalation (Figure 7). In Figure 8, the total amount of deuterated PG in plasma and brain tissue at preselected time points up to 120 min is reported. As can be clearly observed from the graph, the maximum amount of D9-PG is detected in plasma after 15 min (~0.5 μg) and it is significantly higher than the maximum detected in brain tissue after 30 min (~0.0083 μg). Therefore, in vivo results demonstrate that the nanoparticles used in the present study efficiently carried PG into the brain, even though we do not have any evidence concerning the pathway by which PG reaches the brain tissue. NPs may allow PG to directly reach the brain parenchyma via the nose-to-brain olfactory pathway, bypassing the BBB. However, obtained results seem also to indicate that PG released from NPs diffuses from the nasal mucosa into the blood stream, from where it may pass the blood–brain barrier according to its lipophilic nature [26].

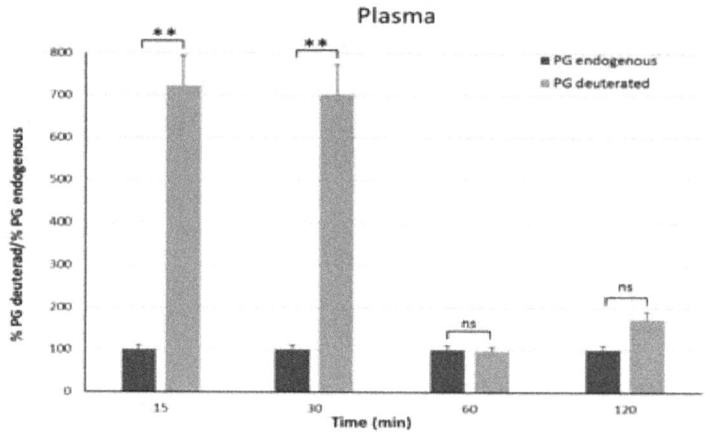

Figure 6. Plasma endogenous and deuterated PG detected on male Sprague–Dawley rats 15 min, 30 min, 1 h, and 2 h after continuous PGNP1D inhalation. The asterisks indicate statistically significant data (** = $p \leq 0.01$), ns indicates not significant data ($p > 0.05$).

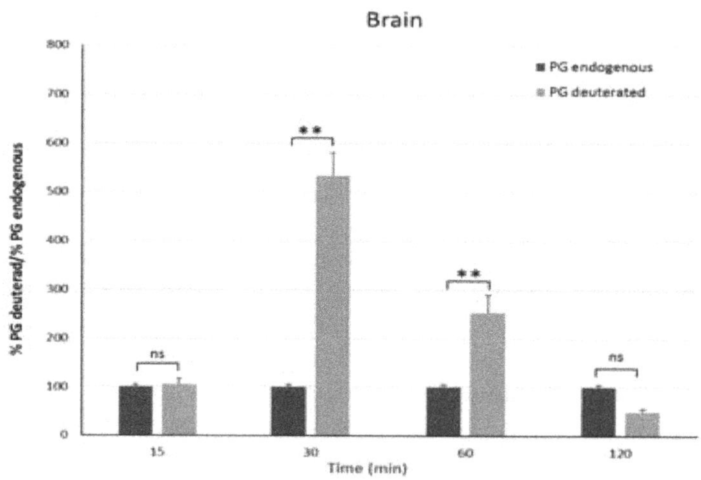

Figure 7. Brain endogenous and deuterated PG detected on male Sprague–Dawley mice 15 min, 30 min, 1 h, and 2 h after continuous PGNP1D inhalation. The asterisks indicate statistically significant data (** = $p \leq 0.01$), ns indicates not significant data ($p > 0.05$).

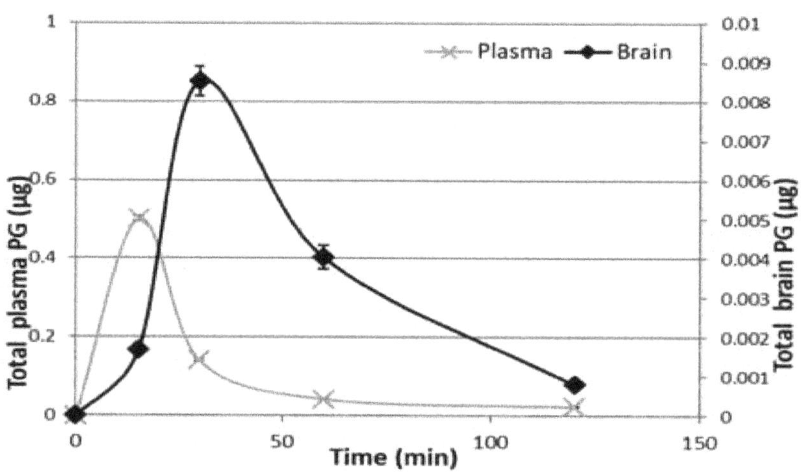

Figure 8. Deuterated PG in plasma and brain 15 min, 30 min, 1 h, and 2 h after continuous PGNP1D inhalation.

4. Conclusions

In this work, NPs loaded with different PG concentrations were obtained from trimethyl chitosan and sodium alginate cross-linked with sodium tripolyphosphate. Among the various prepared NPs, characterization studies allowed us to select the best formulation (PGNP1) in terms of size, stability, and drug release profile. These NPs have been loaded with deuterated PG and tested in vivo on Sprague–Dawley male rats. In vivo results demonstrate that the selected nanoparticles could be an efficient carrier for PG brain delivery useful in the treatment of different neurodegenerative disorders. Further research will be carried out in order to identify the main route involved in PG delivery to the brain tissue.

Author Contributions: Conceptualization, M.C.C., A.R.C., P.C., and C.S.; Data curation, M.C.C., A.M.M., S.E., L.B., and M.C.M.; Formal analysis, M.C.C. and L.B.; Investigation, M.C.C., A.R.C., P.C., A.M.M., S.E., and L.B.; Methodology, P.C. and C.S.; Project administration, A.M.M.; Resources, M.C.C. and M.C.M.; Supervision, A.R.C. and C.S.; Validation, S.E. and F.L.; Visualization, M.C.M.; Writing—original draft, M.C.C., A.R.C., P.C., and F.L.; Writing—review and editing, F.L. and C.S.

Acknowledgments: The author would like to thank Francesca Marongiu for her help.

References

1. Bourque, M.; Morissette, M.; Di Paolo, T. Repurposing sex steroids and related drugs as potential treatment for Parkinson's disease. *Neuropharmacology* **2019**, *147*, 37–54. [CrossRef] [PubMed]
2. Vegeto, E.; Villa, A.; Della Torre, S.; Crippa, V.; Rusmini, P.; Cristofani, R.; Galbiati, M.; Maggi, A.; Poletti, A. The role of sex and sex Hormones in Neurodegenerative Diseases. *Endocr. Rev.* **2019**, in press. [CrossRef] [PubMed]
3. Hirsch, L.; Jette, N.; Frolkis, A.; Steeves, T.; Pringsheim, T. The Incidence of Parkinson's Disease: A Systematic Review and Meta-Analysis. *Neuroepidemiology* **2016**, *46*, 292–300. [CrossRef] [PubMed]
4. Ascherio, A.; Chen, H.; Schwarzschild, M.A.; Zhang, S.M.; Colditz, G.A.; Speizer, F.E. Caffeine, postmenopausal estrogen, and risk of Parkinson's disease. *Neurology* **2003**, *60*, 790–795. [CrossRef] [PubMed]
5. Giatti, S.; Calabrese, D.; Pesaresi, M.; Cermenati, G.; Mitro, N.; Viviani, B.; Garcia-Segura, L.M.; Caruso, D. Levels and actions of progesterone and its metabolites in the nervous system during physiological and pathological conditions. *Prog. Neurobiol.* **2014**, *113*, 56–69.
6. Callier, S.; Morissette, M.; Grandbois, M.; Pélaprat, D.; Di Paolo, T. Neuroprotective properties of 17β-estradiol, progesterone, and raloxifene in MPTP *C57Bl/6 mice*. *Synapse* **2001**, *41*, 131–138. [CrossRef]
7. Bourque, M.; Morissette, M.; Al Sweidi, S.; Caruso, D.; Melcangi, R.C.; Di Paolo, T. Neuroprotective Effect of Progesterone in MPTP-Treated Male Mice. *Neuroendocrinology* **2016**, *103*, 300–314. [CrossRef]
8. Xiao, G.; Wei, J.; Yan, W.; Wang, W.; Lu, Z. Improved outcomes from the administration of progesterone for patients with acute severe traumatic brain injury: A randomized controlled trial. *Crit. Care* **2008**, *12*, R61. [CrossRef]
9. Wright, D.W.; Kellermann, A.L.; Hertzberg, V.S.; Clark, P.L.; Frankel, M.; Goldstein, F.C.; Salomone, J.P.; Dent, L.L.; Harris, O.A.; Ander, D.S.; et al. ProTECT: A Randomized Clinical Trial of Progesterone for Acute Traumatic Brain Injury. *Ann. Emerg. Med.* **2007**, *49*, 391–402. [CrossRef]
10. Wali, B.; Ishrat, T.; Won, S.; Stein, D.G.; Sayeed, I. Progesterone in experimental permanent stroke: A dose-response and therapeutic time-window study. *Brain* **2014**, *137*, 486–502. [CrossRef]
11. Osmanovic-Barilar, J.; Salkovic-Petrisi, M. Evaluating the Role of Hormone Therapy in Postmenopausal Women with Alzheimer's Disease. *Drugs Aging* **2016**, *33*, 787–808. [CrossRef] [PubMed]
12. Unfer, V.; Casini, M.L.; Marelli, G.; Costabile, L.; Gerli, S.; Di Renzo, G.C. Different routes of progesterone administration and polycystic ovary syndrome: A review of the literature. *Gynecol. Endocrinol.* **2005**, *21*, 119–127. [CrossRef] [PubMed]
13. Tavaniotou, A.; Smitz, J.; Bourgain, C.; Devroey, P. Comparison between different routes of progesterone administration as luteal phase support in infertility treatments. *Hum. Reprod. Update* **2000**, *6*, 139–148. [CrossRef] [PubMed]

14. McAuley, J.W.; Kroboth, F.J.; Kroboth, P.D. Oral administration of micronized progesterone: A review and more experience. *Pharmacotherapy* **1996**, *16*, 453–457.
15. Kozlovskaya, L.; Abou-Kaoud, M.; Stepensky, D. Quantitative analysis of drug delivery to the brain via nasal route. *J. Control. Release* **2014**, *189*, 133–140. [CrossRef]
16. Yuba, E.; Kono, K. Nasal Delivery of Biopharmaceuticals. In *Mucosal Delivery of Biopharmaceuticals*; Springer: Boston, MA, USA, 2014; pp. 197–220.
17. Dhuria, S.V.; Hanson, L.R.; Frey, W.H. Intranasal delivery to the central nervous system: Mechanisms and experimental considerations. *J. Pharm. Sci.* **2010**, *99*, 1654–1673. [CrossRef]
18. Bourganis, V.; Kammona, O.; Alexopoulos, A.; Kiparissides, C. Recent advances in carrier mediated nose-to-brain delivery of pharmaceutics. *Eur. J. Pharm. Biopharm.* **2018**, *128*, 337–362. [CrossRef]
19. Mohammed, M.A.; Syeda, J.T.M.; Wasan, K.M.; Wasan, E.K. An Overview of Chitosan Nanoparticles and Its Application in Non-Parenteral Drug Delivery. *Pharmaceutics* **2017**, *9*, 53. [CrossRef]
20. Warnken, Z.N.; Smyth, H.D.C.; Watts, A.B.; Weitman, S.; Kuhn, J.G.; Williams, R.O. Formulation and device design to increase nose to brain drug delivery. *J. Drug Deliv. Sci. Technol.* **2016**, *35*, 213–222. [CrossRef]
21. Marci, L.; Meloni, M.C.; Maccioni, A.M.; Sinico, C.; Lai, F.; Cardia, M.C. Formulation and characterization studies of trimethyl chitosan / sodium alginate nanoparticles for targeted drug delivery. *ChemistrySelect* **2016**, *1*, 669–674. [CrossRef]
22. Kulkarni, A.D.; Patel, H.M.; Surana, S.J.; Vanjari, Y.H.; Belgamwar, V.S.; Pardeshi, C.V. N,N,N-Trimethyl chitosan: An advanced polymer with myriad of opportunities in nanomedicine. *Carbohydr. Polym.* **2017**, *157*, 875–902. [CrossRef] [PubMed]
23. Mourya, V.K.; Inamdar, N.N. Trimethyl chitosan and its applications in drug delivery. *J. Mater. Sci. Mater. Med.* **2009**, *20*, 1057–1079. [CrossRef] [PubMed]
24. Yu, S.; Lee, M.; Shin, S.; Park, J. Apoptosis induced by progesterone in human ovarian cancer cell line SNU. *J. Cell. Biochem.* **2001**, *82*, 445–451. [CrossRef] [PubMed]
25. Nilsson, M.E.; Vandenput, L.; Tivesten, Å.; Norlén, A.K.; Lagerquist, M.K.; Windahl, S.H.; Börjesson, A.E.; Farman, H.H.; Poutanen, M.; Benrick, A.; et al. Measurement of a Comprehensive Sex Steroid Profile in Rodent Serum by High-Sensitive Gas Chromatography-Tandem Mass Spectrometry. *Endocrinology* **2015**, *156*, 2492–2502. [CrossRef]
26. Ducharme, N.; Banks, W.A.; Morley, J.E.; Robinson, S.M.; Niehoff, M.L.; Mattern, C.; Farr, S.A. Brain distribution and behavioral effects of progesterone and pregnenolone after intranasal or intravenous administration. *Eur. J. Pharmacol.* **2010**, *641*, 128–134. [CrossRef]

10

Intestinal Permeation Enhancers for Oral Delivery of Macromolecules: A Comparison between Salcaprozate Sodium (SNAC) and Sodium Caprate (C_{10})

Caroline Twarog [1], Sarinj Fattah [1], Joanne Heade [1], Sam Maher [2], Elias Fattal [3] and David J. Brayden [1,*]

1 UCD School of Veterinary Medicine and UCD Conway Institute, University College Dublin, Belfield, Dublin 4, Ireland; caroline.twarog@ucdconnect.ie (C.T.); sarinj.fattah@ucd.ie (S.F.); joanne.heade@ucdconnect.ie (J.H.)

2 School of Pharmacy, Royal College of Surgeons in Ireland, St. Stephen's Green, Dublin 2, Ireland; sammaher@rcsi.ie

3 School of Pharmacy, Institut Galien, CNRS, Univ. Paris-Sud, Univ. Paris-Saclay, 92290 Châtenay-Malabry, France; elias.fattal@u-psud.fr

* Correspondence: david.brayden@ucd.ie

Abstract: Salcaprozate sodium (SNAC) and sodium caprate (C_{10}) are two of the most advanced intestinal permeation enhancers (PEs) that have been tested in clinical trials for oral delivery of macromolecules. Their effects on intestinal epithelia were studied for over 30 years, yet there is still debate over their mechanisms of action. C_{10} acts via openings of epithelial tight junctions and/or membrane perturbation, while for decades SNAC was thought to increase passive transcellular permeation across small intestinal epithelia based on increased lipophilicity arising from non-covalent macromolecule complexation. More recently, an additional mechanism for SNAC associated with a pH-elevating, monomer-inducing, and pepsin-inhibiting effect in the stomach for oral delivery of semaglutide was advocated. Comparing the two surfactants, we found equivocal evidence for discrete mechanisms at the level of epithelial interactions in the small intestine, especially at the high doses used in vivo. Evidence that one agent is more efficacious compared to the other is not convincing, with tablets containing these PEs inducing single-digit highly variable increases in oral bioavailability of payloads in human trials, although this may be adequate for potent macromolecules. Regarding safety, SNAC has generally regarded as safe (GRAS) status and is Food and Drug Administration (FDA)-approved as a medical food (Eligen®-Vitamin B_{12}, Emisphere, Roseland, NJ, USA), whereas C_{10} has a long history of use in man, and has food additive status. Evidence for co-absorption of microorganisms in the presence of either SNAC or C_{10} has not emerged from clinical trials to date, and long-term effects from repeat dosing beyond six months have yet to be assessed. Since there are no obvious scientific reasons to prefer SNAC over C_{10} in orally delivering a poorly permeable macromolecule, then formulation, manufacturing, and commercial considerations are the key drivers in decision-making.

Keywords: oral macromolecule delivery; oral peptides; sodium caprate; salcaprozate sodium; epithelial permeability; epithelial transport

---

1. Introduction

Despite an increasing trend in drug discovery and development in favor of biologics (macromolecules), poor oral availability remains a major impediment to even more widespread application. One group of macromolecules, peptides and proteins, are especially advocated due to excellent specificity, selectivity, safety, and efficacy. Indeed, a combined ~240 were marketed since the 1980s [1]. Of that list, 12% have <60 amino acids, designating approximately 30 peptides from that total [2]. Over 90% of peptides are injectable formulations, with just 4% delivered orally, and even lower percentages delivered via the skin and airway routes [2]. Recent progress was made toward the development of oral formulations for peptides where there are scientific, patient acceptability, and commercial arguments for non-injectable alternatives, especially for those that are used chronically and require frequent dosing (e.g., glucagon-like peptide 1 (GLP-1) analogs) [3]. The oral route offers greater patient compliance and can generate large market sales for molecules working indirectly on the same overall biological target, even if overall efficacy is lower than parenteral options. This is the case for oral dipeptidyl peptidase 4 (DPP-4) small-molecule inhibitors in competition with injectable GLP-1 peptide analogs [4]. Oral administration of peptides is limited by local conditions within the gastro-intestinal (GI) tract except for two relatively low-molecular-weight (LMW) examples designed for systemic delivery: a microemulsion of cyclosporin (Neoral®, Novartis, Switzerland) and a conventional solid-dose formulation of desmopressin (Minirin®, Ferring, USA) [5]. However, these examples are exceptions based on the atypical macrocycle structures of the two peptides, yielding oral bioavailabilities (BA) of 30–40% for lipophilic cyclosporine in Neoral® and just 0.17% for the highly potent hydrophilic desmopressin, Minirin® [6].

2. Challenges for Oral Delivery of Macromolecules

Oral administration of hydrophilic macromolecules with a molecular weight (MW) above 1000 Da remains a challenge due to susceptibility to pH and gastric/small intestinal enzymes, as well as low intestinal epithelial membrane permeability. The low permeability results from minimal passive or carrier-mediated transcellular permeation across phospholipid bilayers, as well as restricted paracellular transport via tight junctions. If they were small molecules, peptides would likely be assigned to Class III of the biopharmaceutics classification system (BCS), typically exhibiting high aqueous solubility (but not always) and low intestinal permeability. It is noteworthy that, even in the example of cyclosporine where the fraction absorbed (f_{abs}) is high, sensitivity to intestinal cytochrome P450 metabolism and P-glycoprotein efflux reduce the BA [7]; its primary problem is intestinal wall metabolism, not permeability. Other variables also impact the feasibility of oral delivery of macromolecules. If the plasma half-life ($t_{\frac{1}{2}}$) is too short, it will not be economically viable to administer a peptide candidate in multiple daily oral doses, where safety, efficacy, and variability issues would also arise. Similarly, a large therapeutic index (TI) is important in the context of selecting potent macromolecules as oral candidates, since efficacy and safety need to be addressed at the low and variable BA values that may be achieved even with successful oral formulations.

Investigators attempted to address pre-systemic degradation and poor permeation in the same formulation. A common approach is to combine peptidase inhibitors with absorption-modifying excipients (AMEs) or chemical permeation enhancers (PEs). These are usually formulated in enteric-coated dosage forms [6], although those formulated with salcaprozate sodium (SNAC), the leading candidate PE of the Eligen® technology (Emisphere, NJ, USA), do not seem to require coating [8]. In addition to avoiding degradation by gastric enzymes and low pH, enteric-coated capsules and tablets avoid dilution and premature release of both PE and macromolecule in the stomach. Furthermore, coatings can assist in promoting co-release of both in high concentrations at the same region to maximize intestinal permeability [9], a formulation goal to maximize payload delivery. Incorporation of PEs in conventional oral dosage forms is considered a relatively basic technology approach to address macromolecule permeability [10]. However, the ease with which PEs can be incorporated into delivery systems without the need for sophisticated and costly formulation made them more commercially attractive compared to, for example, nanotechnology [11] and device-based systems [12]. The majority of formulations currently in clinical trials for oral peptides are, therefore, based on PEs, whereas most nanotechnology and device-based systems remain in preclinical research [6]. This scenario may change if PE-based formulations only prove efficacious and commercially viable for exceptions: highly potent, stable, long-$t_{\frac{1}{2}}$ molecules of relatively low MW, and with a large TI.

3. Intestinal Permeation Enhancers

Numerous compounds including surfactants, bile salts, bacterial toxins, chelating agents, and medium-chain fatty acids (MCFA) proved to be effective PEs for poorly permeable molecules in in vitro and in vivo studies [10,13]. A comprehensive analysis of the majority of intestinal PEs from these classes that are used with peptides is available [10]. PEs that increase permeability across Caco-2 monolayers, isolated intestinal tissue mucosae, and in rodent models may also improve oral BA in humans, but this is not guaranteed since such studies are predominantly based on admixtures with payloads, not oral formulations. Furthermore, scale-up of the final formulation, PE dose, dilution, spreading, and release of both PE and payload during transit in the human GI tract, as well as the influence of enzymes, bile salts, and lipids in human intestinal fluids, must all be taken into account when attempting to make oral BA predictions for humans from preclinical studies. There are currently over 50 clinical trials in which PEs were shown to increase oral absorption of poorly permeable molecules, mostly achieved using surfactants [14]. The most widely tested PEs in these trials include Eligen® carriers, MCFAs, acyl carnitines, bile salts, and ethylenediaminetetraacetic acid (EDTA) [15]. The MCFA, sodium caprate (C_{10}), and the C_8 derivative, salcaprozate sodium (SNAC), are of particular interest as they had over 20 years of development in proprietary delivery platforms and have been tested in human trials more than any other PEs. C_{10} was originally developed as the main component of an oral solid-dosage form (GIPET™, Gastro-Intestinal Permeation Enhancement Technology) by Elan Pharma (Dublin, Ireland), and then, following licensing, by Merrion Pharmaceuticals (Dublin, Ireland) for oral peptide delivery, and by Ionis Pharmaceuticals (Carlsbad, CA, USA) for oral delivery of antisense oligonucleotides. SNAC was developed by Emisphere (NJ, USA) as the lead agent of its Eligen® carrier technology. Novo Nordisk (Bagsværd, Denmark) licensed both GIPET™ and Eligen® to assess with their insulin and GLP-1 analogs, ultimately opting to focus on an SNAC tablet formulation with their highly potent, stable, long-$t_{\frac{1}{2}}$ (160 h) injectable GLP-1 analog, semaglutide, for advanced clinical development, while abandoning GIPET™, along with further attempts to create an oral insulin.

4. Introducing C_{10}

C_{10} is the sodium salt of capric acid, an aliphatic saturated 10-carbon MCFA (Figure 1A). Fatty acids are ubiquitous nutrients liberated in high quantities during digestion of glycerides in the GI tract. They are also present in low mM concentrations in various nutrient sources, including milk. C_{10} is approved as a food additive in both the United States (US) and European Union (EU) and there are no daily limits on consumption; it was recently concluded that its presence in food should have no impact on human health [16]. C_{10} was a component of an approved rectal suppository of ampicillin (Doktacillin®, Meda, Solna, Sweden) [17]. It was since assessed in clinical trials by Merrion Pharma as oral solid-dosage forms (GIPET™) for the delivery of a wide range of poorly permeable actives, including small molecules (e.g., zoledronic acid, alendronate) and macromolecules (insulin, desmopressin, acyline, and antisense oligonucleotides) [18]. C_{10} is a soluble anionic surfactant, sensitive to changes in pH and ionic strength. At pH values 1–3 units below its pKa (~5) in gastric fluid, it exists in the non-ionized, insoluble, and inactive capric acid form. At acidic pH values, the surfactant can reduce surface tension, but does not exhibit detergent action. At pH values 1–3 units above its pKa (i.e., values that typically occur in the small intestine), C_{10} exists in an ionized soluble form with detergent capacity. Like many other efficient detergents, it does not form micelles efficiently owing to repulsion between the charged hydrophilic head groups. The resulting high concentration of free monomeric surfactant enables epithelial plasma membrane interaction and confers a transcellular element to its mode of action. The critical micellar concentration (CMC) value of C_{10}, like other ionizable surfactants, varies depending on the medium composition. Micelles form at lower concentrations in higher-ionic-strength buffers because the counter-ions in media interact closely with anionic head groups. Thus, varying the ionic strength alters the free monomeric concentration of C_{10} in the small intestine.

5. Introducing SNAC

SNAC is a synthetic *N*-acetylated amino-acid derivative of salicylic acid (Figure 1B). It was discovered as part of a screen to identify carrier-based PEs that could "chaperone" poorly permeable payloads across the intestine [19]. The carrier library of over 1500 compounds was collectively termed Eligen®, and it formed the portfolio of Emisphere Technologies. SNAC is the most extensively tested carrier and the only PE approved in an oral formulation designed to improve oral BA, albeit with a small molecule, cyanocobalamin/SNAC [20]. It is important to note that this oral form of vitamin B_{12} was approved under the regulatory pathway for medical foods, which does not have to meet the standards required for drug approvals, although the regulatory requirements for medical foods are still much higher than those of dietary supplements [21]. Emisphere obtained generally recognized as safe (GRAS) status for SNAC, which was a requirement for developing cyanocobalamin/SNAC for the medical food regulatory pathway. Having GRAS status for this PE may have somewhat mitigated some of the perceived risks associated with the oral semaglutide program at Novo Nordisk. In the 1990s, initial focus on SNAC was aimed at developing an oral formulation of the poorly permeable macromolecule, heparin [22]. In other preclinical studies, it also improved intestinal permeation of peptides (salmon calcitonin (sCT) and insulin) [23], along with poorly permeable small molecules (e.g., cromolyn) [24]. SNAC was tested in many formats: taste-masked liquids, tablets, and soft gelatin capsules. Similar to C_{10}, SNAC can be blended with the active pharmaceutical ingredient (API) using conventional processes, which makes manufacturing uncoated oral tablet dosage forms economic and relatively easy to scale.

It remains unclear if the high concentrations of SNAC required to improve small intestinal epithelial permeation relate to membrane perturbation, membrane fluidization, payload solubility changes, or tight junction openings, or whether it is a chaperone system that improves transcellular permeation via hydrophobization of the payload through non-covalent linkages. Of these factors and, unlike C_{10}, there is less direct evidence for tight junction involvement in the mechanism of SNAC than the other factors; hence, its common designation is as a transcellular PE. Common features are that C_{10} and SNAC are weak acids that display amphiphilicity and surface activity. However, there is a structural difference between them arising from the greater distribution of hydrophilic functional groups in the salicylamide region of SNAC, as evident from its higher polar surface area (89.5 Å^2) compared to C_{10} (40.1 Å^2) [25,26]. It follows that the hydrophobic region of SNAC should be less efficient at inserting into phospholipid membranes than C_{10} [27]. This may be one of the reasons why higher concentrations of SNAC than C_{10} are needed to improve permeation.

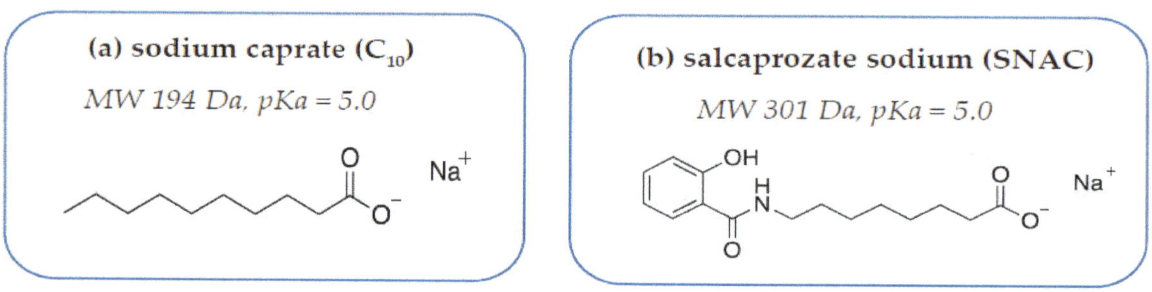

Figure 1. Structures of (**a**) sodium caprate (C_{10}) and (**b**) salcaprozate sodium (SNAC).

6. How Do SNAC and C_{10} Alter GI Permeability?

6.1. Challenges in Determining Mechanism of Action

PEs can improve permeability via a combination of mechanisms. Such mechanisms include opening tight junctions to increase paracellular permeability, decreasing mucus viscosity, inhibition of epithelial efflux pumps, complexation/hydrophobization of payload, increasing membrane fluidity, and (indirectly) via peptidase inhibition. The various mechanisms of action of C_{10} and SNAC were studied using cell biology and physicochemical techniques including membrane fluorescence, Western blotting, electrophoretic mobility, molecular imaging, and physical analysis. More recent approaches to the study of the interactions between PEs and payloads use surface plasmon resonance [28], as well as accelerated capillary electrophoresis, and isothermal titrated calorimetry (ITC) [29]; however, these techniques are mostly restricted to simple physiological buffers rather than bio-relevant intestinal fluids. In particular, a concern is that intricate mechanisms determined in in vitro assays might not reflect the true mechanism, because the PE concentrations used in vitro are typically lower than the efficacious doses used in vivo. There is, therefore, uncertainty regarding the actual local concentrations of PE and payload at the small intestinal epithelial wall in a particular region due to variability in dissolution, spreading, and dilution in the human GI lumen during transit.

6.2. C_{10} Mode of Action

The mode of action of C_{10} was studied at great lengths in a range of delivery models. In summary, concentrations that lead to alteration to permeability coefficients or oral BA are associated with mild mucosal damage and other hallmarks of transcellular perturbation. At low concentrations, increases in permeability of hydrophilic small molecules across Caco-2 monolayers using relatively low concentrations of C_{10} (2.5 mM) can be uncoupled from loss of monolayer integrity, accompanied by reversible reductions in transepithelial electrical potential (TEER) [27,30], indicative of a paracellular mechanism. The higher concentrations required to alter permeability in isolated rat and human intestinal tissue mucosae are associated with transcellular perturbation [31,32]. Mode-of-action studies at higher concentrations (8–13 mM) in Caco-2 monolayers also allude to a paracellular mechanism involving activation of membrane-bound phospholipase C [33–35]. The resulting increase in inositol 1,4,5-triphosphate (IP3) leads to an increase in intracellular calcium (Ca^{2+}), which in turn activates calmodulin and myosin light-chain kinase (MLCK). This event triggers the contraction of the peri-junctional actomyosin ring (PAMR) [36], permitting increased tight junction (TJ) permeability.

Nonetheless, these studies involving pharmacological inhibitors are not definitive proof of a discrete paracellular effect. Impedance spectroscopy in HT29/B6 human intestinal monolayers also supports the dataset showing that C_{10} acts via a paracellular mechanism; this was associated with removal or redistribution of the TJ proteins claudin 5 and tricellulin [37]. However, in the absence of data supporting the absence of transcellular perturbation (a dye uptake assay), the data from this study do not provide conclusive evidence for a paracellular mode of action either. It is impossible to ignore the evidence from a wide range of studies that C_{10} also disrupts cell membranes at 8–13 mM. C_{10} also caused Caco-2 cell leakage of intracellular ATP from Caco-2 cells [33], a likely consequence of plasma membrane perturbation. One interpretation is that cells respond to the initial membrane perturbation challenge by C_{10} with compensating intracellular signaling processes involved in mucosal repair, beginning with disbandment of TJs, and concluded by epithelial resealing [38].

Some of the strongest evidence in favor of a mechanism driven primarily by perturbation, however, comes from high content image analysis in live Caco-2 cells. C_{10} (2.5 mM) increased intracellular Ca^{2+} in Caco-2 cells prior to the plasma membrane permeability changes detected at 8.5 mM [27]. C_{10} (8.5–13 mM) altered both plasma and mitochondrial membrane integrity, indicative of perturbation; importantly, these were the minimum concentrations needed to induce a permeability increase. The elucidation of the primary mode of action as membrane perturbation was clarified by the capacity of C_{10} to preferentially displace claudins 4 and 5 from lipid rafts in MDCK cells, consistent with surfactant properties [39]. Other evidence comes from a recent surfactant screen using isolated rat intestinal mucosae in Ussing chambers, where C_{10} caused a concentration-dependent increase in epithelial histology damage [40]. Given the close association between permeation enhancement and mucosal perturbation in tissue and animal models, it was, therefore, not surprising that the cyto-protectant prostaglandin analog, misoprostol, prevented both the C_{10}-induced increase in flux of hydrophilic markers across Caco-2 monolayers and cell damage [41]. From these arguments, it is likely that the high concentrations of C_{10} used in tablets also cause a degree of mild reversible mucosal perturbation in vivo, not unlike that seen with aspirin, alcohol, and spicy foods [42]. In a study of a human rectal formulation of ampicillin with C_{10}, there was evidence of mild and reversible mucosal perturbation [17], although the data were confounded by the hyper-osmolarity of the formulation. While it is not possible to conclude that mucosal perturbation of the relatively static rectal mucosal compartment extrapolates directly to the small intestine where transit is relatively fast, it is likely that C_{10} causes mild and reversible regional perturbation within a short period at the high concentrations exposed to the small intestinal epithelium prior to its almost complete absorption within minutes.

There is a lack of understanding of the physicochemical aspects of how C_{10} interacts with mixed micelles in the small intestine in the fasted and fed states. Above its CMC of 25 mM in physiological buffer [27], C_{10} forms micelles and there is a distinct ratio of monomer to micellar-bound material, as highlighted in a recent study on alkyl maltosides [43]. In simulated intestinal buffers, it is uncertain whether the payload is incorporated into or adsorbs onto colloidal structures (e.g., mixed micelles, vesicles, lipid droplets), or whether it admixes with the C_{10} monomer. There is resulting confusion over which format the payload permeates. Thus, while one envisages a paracellular permeation route for polar macromolecules due to hydrophilicity, a transcellular pathway may also be available if C_{10}-entrapped vesicles and mixed micelles adsorb payload. Figure 2 is a composite of the possible multiple effects of C_{10} on intestinal epithelia.

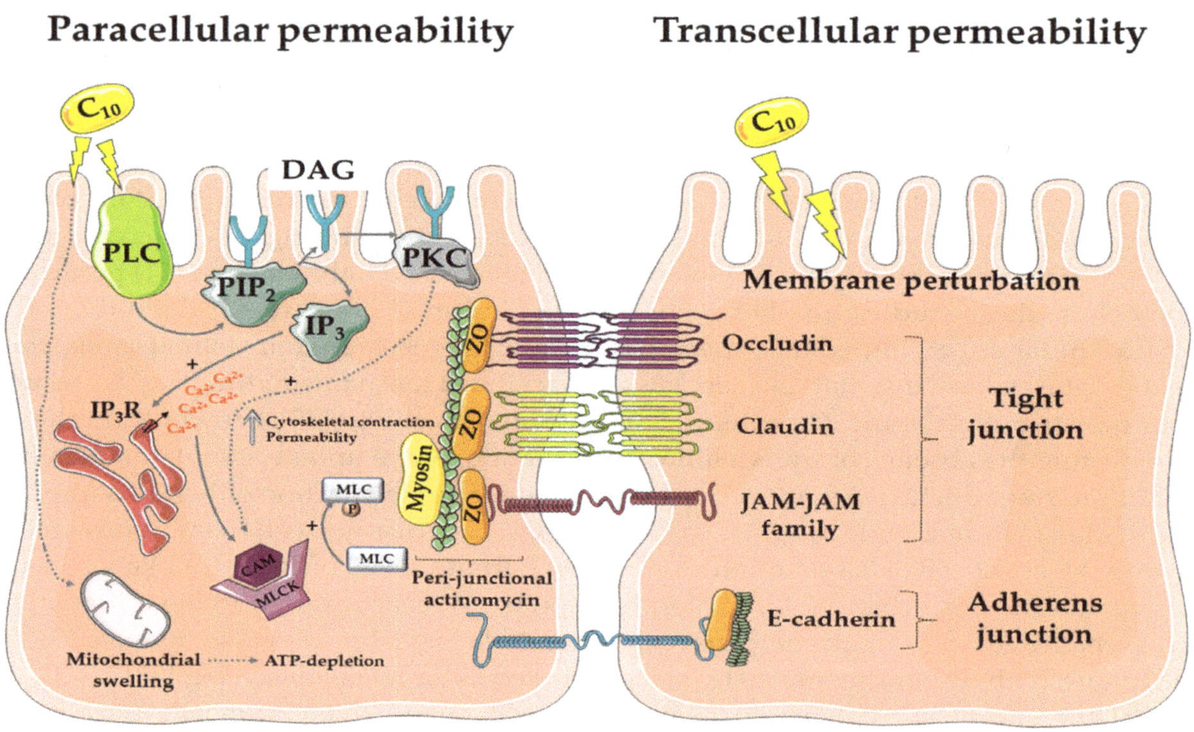

Figure 2. Mode of action of C_{10}. The diagram represents the proposed mechanism of action of C_{10} via paracellular flux (**left**) and transcellular perturbation (**right**) to induce drug permeability across the intestinal mucosa. Abbreviations: PLC: phospholipase C; PIP_2: phosphatidylinositol 4,5-bisphosphate; DAG: di-acyl glycerol; PKC: protein kinase C; IP_3R: inositol triphosphate receptor; MLC: myosin light chain, CAM: calmodulin; ZO: zonula occludens; JAM: junctional adhesion molecule. Image created using a template from Servier Medical Art under a Creative Commons Attribution License.

6.3. SNAC Mode of Action

A different mode of action to that of C_{10} was proposed to explain how SNAC improves intestinal permeability. In the 1990s, Emisphere scientists proposed that SNAC improves passive transcellular permeation via hydrophobization. The hypothesis was that dipole–dipole non-covalent interaction between the carrier and structural moieties of the payload caused a conformational change in the latter, leading to exposure of hydrophobic regions that favor transcellular permeation. The interaction between SNAC and heparin [22,44] and with insulin [45] was, therefore, thought to be based on increased lipophilicity through hydrogen bonding and/or hydrophobic interactions, permitting dissolution of the complex in lipid bilayers. In support of this hypothesis, SNAC at a concentration of 17 mg/mL improved the permeation of insulin, but not that of radiolabeled mannitol across Caco-2 monolayers, suggesting that the effect was neither related to opening tight junctions nor to a decline in barrier integrity, and this interpretation was supported by confocal microscopy [45]. Higher concentrations of SNAC (50 mg/mL) that were more reflective of concentrations used in in vivo studies, however, caused complete loss of TEER and a 36-fold increase in [^{3}H]-mannitol permeability in Caco-2 monolayers [44], data that do not permit definitive conclusions to be made regarding mechanism since such high concentrations compromised the Caco-2 model. In isolated rat jejunal mucosae mounted in Ussing chambers, SNAC (33–66 mM) boosted the flux of a polar marker molecule, 6-carboxy-fluorescein (6-CF), but not that of [^{3}H]-mannitol across the epithelium and without reducing TEER values [46]. The authors argued that SNAC was indeed exploiting a transcellular pathway and not tight junctions to allow permeation of the hydrophilic polar ionized molecule (6-CF) and, somewhat controversially, they suggested that SNAC was reducing the charge on CF, thereby improving the capacity to partition in the epithelium. Similar to the Caco-2 study [44], when SNAC was added to jejunal mucosae at a concentration of 165 mM, TEER dropped and the permeability coefficient (Papp) of [^{3}H]-mannitol was increased [46], denoting a compromising event. Other Caco-2 studies also support a transcellular mechanism; Malkov et al. [47] detected intracellular signal increases ascribed to fluorescently labeled heparin and in the presence of SNAC, whereas immunohistochemistry data indicated that there were no changes of F-actin or the actinomycin ring during heparin flux. Ding et al. [48] used ITC and Fourier-transform infrared (FTIR) spectroscopy to study the interaction between cromolyn and SNAC, and concluded that the aromatic ring of SNAC inserted between those of cromolyn via its 2-hydroxybenzamide motif, leading to an increase in hydrophobicity of the complex and a reduction in cromolyn hydration. Lactate hydrogenase release (LDH) measurements indicated that the increased cromolyn fluxes across Caco-2 monolayers in the presence of SNAC were not associated with cell damage.

Despite the elegance of the purported complex mechanism (Figure 3) of how SNAC might increase transcellular flux of multiple payloads, the hypothesis is problematic in several respects. If Eligen® carriers acted solely using dipole–dipole interactions via hydrophobization (and not an electrostatic interaction), it would be difficult to envisage a significant increase in passive permeation since the retention of ionized functional groups would impede passive movement across phospholipid bilayers.

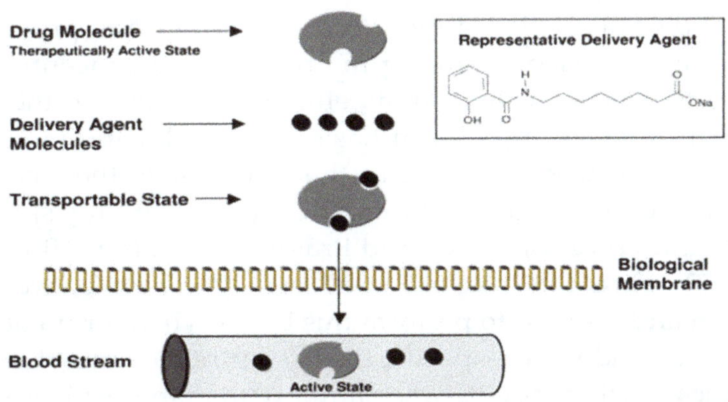

Figure 3. Schematic of Eligen® drug-delivery technology mechanism in intestinal epithelia, as advocated by Emisphere scientists in 2006. "Carrier molecule (delivery agent) associates with drug molecule to create a transportable complex (lipophilic). Because of the weak association, carrier and drug dissociate by simple dilution on entering the blood circulation." Reproduced from Reference [49] under the terms of the Creative Commons Attribution License.

SNAC forms a conjugate base at the pH of the small intestinal lumen, so it can undergo complexation via hydrophobic ion pairing (HIP) with the conjugate acid of basic amino-acid side chains in macromolecules. However, HIP cannot fully account for Eligen®-mediated hydrophobization of anionic payloads including heparin and cromolyn [24]. An alternative interpretation arises from another SNAC study with cromolyn; SNAC increased Caco-2 epithelial cell membrane fluidity as measured by fluorescence anisotropy, consistent with a surfactant-induced membrane perturbation effect, whereas in this study there was no increase in cromolyn's lipophilicity [50]. Still, the overall contribution of transcellular perturbation to the increased flux is not clear since the presence of hydrophilic functional groups in the salicylamide region of SNAC gives rise to inefficient micelle formation (CMC: 56 mM in phosphate-buffered saline (PBS)) [50], and this will not favor membrane insertion. There are a number of other anomalies concerning the original chaperone transcellular mechanism proposed for SNAC (reviewed in Reference [49]). Firstly, since the structure of SNAC comprises MCFA and salicylic-acid moieties, non-specific detergent/surfactant effects on the epithelium should be expected. Secondly, the thermodynamic considerations with respect to the non-covalent linkage between SNAC and payload during epithelial flux are yet to be addressed. Furthermore, there were no calculations on the affinity of SNAC to payloads, except to assert that affinity was weak, now confirmed for exenatide [29]. Thirdly, a transcellular mechanism should account for epithelial endocytosis uptake pathways (e.g., via clathrin- or caveolae-mediated pathways or macropinocytosis), where a template to follow is in place for the other group of transcellular permeability-enhancing agents, the cell-penetrating peptides [51]. Finally, caution must be exercised in making definitive conclusions on mechanism using some of these assays; epithelial TEER values yield information on monolayer integrity, but reveal no direct information about tight junctions. Secondly, the absence of changes in tight-junction-associated antibody imaging for associated proteins is not definitive. Thirdly, fluorescently labeled payloads need to be assessed for their capacity to remain intact during flux. Finally, LDH release from monolayers following exposure to SNAC would not be regarded as a particularly sensitive assay, especially when increased membrane fluidization was observed. In sum, evidence from Caco-2 studies is not yet convincing enough to solely ascribe an exclusive transcellular mechanism for SNAC; moreover, there is little data to directly support the chaperone hypothesis. On the other hand, there are some differences between the mechanism of action of SNAC and those of PEs with mechanisms associated with tight-junction openings (e.g., EDTA).

Recently, Novo Nordisk offered a new mechanism of action for SNAC in its non-enteric coated tablet of the GLP-1 analog, semaglutide ($t_{\frac{1}{2}}$ = 160 h). Using a ligated dog model, they found that systemic delivery was achieved solely from stomach administration of the tablet [52]. The theory is that SNAC forms a complex around the semaglutide in the stomach and causes a transient increase in local pH around the molecule. It is claimed that semaglutide is protected against pepsin by SNAC and that solubility is increased, resulting in an increased concentration-dependent flux of semaglutide across the gastric mucosa, using a transcellular mechanism as the tablet comes in intimate contact with the epithelium. By shifting the emphasis toward elevation in stomach pH away from conformational changes and increased lipophilicity, the theory takes the focus away from membrane perturbation. Moreover, the authors argue that this mechanism is highly specific for semaglutide, in that similar studies with admixtures of SNAC and liraglutide led to no flux increase across in vitro gastric epithelial models [52]. Part of the role of SNAC seemed to be to convert semaglutide to a more permeable monomeric form and it seems to perform this better when formulated in a stomach-specific tablet. Is this payload-specific and region-specific theory entirely compatible with the previous data from small intestinal studies in which SNAC was paired with many payloads of differing structures? With new cell-imaging tools available, along with advanced biophysical methods to decipher the interaction between SNAC and payloads, it is likely that much of the discrepancy surrounding the mechanism of SNAC will be resolved. Figure 4 is a composite of the possible effects that SNAC has in the stomach when formulated with semaglutide.

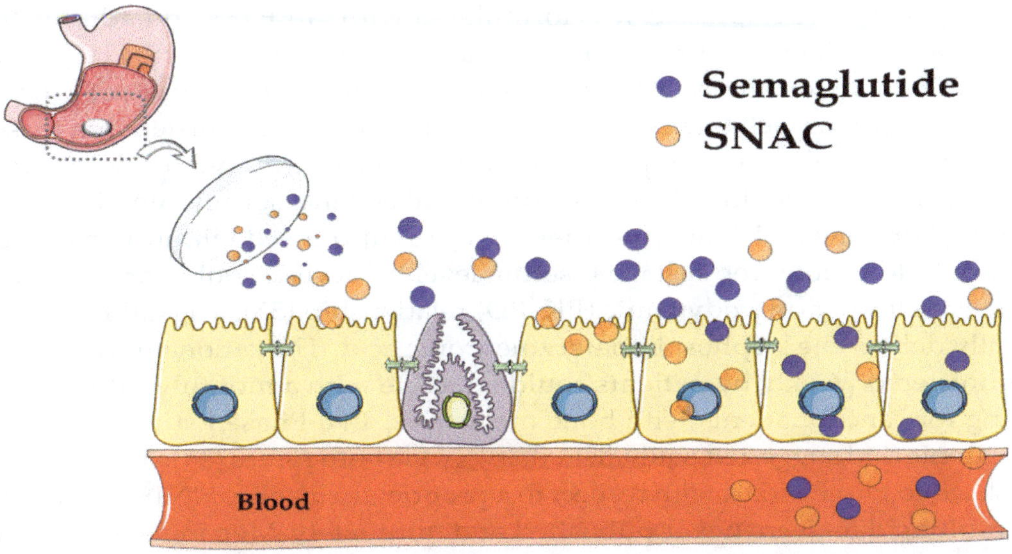

Figure 4. Theory of oral semaglutide absorption, as advocated by Novo Nordisk. Modified from Reference [52]. The diagram represents the proposed mechanism of action of SNAC in inducing transcellular flux of semaglutide across the gastric epithelium of the stomach. The optimum once-daily tablet consists of 14 mg of semaglutide co-formulated with 300 mg of SNAC. After digestion, the tablet erodes rapidly in the stomach, resulting in the release of a highly concentrated amount of SNAC that neutralizes the pH of gastric fluid in the immediate vicinity of the tablet to inactivate pepsin. SNAC is thought to induce semaglutide monomer production and increase gastric epithelial membrane fluidity, but without affecting tight junctions, thereby allowing transcellular passage of semaglutide into systemic circulation. The complex may dissociate at some point in the flux process (Figure 3) due to weak association, but direct evidence for this is scant. Black circles = semaglutide; white circles = SNAC. Image made using a template from Servier Medical Art under a Creative Commons Attribution License.

In sum, the in vitro studies on the mechanism of action of the two agents on cultured intestinal epithelia suggest some common surfactant-based features; however, in contrast to SNAC, there is direct evidence for tight-junction openings induced by C_{10}. The culture models are sub-optimal, however, as they do not discriminate permeation enhancement from perturbation very well, nor do they predict in vivo consequences; the models have difficulty in tolerating both high concentrations of PEs and simulated intestinal fluids.

7. C_{10} and SNAC: Pharmacokinetics and Efficacy in Clinical Trials

7.1. C_{10}

GIPET™ was advanced to clinical testing as enteric-coated tablets containing C_{10} with both peptide and small-molecule payloads [18,42]. Human studies using radiolabeled polyethylene glyol (PEG) revealed that the permeating enhancement effects of GIPET™ were transient and reversible in <1 h [18]. GIPET™ was tested in a range of doses with several poorly absorbed molecules in a total of 16 Phase I studies comprising over 300 subjects [18]. Overall, while oral BA values of >5% were cited for some molecules, the most notable feature was the massive intra-subject variability across all studies, constituting an issue for safety and efficacy.

Pharmacokinetics (PK) analysis of human trials for GIPET™ formulations with low-molecular-weight heparin (LMWH) and desmopressin was described [18]. LMWH–GIPET™ was formulated in tablets containing either 45,000 or 90,000 IU of LMWH at two dose levels of C_{10}. Oral BA was calculated relative to the standard sub-cutaneous (s.c.) dose of 3200 IU following administration to 14–16 subjects. Relative oral BA of 3.9–7.6% was achieved [18]. With a high dose of LMWH combined with a high dose of C_{10}, increased levels of an anti-clotting biomarker were seen in all subjects; the responses were sustained and had a similar time course to the s.c. route. This particular formulation was not progressed clinically (Table 1). When desmopressin was formulated with GIPET™ and administered orally to 18 human subjects, a bioavailability of 2.4% relative to the s.c. route was detected [18], an improvement over the typical 0.2% value for Minirin® tablets. Again, this formulation was not progressed further. The GIPET™ technology was well tolerated even when repeatedly administered in these small Phase I studies [18]. Other clinical trial examples include the gonadotropin-releasing hormone (GnRH) antagonist decapeptide, acyline. In a Phase I study of oral acyline, serum luteinizing hormone (LH), follicle-stimulating hormone (FSH), and testosterone were suppressed within 12 h at the 10-, 20-, and 40-mg single doses tested. However, sustained serum levels of acyline could not be detected, and there was no pharmacokinetic–pharmacodynamic (PK–PD) relationship [53]. The GIPET™ technology was also used to orally deliver the bisphosphonate, zoledronic acid. The rationale was that an oral tablet (Orazol™) administered weekly by patients could compete with a monthly infusion of Zometa® in a hospital setting for cancer patients with bone metastasis. In a Phase I study, urinary excretion of unchanged zoledronic acid suggested equivalent delivery via both routes [54]. The licensing of GIPET™ to Novo Nordisk led to Phase I trials with respect to a proprietary insulin, NN1953, and a GLP-1 analog; however, the resulting data were never published and, ultimately, Merrion's remaining intellectual property (IP) assets were sold to Novo Nordisk, before being liquidated in 2016. Novo Nordisk in turn decided to move away from developing oral insulin to concentrate on its oral GLP-1 analog program. Nonetheless, an important Phase II trial from that time assessing a once-daily long-acting basal insulin (I338) with a $t\frac{1}{2}$ of 70 h in a GIPET™ formulation was published in 2019 by Novo Nordisk [55]. In this study, a relative oral F versus the long-acting s.c.-administered insulin glargine (Lantus®, Sanofi, Paris) of 1.5–2.0% was achieved without evidence of toxicity over eight weeks. Although similar plasma glucose reduction was achieved by the oral GIPET™-based formulation to the s.c. insulin, the rationale for discontinuation was that the dose of I338 was not commercially viable. The GIPET™ journey with oral peptides and poorly permeable small molecules, therefore, ended without generating a product in 2015. As a post-script, a Phase I study was published in 2018 by Biocon (India) in which a C_{10}-based formulation of their alkylated PEGylated fast-acting meal-time insulin (IN-105; Insulin Tregopil) was shown to have no effect on the PK of oral metformin in fasted conditions and it was well tolerated [56]. Therefore, C_{10} continues to be used in oral peptide formulations both in clinical trials and as a comparator for other PEs in preclinical studies.

The other arm of the original Elan licensing of C_{10}-based matrix tablets in the late 1990s continued in parallel with respect to antisense oligonucleotides. The gene medicine specialty Pharma, Ionis Pharmaceuticals (Carlsbad, CA, USA) (formerly Isis Pharma) developed a number of oral antisense oligonucleotide formulations containing C_{10} for clinical testing against RNA targets. One candidate that progressed to Phase I was ISIS 104838, a tumor necrosis factor (TNF)-α inhibitor. Oral administration of a C_{10}-based tablet to dogs resulted in average absolute oral BA of 1.4% [57]. Tissue histology of the small intestine and large intestine of the dogs indicated no changes following once-daily dosing of tablets containing ~1 g of C_{10} over seven consecutive days. A subsequent Phase I trial examined ISIS 104838 (100 or 140 mg) formulated with C_{10} (660 mg) in immediate-release mini-tablets packaged in enteric-coated gelatin capsules, with or without a second mini-tablet containing only C_{10}. The second group of mini-tablets was coated with different layers of Eudragit® RS30D to allow for subsequent further release of the C_{10} following erosion of the first tablet containing ISIS 104838 [58]. The goal was to create a greater window for absorption by prolonging the time C_{10} was in contact with the epithelium, given that it is rapidly absorbed with a T_{max} of 7 min. All formulations together yielded an average oral BA of 9.5% relative to s.c. injection, with the formulation designed for additional immediate release of C_{10} giving a value of 12%; however, the intra-subject variability ranged from 2–28% [58]. In 2017, Ionis advanced an oral antisense molecule IONIS-JBI1-2.5Rx, aimed at an RNA target associated with a GI autoimmune disorder, to Phase I trials in collaboration with Janssen (Beerse, Belgium) [59]; however, it is unlikely that the formulation contains C_{10} as it is designed for local colonic delivery. Table 1 summarizes the clinical data reported for a range of poorly permeable molecules with C_{10}. Of these, there are only four peer-reviewed original research papers for GIPET™ tablets.

Table 1. Summary of data from selected studies in humans reported for a range of poorly permeable molecules formulated with sodium caprate (C_{10}).

Description	Treatment	Outcome	Reference
Ampicillin with C_{10} in healthy subjects (n = 12).	Rectal suppository containing 250 mg of ampicillin and 25 mg of C_{10}.	C_{max} increased 2.6-fold compared to ampicillin alone and BA increased 1.8-fold. Some local tissue damage not ascribed to C_{10}.	[17]
Phenoxymethylpenicillin, antipyrine with C_{10} in healthy subjects (n = 6).	Rectal perfusion containing 2 g of phenoxymethylpenicillin, 8 mg of antipyrine, and 0.7 g of C_{10}. Two treatments (T), T1: pH 6 and T2: pH 7.4. Each subject received control (no C_{10}) and treatment.	C_{10} was ineffective at increasing permeability across rectal epithelium.	[60]
GIPET™: oral acyline in healthy subjects (n = 8).	3 oral tablet doses of acyline: 10, 20, and 40 mg. Subjects received all doses, 1 week apart, under fasting conditions.	Significant reduction in LH, FSH, and testosterone. No serious treatment related adverse effects.	[53]
GIPET™: oral zoledronic acid in prostate cancer patients with bone metastasis (n = 30).	Once-weekly enteric-coated Orazol™ tablets containing 20 mg of zoledronic acid versus weekly Zometa® (4 mg) i.v. infusion over 49 days.	Equivalent urine output biomarkers; claim of 5% bioavailability (BA) in patent.	[54]
Antisense oligonucleotide with C_{10} (ISIS 104838) in healthy subjects (n = 15).	Enteric-coated tablets, four formulations, and one after a high-fat meal. Subjects received all treatments.	9.5% bioavailability compared to s.c. No study-related adverse effects.	[58]
Basal insulin in C_{10} formulation versus insulin glargine in Type 2 diabetics (s.c.) (n = 25).	Daily tablets of a long-acting insulin (I338) over 8 weeks.	1.5–2.0% bioavailability compared to s.c. Comparable reductions in plasma glucose.	[55]
Insulin tregopil (IN-105) in C_{10} tablets in healthy subjects.	Single treatments of insulin along with metoformin over 4 periods of 2 days.	No effects on the pharmacokinetics (PK) of metformin; good safety.	[56]

LH, luteinizing hormone; FSH, follicle-stimulating hormone; s.c., sub-cutaneous; i.v., intravenous. The Phase II study [55] is the most comprehensive of these studies.

7.2. SNAC

SNAC was in a succession of clinical trials in oral formulations with poorly permeable actives since the late 1990s, culminating with approval for cyanocobalamin as a medical food for vitamin B_{12}-deficient anemic subjects in 2014 [20,21]. The initial clinical trials were carried out using unfractionated heparin in 1998 [61]. In the first Phase I study, 2.25 g of taste-masked SNAC was combined with 30,000–150,000 IU of heparin and administered to subjects via gavage; the formulation achieved increases in outputs associated with anti-coagulation efficacy: activated partial thromboplastin time (aPTT) and production of anti-factor Xa. This led to subsequent Phase I and II trials with taste-masked 10–15-mL liquid formulations in patients undergoing total hip replacements; oral heparin was dosed at either 60,000 or 90,000 IU with 1.5 or 2.25 g of SNAC respectively, and results were compared to s.c. administration of 5000 IU of heparin [62]. The oral dosing regimen comprised 12–16 doses over a four-day period after surgery. Data from the second Phase I study showed that the oral heparin liquid formulation induced anti-factor Xa activity similar to s.c. heparin. In the Phase II trial, major bleeding events were similar between oral and s.c. heparin groups, thereby offering encouragement on the safety front. In 2002, the oral liquid heparin formulation ultimately missed its primary efficacy end-point in a Phase III trial (PROTECT) comparing oral heparin (either 60,000 IU/1.5 g SNAC or 90,000 IU/2.25 g SNAC three times a day) to s.c. LMWH (enoxaparin) over a 30-day period with assessment for deep vein thrombosis as the read-out. The study comprised over 2000 patients undergoing elective hip replacement, a study that was associated with poor compliance due to the bitter taste of the solution [49]. Direct leveraging from a taste-masked drink to a solid dosage form was not possible, due to the high quantities of SNAC and heparin. Subsequently, a new Phase I PK–PD study was eventually carried out in 2007 in 16 subjects receiving a 75,000 IU heparin/500 mg

SNAC total dose in soft gel capsules [63]. It confirmed the effect on aPTT and the orally delivered heparin had a C_{max} of 58 min. Ultimately, a solid dose formulation of oral heparin/SNAC never reached Phase III and was abandoned, perhaps in part because of the advantages of LMWH over unfractionated heparin, as well as the advent of alternative oral anti-thrombotics.

In relation to other payloads and Eligen® carriers, a caprylic-acid derivative, possibly SNAC, was also formulated with sCT, and a Phase I study in eight volunteers was published in 2002, with a comprehensive analysis of PK [64]. This benchmark study described tablets of 0.4 mg of sCT with 225 mg of SNAC that were dosed singly, in duplicate, or in triplicate to present individual doses of 0.4, 0.8, and 1.2 mg of sCT. The resulting absolute oral BA values versus an intravenous (i.v.) dose of 10 μg ranged from 0.5–1.4%. An Eligen® formulation of insulin was also assessed in a 2010 trial in 14 Type 2 diabetics (T2D) where the carrier was monosodium *N*-(4-chlorosalicyloyl)-4-aminobutyrate (4-CNAB). An oral BA of 7 ± 4% was achieved from a 300-IU dose (with 200–400 mg of 4-CNAB) versus an s.c. dose of 15 IU in fasting subjects [65]. Such large variability would not be acceptable for this low-therapeutic-index drug. A third related Eligen® carrier, 8-(*N*-2-hydroxy-5-chloro-benzoyl)-amino-caprylic acid (5-CNAC), was also evaluated by Novartis (Switzerland) and Nordic Biosciences (Herlev, Denmark) in three large Phase III trials for oral sCT: two for osteoarthritis [66] (NCT00486434 and NCT00704847) and one for osteoporosis [67] (NCT00525798). The dosing to several thousand patients across the three trials comprised one tablet (0.8 mg sCT with 200 mg of 5-CNAC) in a tablet administered twice a day with 50 mL of water approximately 30 min ahead of meals. These studies lasted 24 months for the osteoarthritis trials and 36 months for the osteoporosis trial. Although these trials missed their primary efficacy end-points, interesting assessments concerning dosing formats and regimes were published with conclusions that may have relevance for SNAC trials [68]. Differences in sCT absorption and effects on bone biomarkers occurred depending on the volume of water, proximity to a meal, and the time of day (reflecting circadian rhythms in bone turnover). Table 2 summarizes the clinical trial performance of oral SNAC and related Emisphere carrier formulations across a range of poorly permeable molecules.

Table 2. Summary of data from selected studies in humans reported for a range of poorly permeable molecules formulated with either salcaprozate sodium (SNAC), monosodium *N*-(4-chlorosalicyloyl)-4-aminobutyrate (4-CNAB), or 8-(*N*-2-hydroxy-5-chloro-benzoyl)-amino-caprylic acid (5-CNAC). T2D—type 2 diabetes; sCT—salmon calcitonin.

Description	Treatment	Outcome	Reference
Vitamin B_{12} with SNAC in tablets in healthy subjects (n = 20). Medical food clinical study.	(A) Two tablets, each with 5 mg of vitamin B_{12} with 100 mg of SNAC (B) One tablet: 5 mg of vitamin B_{12} with 100 mg of SNAC (C) One commercial tablet: 5 mg of vitamin B_{12} (D) 1 mg of vitamin B_{12} via i.v. injection.	Treatment (B) achieved 3% higher absolute BA compared to the commercial oral formulation. No adverse effects.	[20]
Heparin with SNAC in hip replacement patients, (n = 123). Phase II.	Two studies: one dose every 8 h (max 16 doses), and two doses every 8 h (max 12 doses).	Achieved anti-factor Xa activity comparable to s.c. heparin. No change in major bleeding events compared to s.c.	[62]
Insulin with 4-CNAB in untreated T2D (n = 10). Phase II.	300 mg of insulin with 400 mg of 4-CNAB, or 15 IU of insulin s.c. Performed under fasting conditions.	C_{max} was higher and was reached faster compared to s.c. Shorter duration and high subject variability. No adverse effects.	[65]
sCT with 5-CNAC in osteoarthritic patients over 24 months (n = 1176 and n = 1030) Phase III.	0.8 mg of sCT in tablets twice daily for 24 months.	No significant effect compared to placebo.	[66]
sCT with 5-CNAC in postmenopausal women with osteoporosis (n = 4665). Phase III.	0.8 mg or placebo in tablets daily, together with vitamin D and calcium for 36 months.	No beneficial effect on fractures was observed. No change in quality of life.	[6]

Recent focus, however, shifted entirely to the clinical development of the oral semaglutide/SNAC tablet by Novo Nordisk. Once-daily oral semaglutide with 300 mg of SNAC resulted in improved glycemic control and greater reductions in body weight than placebo in a 26-week Phase II dose-escalation study in doses ranging from 2.5–40 mg of semaglutide per day in over 600 patients with T2D [69]. Daily oral administration of semaglutide (20 mg and 40 mg) with SNAC lowered glycated hemoglobin (HbA1c) by over 1.4% and these data were comparable with that seen with weekly s.c. administration of semaglutide (1 mg). For oral semaglutide with SNAC, the oral BA is likely to be ~1%, although the focus of the publications was on the PD effect and biomarkers. Clues come from Beagle dog studies where tablets containing 300 mg of SNAC with 5–20 mg of semaglutide gave oral BA values of 1.22 ± 0.25% following oral administration [52,70]. Novo Nordisk completed ten Phase IIIa PIONEER trials in 2018. Top-line data from PIONEER 1 achieved significance with respect to a reduction in HbA1c of 1.5% with a 14-mg semaglutide dose in T2D, along with evidence of some weight loss [71]. Recent trials also revealed that renal impairment did not affect PK parameters of 5 mg and 10 mg of semaglutide formulated with 300 mg of SNAC over a short time frame in diabetics [72]. This design was repeated in diabetic patients with hepatic impairment with the same outcome in that PK values were not altered and, therefore, no dose adjustment was needed in these patients [73]. The question of the impact of omeprazole on PK was also assessed, as elevation of bulk stomach pH might have confounded the purported mechanism of SNAC. Using a 5-mg semaglutide dose in patients taking 40 mg of omeprazole over a 10-day period with a follow-up period out to 21 days, overall PK values for both semaglutide and SNAC were unchanged, leading to a conclusion that dose adjustment would be also unnecessary in patients on concomitant omeprazole [74]. The implications of these findings would support the determination that the pH increase created by SNAC in the stomach must be at the semaglutide tablet surface [52] and does not impact bulk stomach pH; otherwise, a large effect of omeprazole on PK would have been expected. The PIONEER 6 Phase III study enrolled diabetics with cardiovascular disease in order to exam oral semaglutide PK and PD in this cohort to see if the daily 14-mg formulation increases cardiovascular risk [75]. Selected oral semaglutide clinical data are summarized in Table 3. It will be interesting to examine patient compliance with the current rather inconvenient dosing regime, especially in post-marketing studies if oral semaglutide is approved, since the daily tablet must be taken at least 30 min before meals in the morning in order to avoid food interference with formulation performance.

Table 3. Selected clinical trial data with an emphasis on peer-reviewed literature from the daily semaglutide/SNAC oral tablet formulation from Novo Nordisk in T2D patients.

Description	Parameters	Comment	Reference
Phase II dose-ranging 26-week study in patients (*n* = 632) (NCT01923181).	0.7–1.9% reduction in glycated hemoglobin (HbA1c); some weight reduction; mild gastro-intestinal (GI) side effects common.	The key trial which supported moving to Phase III.	[69]
PIONEER-1 Phase IIIa 26-week study in patients (*n* = 703) (NCT02906930).	Mean 1.5% reduction in HbA1c confirmed with 14-mg dose; 4.1-kg weight reduction; mild–moderate nausea in 16% versus 6% in placebo.	14 mg established as semaglutide dose with 300 mg of SNAC in all studies.	[71]
PIONEER 5 Phase IIIa in renal-impaired patients (*n* = 71) (NCT02014259).	5 mg of semaglutide for 5 days; 10 mg for 5 days, assessed up to 21 days after; no change in PK overall.	Area under curve (AUC) and half-life ($t_{\frac{1}{2}}$) similar to regular T2D patients, no need to change dose regime.	[72]
Trial in hepatic-impaired patients (*n* = 56) (NCT02016911).	Design as for PIONEER-5.	AUC, C_{max}, and $t_{\frac{1}{2}}$ unchanged, no need to change in dose regime.	[73]

Table 3. *Cont.*

Description	Parameters	Comment	Reference
Trial in healthy subjects [1] taking omeprazole (n = 54) (NCT02249871).	5 mg for 5 days, followed by 10 mg for 5 days) ± 40 mg omeprazole.	AUC and stomach pH slightly higher in semaglutide/omeprazole group, but no need to change dose regime.	[74]
PIONEER-6 Phase IIIa assessed cardiovascular (CV) risk in T2D patients (n = 3183) (NCT02692716).	Primary end-points: reduction in major CV events over median 16-month period.	Cardiovascular (CV) outcomes not different from placebo, but suggestion of a mortality benefit of oral tablet.	[75]

[1.] All studies in T2D patients except for the omeprazole study. [2.] PIONEER Phase III 10 study designs are available at https://pharmaintelligence.informa.com/resources/product-content/novos-oral-semaglutide-passes-pioneer-2-but-weight-loss-result-a-bit-disappointing (accessed 12 February 2019). Details of all oral semaglutide trials are available at www.clinicaltrials.gov.

8. Safety of SNAC and C_{10} in Preclinical and Clinical Studies

Although C_{10} was previously marketed in a rectal product, this has limited relevance to the safety of an orally delivered tablet formulation. The approval of SNAC in an oral vitamin-B_{12} medical food product, though encouraging, is also only partially informative. Nonetheless, the clinical trial experience with both PEs in hundreds of subjects over more than 20 years suggest that only very low numbers of subjects experienced side-effects that caused drop out from trials, and the majority of reports were related to mild GI effects including nausea and diarrhea for GIPET™ [18,42] and SNAC [69]. Reversibility studies performed with C_{10} in humans using the lactulose:mannitol urinary excretion ratio (LMER) assay showed that, following intra-jejunal administration to human subjects, the enhancer only increased permeability in a 20-min window [42]. It seems that dilution, spreading, and rapid intestinal absorption of both C_{10} and SNAC prevents prolonged exposure in vivo. There is no direct evidence, even from studies with a duration as long as six months, that stomach or duodenal ulcers are caused by these PEs, nor that pathogens can gain entry across a compromised intestinal epithelium. Still, post-marketing surveillance will provide more safety data in the context of daily administration over several years, at least in the case of SNAC with both vitamin B_{12} and semaglutide in the event of Food and Drug Administration (FDA) approval. Additional safety experience for SNAC will be ascertained from extensive Phase III oral semaglutide trials, which will fully report in 2019.

In terms of preclinical safety data, the experience for both molecules is extensive. Numerous studies reveal little toxicity of high doses of C_{10} in rats, dogs, and pigs following oral administration alone and in combination with payloads [18,42,76]. In a study of the acute effects of a C_{10}-based dosage form (Orasense™) in Beagles, Raoof et al. provided evidence of the safety of oral hydroxypropyl methyl cellulose-coated C_{10}/antisense tablets [57]. Several hundred milligrams of C_{10} were used in each tablet and dogs received treatment three times per day for seven days. Clinical chemistry and blood biochemistry parameters were normal; the dogs tolerated the formulation and there was normal weight gain. Canine intestinal issues were also adjudged normal following macroscopic examination post mortem. Five separate canine daily tolerance studies revealed encouraging safety data for selected components of the GIPET I and II technology [42]. Similar studies were also carried out intra-intestinal catheterized pigs where C_{10} was formulated with antisense oligonucleotides at doses up to 100 mg/kg of the MCFA; it was well tolerated following multiple doses and with little evidence of intestinal epithelial damage post mortem [77].

For SNAC, Riley et al. carried out a sub-chronic oral toxicity test of SNAC in rats and found a no observed adverse effect (NOAEL) level of 1 g/kg/day in rats for up to 13 weeks; it was only a massive dose of 2 g/kg/day that eventually caused significant mortality [78]. It was also examined for gestational toxicity in pregnant rats at oral doses up to 1 g/kg/day where slight weight loss was seen; there was no effect on growth of pups, but some evidence of a small increase in the still-birth rate was noted [79]. Some GI effects including emesis and diarrhea were observed in studies involving monkeys at a dose of $\geq$1.8 g/kg/day [80]. SNAC ultimately achieved provisional GRAS status as a food additive. The safety data from clinical and preclinical studies, therefore, raised no red flags for either agent in oral dosage forms at high concentrations with a wide range of actives tested to date. An important safety consideration is the high inter-subject variability typically associated with the low oral bioavailability values for all payloads tested with both PEs to date; formulation with these PEs will, therefore, not be suitable for molecules with low therapeutic indices.

It is clear that surfactant-based PEs cause a mild degree of reversible perturbation of the intestinal mucosa. The small intestinal epithelium is entirely renewed every 72 h [81]; there is a high rate of cellular turnover and the intestine has a high capacity to replace cells, due to migrating stem cells from the intestinal crypt. There is also a reserve of stem cells that are dormant until epithelial injury occurs, at which point they are recruited to assist with restoration [82]. The capacity of the intestinal mucosa to repair is also associated with secretion of mucus, prostaglandins, and bicarbonate [80]. For a comprehensive review of repair and restoration of the intestinal barrier, see Blikslager et al. [38]. The capacity for epithelial repair following C_{10} exposure was investigated in rat jejunal instillations, where full restitution was seen within 60 min of exposure [83]. These data were similar to that seen in rat models with other PEs including bile salts [84] and sodium dodecyl sulfate (SDS) [85]. Since C_{10} and SNAC are rapidly and completely absorbed, one interpretation is that, following local and transient mucosal perturbation leading to a transient increase in permeability, the epithelium recovers due to gradual dilution of the PE.

Another concern over routine use of PEs is based on their potential capacity to promote microbiome changes and absorption of microorganisms, antigens, and toxins leading to local inflammation, autoimmune disease, and sepsis [86]. Surfactants may impair the protective mucus layer, facilitating the diffusion of luminal bacteria to the intestinal epithelium and ultimately disturbing the host microbiota [87]. In a recent study which generated much debate, evidence was provided that the approved excipient emulsifiers, polysorbate-80 and carboxymethyl cellulose, disturb microbiota composition and induce obesity in mice [88]. Whether these data have any true significance for humans is not known at this point, but it is clear that intestinal microbiome research is going to become more relevant in toxicology profiling of oral formulations. A second concern that is continually raised is the potential increase in permeability of bystander molecules arising from tissue damage induced by PEs [89,90]. Taking into account the precise conditions required for permeation enhancement (high concentrations of payload and PE contemporaneously at the intestinal epithelium), as well as the marked difference in the MW of candidate payloads (<10 kDa) compared to that of typical bacteria, viruses, and bacterial lipopolysaccharide (LPS) (>100 kDa), this concern may be overstated. Nonetheless, clinical pharmacology data from binge-drinking human subjects suggests that alcohol can permit absorption of endotoxins and can promote elevation of type 1 cytokines in plasma, akin to a low-grade infection [91]; thus, together with the study of relevant microbiome changes, more research is needed to filter the true toxicological risks of orally delivered PEs following chronic exposure.

Several studies describe an anti-microbial effect of C_{10} at high concentrations. Cox et al. [92] demonstrated the bactericidal property of C_{10} against *Salmonella typhimurium*, and it also prevented its attachment to intestinal epithelia. Moreover, there was no evidence from the same study that C_{10} promoted permeation of this gut pathogen across isolated rat intestinal mucosa. At low mM concentrations, C_{10} is also bactericidal against *Helicobacter pylori* [93]. In an in vivo study with chickens, incorporation of C_{10} in feed at a level of 3 g/kg protected them from colonization by *Salmonella enterica* [94]. Finally, capric acid has antifungal activities on *Microsporium gypsum* mycelia and spores in vitro [95]. These data are consistent with the well-known anti-microbial actions of MCFAs [96]. Although, to our knowledge, similar data are not reported for SNAC, it would be surprising if, upon examining its structure, it did not have similar anti-microbial actions.

9. Conclusions

In comparing the safety and efficacy of C_{10} and SNAC as PEs in preclinical and clinical studies, examination of 20–30 years of literature would suggest that several of the key parameters are similar. Both can permit oral bioavailability of a range of macromolecular payloads by <5%, with mean values closer to ~1%. The SNAC clinical PK data with semaglutide seem to be on a par with previous performance, for example, with sCT; however, it is due to its formulation with a potent peptide with a long $t_{\frac{1}{2}}$ and high TI that is of particular interest. It is the long $t_{\frac{1}{2}}$ that can compensate for large intra-subject variability [52]. Aspects that tip the balance to SNAC compared to C_{10} include the following: broader clinical experience and an approved vitamin B_{12} product, more extensive toxicology studies and GRAS status, and the lack of requirement for protection against stomach acid. There is still controversy over the mechanism of action of SNAC; techniques including surface plasmon resonance and ITC are now providing data that suggest that the non-covalent interaction of peptides with either SNAC or C_{10} is low affinity and quite similar for each agent. Moreover, while the literature seems to offer a consensus that C_{10} (at low concentrations) acts on tight junctions via intracellular events, and at high concentrations via transcellular perturbation arising from its surfactant effect, there is not the same consensus concerning the mechanism of action of SNAC. The 1990s theory of an exclusive transcellular action arising from increased lipophilicity of a non-covalent complex between SNAC and the payload was not convincing. The new mechanism suggested for SNAC arising from ligated dog studies argues for a local increase in stomach pH around semaglutide, a mechanism that appears to be specific for this molecule. Finally, the main argument advanced for oral peptide delivery is improved convenience over needles leading to better compliance. Patients will, however, be required to wait 30 min before eating and drinking after taking tablets of semaglutide/SNAC each morning; thus, patients will ultimately decide if this is an inconvenience preferable to a once-a-week injection.

Author Contributions: All authors contributed conceptually, to drafting, to figure and table designs, and to the final editing.

References

1. Fosgerau, K.; Hoffmann, T. Peptide therapeutics: Current status and future directions. *Drug Discov. Today* **2015**, *20*, 122–128. [CrossRef] [PubMed]
2. Usmani, S.S.; Bedi, G.; Samuel, J.S.; Singh, S.; Kalra, S.; Kumar, P.; Ahuja, A.A.; Sharma, M.; Gautam, A.; Raghava, G.P.S. THPdb: Database of FDA-approved peptide and protein therapeutics. *PLoS ONE* **2017**, *12*, e0181748. [CrossRef] [PubMed]
3. Lakkireddy, H.R.; Urmann, M.; Besenius, M.; Werner, U.; Haack, T.; Brun, P.; Alié, J.; Illel, B.; Hortala, L.; Vogel, R.; et al. Oral delivery of diabetes peptides—Comparing standard formulations incorporating functional excipients and nanotechnologies in the translational context. *Adv. Drug Deliv. Rev.* **2016**, *106*, 196–222. [CrossRef] [PubMed]
4. Cowan Report. *Therapeutic Categories Outlook: Comprehensive Study*; Cowan & Co.: New York, NY, USA, 2014.
5. Lewis, A.L.; Richard, J. Challenges in the delivery of peptide drugs: An industry perspective. *Ther. Deliv.* **2015**, *6*, 149–163. [CrossRef]
6. Aguirre, T.A.; Teijeiro-Osorio, D.; Rosa, M.; Coulter, I.S.; Alonso, M.J.; Brayden, D.J. Current status of selected oral peptide technologies in advanced preclinical development and in clinical trials. *Adv. Drug Deliv. Rev.* **2016**, *106*, 223–241. [CrossRef] [PubMed]
7. Benet, L.Z. The drug transporter-metabolism alliance: Uncovering and defining the interplay. *Mol. Pharm.* **2009**, *6*, 631–643. [CrossRef] [PubMed]
8. Eligen® Technology: Summary and Value Proposition. Available online: https://www.emisphere.com/wp-content/uploads/2017/02/Eligen-Technology-Presentation_2.15-Update.pdf (accessed on 12 February 2019).
9. Baluom, M.; Friedman, M.; Assaf, P.; Haj-Yehia, A.I.; Rubinstein, A. Synchronized release of sulpiride and sodium decanoate from HPMC matrices: A rational approach to enhance sulpiride absorption in the rat intestine. *Pharm. Res.* **2000**, *17*, 1071–1076. [CrossRef] [PubMed]

10. Maher, S.; Mrsny, R.J.; Brayden, D.J. Intestinal permeation enhancers for oral peptide delivery. *Adv. Drug Deliv. Rev.* **2016**, *106*, 277–319. [CrossRef] [PubMed]
11. Card, J.W.; Magnuson, B.A. A review of the efficacy and safety of nanoparticle-based oral insulin delivery systems. *Am. J. Physiol. Gastrointest. Liver Physiol.* **2011**, *301*, G956–G967. [CrossRef]
12. Banerjee, A.; Mitragotri, S. Intestinal patch systems for oral drug delivery. *Curr. Opin. Pharmacol.* **2017**, *36*, 58–65. [CrossRef] [PubMed]
13. Whitehead, K.; Karr, N.; Mitragotri, S. Safe and effective permeation enhancers for oral drug delivery. *Pharm. Res.* **2008**, *25*, 1782–1788. [CrossRef] [PubMed]
14. Maher, S.; Ryan, B.; Duffy, A.; Brayden, D.J. Formulation strategies to improve oral peptide delivery. *Pharm. Pat. Anal.* **2014**, *3*, 313–336. [CrossRef] [PubMed]
15. Aungst, B.J. Absorption enhancers: Applications and advances. *AAPS J.* **2012**, *14*, 10–18. [CrossRef] [PubMed]
16. EFSA Panel on Food Additives and Nutrient Sources added to Food (ANS); Younes, M.; Aggett, P.; Aguilar, F.; Crebelli, R.; Dusemund, B.; Filipič, M.; Frutos, M.J.; Galtier, P.; Gott, D.; et al. Re-evaluation of sodium, potassium and calcium salts of fatty acids (E 470a) and magnesium salts of fatty acids (E 470b) as food additives. *EFSA J.* **2018**. [CrossRef]
17. Lindmark, T.; Söderholm, J.D.; Olaison, G.; Alván, G.; Ocklind, G.; Artursson, P. Mechanism of absorption enhancement in humans after rectal administration of ampicillin in suppositories containing sodium caprate. *Pharm. Res.* **1997**, *14*, 930–955. [CrossRef] [PubMed]
18. Walsh, E.; Adamczyk, B.; Chalasani, K.B.; Maher, M.; O'Toole, E.B.; Fox, J.; Leonard, T.W.; Brayden, D.J. Oral delivery of macromolecules: Rationale underpinning Gastrointestinal Permeation Enhancement Technology (GIPET®). *Ther. Deliv.* **2011**, *2*, 1595–1610. [CrossRef]
19. Leone-Bay, A.; Santiago, N.; Achan, D.; Chaudhary, K.; DeMorin, F.; Falzarano, L.; Haas, S.; Kalbag, S.; Kaplan, D.; Leipold, H.; et al. N-acylated alpha amino acids as novel oral delivery agents for proteins. *J. Med. Chem.* **1995**, *38*, 4263–4269. [CrossRef]
20. Castelli, M.C.; Wong, D.F.; Friedman, K.; Riley, M.G. Pharmacokinetics of oral cyanocobalamin formulated with sodium N-[8-(2-hydroxybenzoyl)amino]caprylate (SNAC): An open-label, randomized, single-dose, parallel-group study in healthy male subjects. *Clin. Ther.* **2011**, *33*, 934–945. [CrossRef]
21. Smith, L.; Mosley, J.; Ford, M.; Courtney, J. Cyanocobalamin/Salcaprozate Sodium: A novel way to treat vitamin B_{12} deficiency and anemia. *J. Hematol. Oncol. Pharm.* **2016**, *6*, 42–45.
22. Leone-Bay, A.; Paton, D.R.; Variano, B.; Leipold, H.; Rivera, T.; Miura-Fraboni, J.; Baughman, R.A.; Santiago, N. Acylated non-alpha-amino acids as novel agents for the oral delivery of heparin sodium, USP. *J. Control. Release* **1998**, *50*, 41–49. [CrossRef]
23. Goldberg, M. Gomez-Orellana I. Challenges for the oral delivery of macromolecules. *Nat. Rev. Drug Discov.* **2003**, *2*, 289–295. [CrossRef] [PubMed]
24. Leone-Bay, A.; Leipold, H.; Sarubbi, D.; Variano, B.; Rivera, T.; Baughman, R.A. Oral delivery of sodium cromolyn: Preliminary studies in vivo and in vitro. *Pharm. Res.* **1996**, *13*, 222–226. [CrossRef] [PubMed]
25. Anonymous, Sodium Decanoate, PubChem ID 16211937. Available online: https://pubchem.ncbi.nlm.nih.gov/compound/16211937 (accessed on 12 February 2019).
26. Anonymous, Sodium Caprozate PubChem ID 22669833. Available online: https://pubchem.ncbi.nlm.nih.gov/compound/23669833 (accessed on 12 February 2019).
27. Brayden, D.J.; Gleeson, J.; Walsh, E. A head-to-head multi-parametric high content analysis of a series of medium chain fatty acid intestinal permeation enhancers in Caco-2 cells. *Eur. J. Pharm. Biopharm.* **2014**, *88*, 830–839. [CrossRef] [PubMed]
28. Khafagy, E.S.; Morishita, M.; Takayama, K. The role of intermolecular interactions with penetratin and its analogue on the enhancement of absorption of nasal therapeutic peptides. *Int. J. Pharm.* **2010**, *388*, 209–212. [CrossRef]
29. Twarog, C.; Hillaireau, H.; Taverna, M.; Noiray, M.; Illel, B.; Vogel, R.; Brayden, D.J.; Fattal, E. Oral peptide delivery: Understanding interactions between a peptide and permeation enhancers. In Proceedings of the 11th World Meeting on Pharmaceutics, Biopharmaceutics and Pharmaceutical Technology, Granada, Spain, 19–22 March 2018.

30. Lindmark, T.; Nikkila, T.; Artursson, P. Mechanisms of absorption enhancement by medium chain fatty acids in intestinal epithelial Caco-2 cell monolayers. *J. Pharmacol. Exp. Ther.* **1995**, *275*, 958–964.
31. Sawada, T.; Ogawa, T.; Tomita, M.; Hayashi, M.; Awazu, S. Role of paracellular pathway in nonelectrolyte permeation across rat colon epithelium enhanced by sodium caprate and sodium caprylate. *Pharm. Res.* **1991**, *8*, 1365–1371. [CrossRef]
32. Maher, S.; Kennelly, R.; Bzik, V.A.; Baird, A.W.; Wang, X.; Winter, D.; Brayden, D.J. Evaluation of intestinal absorption enhancement and local mucosal toxicity of two promoters. I. Studies in isolated rat and human colonic mucosae. *Eur. J. Pharm. Sci.* **2009**, *38*, 291–300. [CrossRef]
33. Tomita, M.; Hayashi, M.; Awazu, S. Absorption-enhancing mechanism of EDTA, caprate, and decanoylcarnitine in Caco-2 cells. *J. Pharm. Sci.* **1996**, *85*, 608–611. [CrossRef]
34. Lindmark, T.; Kimura, Y.; Artursson, P. Absorption enhancement through intracellular regulation of tight junction permeability by medium chain fatty acids in Caco-2 cells. *J. Pharmacol. Exp. Ther.* **1998**, *284*, 362–369.
35. Feighery, L.M.; Cochrane, S.W.; Quinn, T.; Baird, A.W.; O'Toole, D.; Owens, S.E.; O'Donoghue, D.; Mrsny, R.J.; Brayden, D.J. Myosin light chain kinase inhibition: Correction of increased intestinal epithelial permeability in vitro. *Pharm. Res.* **2008**, *2*, 1377–1386. [CrossRef]
36. Shimazaki, T.; Tomita, M.; Sadahiro, S.; Hayashi, M.; Awazu, S. Absorption-enhancing effects of sodium caprate and palmitoyl carnitine in rat and human colons. *Dig. Dis. Sci.* **1998**, *43*, 641–645. [CrossRef] [PubMed]
37. Krug, S.M.; Amasheh, M.; Dittmann, I.; Christoffel, I.; Fromm, M.; Amasheh, S. Sodium caprate as an enhancer of macromolecule permeation across tricellular tight junctions of intestinal cells. *Biomaterials* **2013**, *34*, 275–282. [CrossRef] [PubMed]
38. Blikslager, A.T.; Moeser, A.J.; Gookin, J.L.; Jones, S.L.; Odle, J. Restoration of barrier function in injured intestinal mucosa. *Physiol. Rev.* **2007**, *87*, 545–564. [CrossRef]
39. Sugibayashi, K.; Onuki, Y.; Takayama, K. Displacement of tight junction proteins from detergent-resistant membrane domains by treatment with sodium caprate. *Eur. J. Pharm. Sci.* **2009**, *36*, 46–253. [CrossRef]
40. Maher, S.; Heade, J.; McCartney, F.; Waters, S.; Bleiel, S.B.; Brayden, D.J. Effects of surfactant-based permeation enhancers on mannitol permeability, histology, and electrogenic ion transport responses in excised rat colonic mucosae. *Int. J. Pharm.* **2018**, *539*, 11–22. [CrossRef] [PubMed]
41. Brayden, D.J.; Maher, S.; Bahar, B.; Walsh, E. Sodium caprate-induced increases in intestinal permeability and epithelial damage are prevented by misoprostol. *Eur. J. Pharm. Biopharm.* **2015**, *94*, 194–206. [CrossRef]
42. Leonard, T.W.; Lynch, J.; McKenna, M.J.; Brayden, D.J. Promoting absorption of drugs in humans using medium-chain fatty acid-based solid dosage forms: GIPET. *Exp. Opin. Drug Deliv.* **2006**, *3*, 685–692. [CrossRef]
43. Gradauer, K.; Nishiumi, A.; Unrinin, K.; Higashino, H.; Kataoka, M.; Pedersen, B.L.; Buckley, S.T.; Yamashita, S. Interaction with mixed micelles in the intestine attenuates the permeation enhancing potential of alkyl-maltosides. *Mol. Pharm.* **2015**, *12*, 2245–2253. [CrossRef]
44. Brayden, D.; Creed, E.; O'Connell, A.; Leipold, H.; Agarwal, R.; Leone-Bay, A. Heparin absorption across the intestine: Effects of sodium N-[8-(2-hydroxybenzoyl)amino]caprylate in rat in situ intestinal instillations and in Caco-2 monolayers. *Pharm. Res.* **1997**, *14*, 1772–1779. [CrossRef]
45. Malkov, D.; Angelo, R.; Wang, H.Z.; Flanders, E.; Tang, H.; Gomez-Orellana, I. Oral delivery of insulin with the eligen technology: Mechanistic studies. *Curr. Drug Deliv.* **2005**, *2*, 191–197. [CrossRef]
46. Hess, S.; Rotshild, V.; Hoffman, A. Investigation of the enhancing mechanism of sodium N-[8-(2-hydroxybenzoyl)amino]caprylate effect on the intestinal permeability of polar molecules utilizing a voltage clamp method. *Eur. J. Pharm. Sci.* **2005**, *25*, 307–312. [CrossRef] [PubMed]
47. Malkov, D.; Wang, H.Z.; Dinh, S.; Gomez-Orellana, I. Pathway of oral absorption of heparin with sodium N-[8-(2-hydroxybenzoyl)amino] caprylate. *Pharm. Res.* **2002**, *19*, 1180–1184. [CrossRef] [PubMed]
48. Ding, X.; Rath, P.; Angelo, R.; Stringfellow, T.; Flanders, E.; Dinh, S.; Gomez-Orellana, I.; Robinson, J.R. Oral absorption enhancement of cromolyn sodium through noncovalent complexation. *Pharm. Res.* **2004**, *21*, 2196–2206. [CrossRef] [PubMed]
49. Arbit, E.; Goldberg, M.; Gomez-Orellana, I.; Majuru, S. Oral heparin: Status review. *Thromb. J.* **2006**, *4*, 6. [CrossRef] [PubMed]

50. Alani, A.W.; Robinson, J.R. Mechanistic understanding of oral drug absorption enhancement of cromolyn sodium by an amino acid derivative. *Pharm. Res.* **2008**, *25*, 48–54. [CrossRef] [PubMed]
51. Rehmani, S.; Dixon, J.E. Oral delivery of anti-diabetes therapeutics using cell penetrating and transcytosing peptide strategies. *Peptides* **2018**, *100*, 24–35. [CrossRef] [PubMed]
52. Buckley, S.T.; Bækdal, T.A.; Vegge, A.; Maarbjerg, S.J.; Pyke, C.; Ahnfelt-Rønne, J.; Madsen, K.G.; Schéele, S.G.; Alanentalo, T.; Kirk, R.K.; et al. Transcellular stomach absorption of a derivatized glucagon-like peptide-1 receptor agonist. *Sci. Transl. Med.* **2018**, *10*. [CrossRef]
53. Amory, J.K.; Leonard, T.W.; Page, S.T.; O'Toole, E.; McKenna, M.J.; Bremner, W.J. Oral administration of the GnRH antagonist acyline, in a GIPET-enhanced tablet form, acutely suppresses serum testosterone in normal men: Single-dose pharmacokinetics and pharmacodynamics. *Cancer Chemother. Pharmacol.* **2009**, *64*, 641–645. [CrossRef]
54. Leonard, T.W. Composition and Drug Delviery of Bisphosphonates. U.S. Patent 0,215,743 A1, 26 August 2010.
55. Halberg, I.B.; Lyby, K.; Wassermann, K.; Heise, T.; Zijlstra, E.; Plum-Morchel, L. Efficacy and safety of oral basal insulin versus subcutaneous insulin in type 2 diabetes: A randomised, double-blind Phase II trial. *Lancet Diabetes Endocrinol.* **2019**. [CrossRef]
56. Khedkar, A.; Lebovitz, H.; Fleming, A.; Cherrington, A.; Jose, V.; Athalye, S.N.; Vishweswaramurthy, A. Impact of insulin tregopil and its permeation enhancer on pharmacokinetics of metformin in healthy volunteers: Randomized, open-label, placebo-controlled, crossover study. *Clin. Transl. Sci.* **2018**. [CrossRef]
57. Raoof, A.A.; Chiu, P.; Ramtoola, Z.; Cumming, I.K.; Teng, C.; Weinbach, S.P.; Hardee, G.E.; Levin, A.A.; Geary, R.S. Oral bioavailability and multiple dose tolerability of an antisense oligonucleotide tablet formulated with sodium caprate. *J. Pharm. Sci.* **2004**, *93*, 1431–1439. [CrossRef] [PubMed]
58. Tillman, L.G.; Geary, R.S.; Hardee, G.E. Oral delivery of antisense oligonucleotides in man. *J. Pharm. Sci.* **2008**, *97*, 225–236. [CrossRef] [PubMed]
59. Available online: http://ir.ionispharma.com/news-releases/news-release-details/ionis-pharmaceuticals-licenses-first-oral-antisense-drug-acting (accessed on 12 February 2019).
60. Lennernäs, H.; Gjellan, K.; Hallgren, R.; Graffner, C. The influence of caprate on rectal absorption of phenoxymethylpenicillin: Experience from an in-vivo perfusion in humans. *J. Pharm. Pharmacol.* **2002**, *54*, 499–508. [CrossRef] [PubMed]
61. Baughman, R.A.; Kapoor, S.C.; Agarwal, R.K.; Kisicki, J.; Catella-Lawson, F.; FitzGerald, G.A. Oral delivery of anticoagulant doses of heparin. A randomized, double-blind, controlled study in humans. *Circulation* **1998**, *98*, 1610–1615. [CrossRef] [PubMed]
62. Berkowitz, S.D.; Marder, V.J.; Kosutic, G.; Baughman, R.A. Oral heparin administration with a novel drug delivery agent (SNAC) in healthy volunteers and patients undergoing elective total hip arthroplasty. *J. Thromb. Haemost.* **2003**, *1*, 1914–1919. [CrossRef] [PubMed]
63. Mousa, S.A.; Zhang, F.; Aljada, A.; Chaturvedi, S.; Takieddin, M.; Zhang, H.; Chi, L.; Castelli, M.C.; Friedman, K.; Goldberg, M.M.; et al. Pharmacokinetics and pharmacodynamics of oral heparin solid dosage form in healthy human subjects. *J. Clin. Pharmacol.* **2007**, *47*, 1508–1520. [CrossRef] [PubMed]
64. Buclin, T.; Cosma Rochat, M.; Burckhardt, P.; Azria, M.; Attinger, M. Bioavailability and biological efficacy of a new oral formulation of salmon calcitonin in healthy volunteers. *J. Bone Miner. Res.* **2002**, *17*, 1478–1485. [CrossRef] [PubMed]
65. Kapitza, C.; Zijlstra, E.; Heinemann, L.; Castelli, M.C.; Riley, G.; Heise, T. Oral insulin: A comparison with subcutaneous regular human insulin in patients with type 2 diabetes. *Diabetes Care* **2010**, *33*, 1288–1290. [CrossRef] [PubMed]
66. Karsdal, M.A.; Byrjalsen, I.; Alexandersen, P.; Bihlet, A.; Andersen, J.R.; Riis, B.J.; Bay-Jensen, A.C.; Christiansen, C.; CSMC021C2301/2 investigators. Treatment of symptomatic knee osteoarthritis with oral salmon calcitonin: Results from two phase 3 trials. *Osteoarthr. Cartil.* **2015**, *23*, 532–543. [CrossRef]
67. Henriksen, K.; Byrjalsen, I.; Andersen, J.R.; Bihlet, A.R.; Russo, L.A.; Alexandersen, P.; Valter, I.; Qvist, P.; Lau, E.; Riis, B.J.; et al. SMC021 investigators., A randomized, double-blind, multicenter, placebo-controlled study to evaluate the efficacy and safety of oral salmon calcitonin in the treatment of osteoporosis in postmenopausal women taking calcium and vitamin D. *Bone* **2016**, *91*, 122–129. [CrossRef]
68. Karsdal, M.A.; Henriksen, K.; Bay-Jensen, A.C.; Molloy, B.; Arnold, M.; John, M.R.; Byrjalsen, I.; Azria, M.;

Riis, B.J.; Qvist, P.; et al. Lessons learned from the development of oral calcitonin: The first tablet formulation of a protein in phase III clinical trials. *J. Clin. Pharmacol.* **2011**, *51*, 460–471. [CrossRef] [PubMed]

69. Davies, M.; Pieber, T.R.; Hartoft-Nielsen, M.L.; Hansen, O.K.H.; Jabbour, S.; Rosenstock, J. Effect of oral semaglutide compared with placebo and subcutaneous semaglutide on glycemic control in patients with Type 2 diabetes: A Randomized Clinical Trial. *JAMA* **2017**, *318*, 1460–1470. [CrossRef] [PubMed]
70. Bjerregaard, S.; Nielsen, F.S.; Sauerberg, P. Solid Compositions Comprising a GLP-1 Agonist and a Salt of n-(8-(2-Hydroxybenzoyl)Amino)Caprylic Acid. U.S. Patent WO2012080471A1, 8 March 2016.
71. Available online: https://globenewswire.com/news-release/2018/02/22/1379640/0/en/Novo-Nordisk-successfully-completes-the-first-phase-3a-trial-PIONEER-1-with-oral-semaglutide.html (accessed on 28 November 2018).
72. Granhall, C.; Søndergaard, F.L.; Thomsen, M.; Anderson, T.W. Pharmacokinetics, safety and tolerability of oral semaglutide in subjects with renal impairment. *Clin. Pharm.* **2018**, *57*, 1571–1580. [CrossRef] [PubMed]
73. Baekdal, T.A.; Thomsen, M.; Kupčová, V.; Hansen, C.W.; Anderson, T.W. Pharmacokinetics, safety, and tolerability of oral semaglutide in subjects with hepatic impairment. *J. Clin. Pharmacol.* **2018**, *58*, 1314–1323. [CrossRef] [PubMed]
74. Bækdal, T.A.; Breitschaft, A.; Navarria, A.; Hansen, C.W. A randomized study investigating the effect of omeprazole on the pharmacokinetics of oral semaglutide. *Expert Opin. Drug Metab. Toxicol.* **2018**, *14*, 869–877. [CrossRef] [PubMed]
75. Bain, S.C.; Mosenzon, O.; Arechavaleta, R.; Bogdański, P.; Comlekci, A.; Consoli, A.; Deerochanawong, C.; Dungan, K.; Faingold, M.C.; Farkouh, M.E.; et al. Cardiovascular safety of oral semaglutide in patients with type 2 diabetes: Rationale, design and patient baseline characteristics for the PIONEER 6 trial. *Diabetes Obes. Metab.* **2018**. [CrossRef]
76. Maher, S.; Leonard, T.W.; Jacobsen, J.; Brayden, D.J. Safety and efficacy of sodium caprate in promoting oral drug absorption: From in vitro to the clinic. *Adv. Drug Deliv. Rev.* **2009**, *61*, 1427–1449. [CrossRef]
77. Raoof, A.A.; Ramtoola, Z.; McKenna, B.; Yu, R.Z.; Hardee, G.; Geary, R.S. Effect of sodium caprate on the intestinal absorption of two modified antisense oligonucleotides in pigs. *Eur. J. Pharm. Sci.* **2002**, *17*, 131–138. [CrossRef]
78. Riley, M.G.; Castelli, M.C.; Paehler, E.A. Subchronic oral toxicity of salcaprozate sodium (SNAC) in Sprague-Dawley and Wistar rats. *Int. J. Toxicol.* **2009**, *28*, 278–293. [CrossRef]
79. Riley, M.G.; York, R.G. Peri-and postnatal developmental toxicity of salcaprozate sodium (SNAC) in Sprague-Dawley rats. *Int. J. Toxicol.* **2009**, *28*, 266–277. [CrossRef]
80. McCartney FGleeson, J.; Brayden, D.J. Safety concerns over the use of intestinal permeation enhancers: A mini-review. *Tissue Barriers* **2016**, *4*, e1176822. [CrossRef] [PubMed]
81. Van der Flier, L.G.; Clevers, H. Stem cells, self-renewal, and differentiation in the intestinal epithelium. *Annu. Rev. Physiol.* **2009**, *71*, 241–260. [CrossRef]
82. Laine, L.; Takeuchi, K.; Tarnawski, A. Gastric mucosal defense and cytoprotection: Bench to bedside. *Gastroenterology* **2008**, *135*, 41–60. [CrossRef] [PubMed]
83. Wang, X.; Maher, S.; Brayden, D.J. Restoration of rat colonic epithelium after in situ intestinal instillation of the absorption promoter, sodium caprate. *Ther. Deliv.* **2010**, *1*, 75–82. [CrossRef]
84. Gookin, J.L.; Galanko, J.A.; Blikslager, A.T.; Argenzio, R.A. PG-mediated closure of paracellular pathway and not restitution is the primary determinant of barrier recovery in acutely injured porcine ileum. *Am. J. Physiol.* **2003**, *285*, G967–G979. [CrossRef] [PubMed]
85. Narkar, Y.; Burnette, R.; Bleher, R.; Albrecht, R.; Kandela, A.; Robinson, J.R. Evaluation of mucosal damage and recovery in the gastrointestinal tract of rats by a penetration enhancer. *Pharm. Res.* **2008**, *25*, 25–38. [CrossRef] [PubMed]
86. König, J.; Wells, J.; Cani, P.D.; García-Ródenas, C.L.; MacDonald, T.; Mercenier, A.; Whyte, J.; Troost, F.; Brummer, R.J. Human intestinal barrier function in health and disease. *Clin. Transl. Gastroenterol.* **2016**, *7*, e196. [CrossRef]
87. Cani, P.D. Human gut microbiome: Hopes, threats and promises. *Gut* **2018**, *67*, 1716–1725. [CrossRef]
88. Chassaing, B.; Koren, O.; Goodrich, J.K.; Poole, A.C.; Srinivasan, S.; Ley, R.E.; Gewirtz, A.T. Dietary emulsifiers impact the mouse gut microbiota promoting colitis and metabolic syndrome. *Nature* **2015**, *519*, 92–96. [CrossRef]

89. Choonara, B.F.; Choonara, Y.E.; Kumar, P.; Bijukumar, D.; du Toit, L.C.; Pillay, V. A review of advanced oral drug delivery technologies facilitating the protection and absorption of protein and peptide molecules. *Biotechnol. Adv.* **2014**, *32*, 1269–1282. [CrossRef]
90. Tscheik, C.; Blasig, I.E.; Winkler, L. Trends in drug delivery through tissue barriers containing tight junctions. *Tissue Barriers* **2013**, *1*, e24565. [CrossRef] [PubMed]
91. Bala, S.; Marcos, M.; Gattu, A.; Catalano, D.; Szabo, G. Acute binge drinking increases serum endotoxin and bacterial DNA levels in healthy individuals. *PLoS ONE* **2014**, *9*, e96864. [CrossRef] [PubMed]
92. Cox, A.B.; Rawlinson, L.; Baird, A.W.; Bzik, V.; Brayden, D.J. In vitro interactions between the oral absorption promoter, sodium caprate (C10) and S. typhimurium in rat intestinal ileal mucosae. *Pharm. Res.* **2008**, *25*, 114–122. [CrossRef] [PubMed]
93. Petschow, B.W.; Batema, R.P.; Ford, L.L. Susceptibility of *Helicobacter pylori* to bactericidal properties of medium-chain monoglycerides and free fatty acids. *Antimicrob. Agents Chemother.* **1996**, *40*, 302–306. [CrossRef]
94. Van Immerseel, F.; De Buck, J.; Boyen, F.; Bohez, L.; Pasmans, F.; Volf, J.; Sevcik, M.; Rychlik, I.; Haesebrouck, F.; Ducatelle, R. Medium-chain fatty acids decrease colonization and invasion through hilA suppression shortly after infection of chickens with *Salmonella enterica* serovar *Enteritidis*. *Appl. Environ. Microbiol.* **2004**, *70*, 3582–3587. [CrossRef] [PubMed]
95. Chadeganipour, M.; Haims, A. Antifungal activities of pelargonic and capric acid on *Microsporum gypseum*. *Mycoses* **2001**, *44*, 109–112. [CrossRef] [PubMed]
96. Huang, C.B.; Alimova, Y.; Myers, T.M.; Ebersole, J.L. Short and medium-chain fatty acids exhibit antimicrobial activity for oral microorganisms. *Arch. Oral Biol.* **2011**, *56*, 650–654. [CrossRef]

11

Delivery of Nanoparticles across the Intestinal Epithelium via the Transferrin Transport Pathway

Jing M. Yong, Julia Mantaj, Yiyi Cheng and Driton Vllasaliu *

School of Cancer and Pharmaceutical Sciences, Faculty of Life Sciences & Medicine, King's College London, London SE1 9NH, UK

* Correspondence: driton.vllasaliu@kcl.ac.uk

Abstract: The aim of this study was to probe whether the transferrin (Tf) transport pathway can be exploited for intestinal delivery of nanoparticles. Tf was adsorbed on 100 nm model polystyrene nanoparticles (NP), followed by size characterisation of these systems. Cell uptake of Tf and Tf-adsorbed NP was investigated in intestinal epithelial Caco-2 cells cultured on multi-well plates and as differentiated polarised monolayers. Tf-NP demonstrated a remarkably higher cell uptake compared to unmodified NP in both non-polarised (5-fold) and polarised cell monolayers (16-fold difference). Application of soluble Tf significantly attenuated the uptake of Tf-NP. Notably, Tf-NP displayed remarkably higher rate (23-fold) of epithelial transport across Caco-2 monolayers compared to unmodified NP. This study therefore strongly suggests that the Tf transport pathway should be considered as a candidate biological transport route for orally-administered nanomedicines and drugs with poor oral bioavailability.

Keywords: Caco-2; intestinal absorption; nanomedicine; nanoparticle; oral delivery; transferrin

1. Introduction

The oral drug administration route offers the ultimate patient convenience, preference and therefore adherence to drug therapy. However, with a few exceptions, oral administration is currently an option only for small drug molecules that show acceptable intestinal absorption. As a rapidly expanding class of drugs, biologics are presently predominantly given by injection. Significant research efforts over a number of decades have explored technologies to enable oral delivery of biologics, but progress has been relatively poor. Drug delivery strategies in this area mostly utilise absorption or permeation enhancers and focus on smaller biologics, such as glucagon-like peptide 1 (GLP-1) analogues [1]. However, safety concerns, including those related to many surfactants [2], have hindered the clinical translation of these approaches. Recent progress in this area seeks to utilise advances in materials, engineering and electronics, leading to swallowable "devices", such as mucoadhesive patches [3] and the microneedle "robotic pill" [4].

The key challenge in the field of oral delivery of macromolecular biologics concerns the difficulty in overcoming the formidable intestinal epithelial barrier, rather than additional barriers such as the stomach acid and mucosal enzymes, which can be addressed via relatively established technologies. A key requirement for technologies enabling therapeutically-relevant oral delivery of biologics is safety. Rather than disrupting and increasing the permeability of the intestinal epithelium non-selectively (i.e., an effect that a classical permeation enhancer would display), it is desirable to engineer delivery systems that selectively permeate the intestinal mucosa. This can be achieved by targeting and hijacking the natural, physiological transport processes present in the intestinal epithelium. This approach usually requires a ligand or transport-enabling entity capable of intestinal translocation, which is linked (e.g., conjugated or fused) to the biotherapeutic. Alternatively, the ligand can be presented on the surface of drug carriers, particularly nanocarriers [5–7], which may also serve to protect the drug against mucosal enzymatic degradation or enable targeted delivery post absorption.

Transferrin (Tf) has been explored as a potential ligand to enable drug targeting and delivery across biological barriers, particularly the blood-brain barrier (BBB) [8,9], because of its high expression in BBB endothelium [10]. The transferrin receptor (TfR) is expressed in the human gastrointestinal epithelial cells [11]. Furthermore, TfR is overexpressed in colon cancer (similarly to other types of cancer) [12] and the inflamed colon; it was detected in both basolateral and apical sides of enterocytes from the colon tissue biopsies of inflammatory bowel disease (IBD) patients and rats with colitis [13]. Therefore, TfR and TfR-mediated transcytosis could be exploited as a biological system for systemic delivery of biologics, in addition to its potential as a targeting receptor for local delivery in intestinal cancer or IBD.

However, it must be noted that it is currently unclear whether TfR-mediated transcytosis offers opportunity for improving intestinal delivery of biologics in the context of systemic delivery, or local, targeted delivery to the intestinal diseased tissue. This is because of predominant distribution of TfR on the basolateral surface in polarised cells, which presents an obvious obstacle for receptor-mediated mucosal delivery [14]. There are however reports of TfR-mediated transcytosis being explored for oral delivery of biologics via a Tf recombinant fusion protein approach [15] or Tf conjugation to therapeutic macromolecule [16]—both these approaches have shown evidence and potential for the use of TfR-mediated transport as a strategy to enhance the intestinal absorption (i.e., in the apical-to-basolateral direction) of biologics. Importantly, a recent landmark study clearly showed a complete and enhanced apical-to-basolateral transcytosis of Tf-functionalised nanogranules in Caco-2 cells, with Tf modification upregulating the expression of trafficking-related (endocytosis and transcytosis) proteins [17].

This study probed the possibility of improving the intestinal epithelial delivery of nanoparticles (NP), as potentially useful carriers of biologics, by targeting TfR-mediated transcytosis. A fundamental study of this nature is imperative to assess the possibility that TfR-mediated transcytosis may be utilised to facilitate intestinal translocation of nanomedicines. This is important as, with the exception of two studies [17,18], TfR-mediated transcytosis has not been investigated for intestinal delivery of nanosystems. We show here that TfR targeting of NP significantly improves their uptake into intestinal epithelial cells (Caco-2), as well as translocation across cell monolayers serving as an in vitro intestinal model.

2. Materials and Methods

2.1. Materials

Hank's balanced salt solution (HBSS; with sodium bicarbonate, without phenol red), Dulbecco's Modified Eagle's Medium (DMEM) and all other reagents (including cell culture media supplements, antibiotic-antimycotic solution and foetal bovine serum), unless otherwise stated, were purchased from Sigma-Aldrich (Poole, UK). Fluorescently-labelled ("fluospheres"), carboxylate-modified polystyrene microspheres of 0.1 μm diameter (referred to as "NP") and multiwell cell culture plates were purchased from Thermo Fisher Scientific (Waltham, MA, USA). Human holotransferrin (Tf) was purchased from LEE biosolutions (Maryland Heights, MO, USA), while fluorescently-labelled human Tf-CF®488A dye conjugate was purchased from Biotium (Fremont, CA, USA). Transwell permeable inserts of 12 mm diameter and polycarbonate filters and 0.4μm pore size were obtained from Corning (Corning, NY, USA).

2.2. Adsorption of Tf to Nanoparticles

Tf-adsorbed nanoparticles (Tf-NP) were prepared based on a procedure that was previously reported [19]. A 1:2 Tf to NP mass ratio (1.1 mg/mL Tf and 2.2 mg/mL carboxylic-modified NPs) was used, with adsorption achieved by incubation in 50mM 2-(*N*-morpholino)ethanesulfonic acid (MES) buffer at pH 5.9 for 2 h at 20 °C. A previous study characterising Tf adsorption to latex NP reported the

1:1 mass ratio to produce full surface coverage on the same NP systems [19]. Given that we used a lower amount of Tf (below adsorption saturation), the presence of unadsorbed Tf was assumed to be very low and dialysis was not carried out.

2.3. Nanoparticle Characterisation

Average hydrodynamic size (dynamic light scattering, DLS), polydispersity and zeta potential of NP before and post Tf adsorption were measured by using a Malvern zetasizer (Malvern Instruments Ltd., Malvern, UK). Unmodified and Tf-NP were diluted in HBSS (biological buffer used in cell experiments). Measurements were conducted at a scattering angle $\theta = 173$ and at a temperature of 25 °C. For DLS, each measurement was an average of 12 repetitions of 10 s each. Both DLS and zeta potential measurements were repeated three times.

2.4. Cell Culture

Caco-2 cells were cultured on 24-well plates for two days as undifferentiated system and Transwell inserts as differentiated monolayers, following plating at 10^5 cells/cm^2 using DMEM. Cells were cultured on inserts for at least 21 days prior to the experiments, with culture medium replaced every other day. For differentiated Caco-2 system, transepithelial electrical resistance (TEER) was measured periodically and before uptake and transport experiments to ensure integrity of the monolayer and tight junction formation (polarisation). Prior to cell uptake and transport experiments, both undifferentiated and differentiated Caco-2 cells were equilibrated in HBSS for 45 min to minimise the potential impact of media change on cell uptake and transport studies.

2.5. Cell Uptake of Tf

Human Tf CF488A conjugate was applied to Caco-2 cells (cultured on 24-well plates) at 50 µg/mL and cells incubated at 37 °C for two hours. This was followed by removing the applied sample and repeated cell washing using HBSS. Triton X-100 (1% *v*/*v*) was applied to cells for 10 min to permeabilise and detach the cells. Permeabilised cells were then centrifuged and the supernatant harvested. Tf CF488A conjugate was quantified by measuring the fluorescence of supernatant using a Tecan Fluorescence Plate Reader (Tecan Trading AG, Männedorf, Switzerland) at 515 nm emission/490 nm excitation. Quantitation of samples was carried out via a calibration curve.

2.6. Cell Uptake of Tf-NP

Tf-NPs (1:2 mass ratio) were applied to Caco-2 cells cultured on 24-well plates at 40 µg/mL. Cells were incubated with the samples at 37 °C for two hours, following washing with HBSS. Cells were then permeabilised via the application of Triton X-100 (1% *v*/*v* in HBSS). Cells were then harvested and transferred to 1 mL vials for centrifugation. Tf-NPs were quantified by measuring NP fluorescence following centrifugation of permeabilised cells and measurement of fluorescence of the supernatant using a Tecan fluorescence plate reader at 590 nm/645 nm (excitation/emission).

2.6.1. Competition Studies

For competition studies, cells were pre-treated with 10 µg/mL of Tf, shortly followed by application of Tf-NP. Cell uptake was examined as above.

2.6.2. Uptake in Differentiated Monolayers

In addition to examining uptake of Tf-NP in multiwell plate-grown Caco-2 cells, we also tested cell internalisation of these systems in differentiated Caco-2 cells (i.e., following culture on Transwell inserts). Only cell monolayers displaying TEER ≥ 500 Ωcm^2 were used in the experiments (given the typical range observed in our work of 700–1400 Ωcm^2). Application of Tf-NP and cell monolayer permeabilisation was conducted in the same manner as above.

2.7. *Transport of Tf-NP across Differentiated Caco-2 Monolayers*

Caco-2 cells were cultured as polarised monolayers on Transwell inserts as described above. Prior to the transport study, cells were equilibrated in HBSS. Tf-NP (1:2 ratio) were then applied to the apical side of Caco-2 cells at 40 μg/mL for two hours. Unmodified NPs were also applied at equivalent concentration. Cells were incubated with the samples at 37 °C for two hours, with periodic sampling of the basolateral solution every 20 min (this was replaced with fresh HBSS). Samples were transferred onto a black 96-well plate for NP fluorescence quantitation as above.

2.8. *Statistical Analysis*

Unpaired, unequal variance t test (or Welch t test) was performed for comparisons of two group means, while one-way analysis of variance (ANOVA) was utilised for comparison of three or more group means. p value of <0.05 was considered statistically significant. ***, ** and * indicate $p < 0.001$, $p < 0.01$ and $p < 0.05$, respectively, whereas "ns" denotes nonsignificant. Statistical analysis was conducted using GraphPad Prism® Software.

3. Results

This study examined whether TfR-mediated transcytosis may be utilised as a biological transport route to facilitate intestinal delivery of nanomedicines (Figure 1).

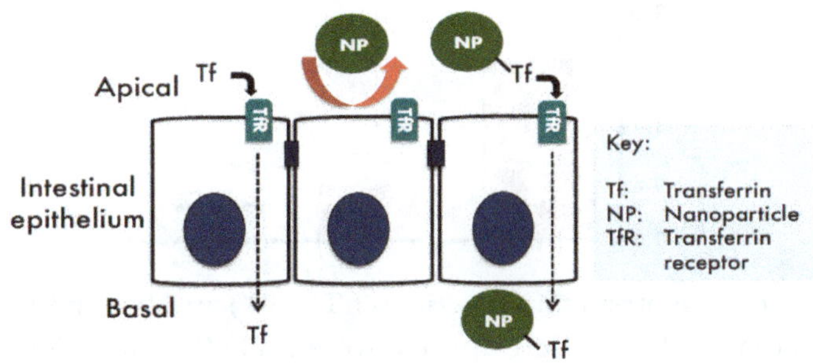

Figure 1. Transferrin transcytosis pathway as a potential route for intestinal delivery of nanomedicines.

3.1. *Nanoparticle Characterisation*

To assess the effect of physical adsorption of Tf to NP on their size, we conducted size characterisation of bare NP and Tf-NP. Data shown in Figure 2 highlight that adsorption of Tf on model polystyrene NP produced an increase in the hydrodynamic diameter of the NP (measured by DLS) from approximately 130 nm to 176 nm, indicating the formation of an adsorbed Tf surface layer of about 23 nm.

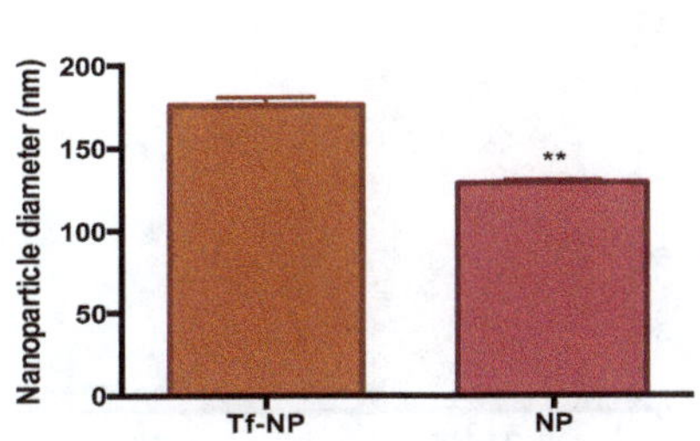

Figure 2. Hydrodynamic size of bare nanoparticles (NP) and transferrin-adsorbed systems (Tf-NP). Size was characterised by dynamic light scattering (DLS), with systems suspended in Hank's Balanced Salt Solution (HBSS). Measurements were done at scattering angle $\theta = 173$ and at a temperature of 25 °C. Data shown as mean ± SD. Each measurement was an average of 12 repetitions of 10 s each and repeated three times. ** denotes $p < 0.01$.

In terms of surface charge, the zeta potential of unmodified NP was −35.7 (± 1.57), whereas for Tf-NP this amounted to −14.3 (± 1.03), resulting in a statistically significant reduction of negative surface charge post Tf adsorption ($p = 0.0001$).

3.2. Cell Uptake of Tf

Uptake of Tf by multiwell-cultured (undifferentiated) Caco-2 cells following application at 50 µg/mL (at 37 °C for two hours) was 0.18 µg/well (24-well plate).

3.3. Cell Uptake of Tf-NP

The internalisation of Tf-NP by intestinal Caco-2 cells was tested under different conditions in non-polarised, multiwell-cultured cells (Figure 3), prior to subsequent examination in differentiated cell monolayers (Figure 4). Considering the multiwell-cultured cells, Figure 2 shows the internalisation of Tf-NP after application alone, or following treatment with soluble Tf ('+Tf'). The figure also depicts the uptake of bare NP. The data highlight more than five-fold higher cell uptake of Tf-NP compared to bare NP. Importantly, following cell treatment of Tf-NP in conjunction with excess free Tf, cell internalisation of the former was attenuated by more than three-fold.

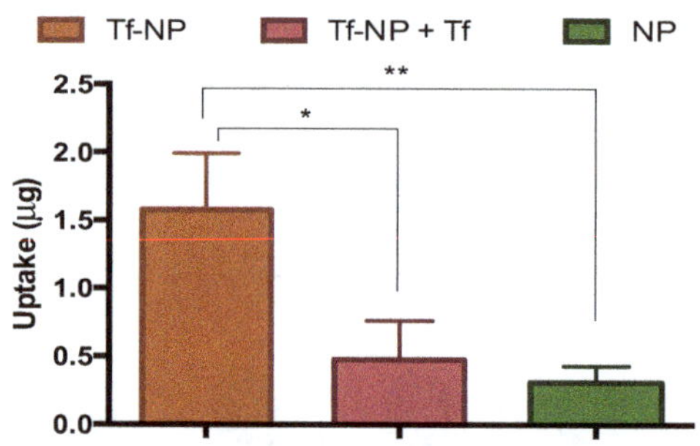

Figure 3. Uptake of transferrin-adsorbed nanoparticles ('Tf-NP') and bare nanoparticles (NP) by Caco-2 cells cultured on multiwell plates. Tf-NP were applied to cells at 40 µg/mL alone or just after application of 10 µg/mL soluble Tf ('Tf-NP + Tf'). Cells were incubated with the samples at 37 °C for two hours. Cell internalisation was measured following permeabilization with Triton X-100 (1% *v/v* in Hank's Balanced Salt Solution), centrifugation and measurement of nanoparticle fluorescence. Data shown as the mean ± SD ($n = 3$). ** and * denote $p < 0.01$ and $p < 0.05$, respectively.

3.4. NP-Tf Uptake in, and Transport across, Differentiated Monolayers

Cell uptake of Tf-NP in differentiated Caco-2 monolayers is depicted in Figure 4. The data demonstrate more than 16-fold higher cell uptake of Tf-NP compared to bare NP.

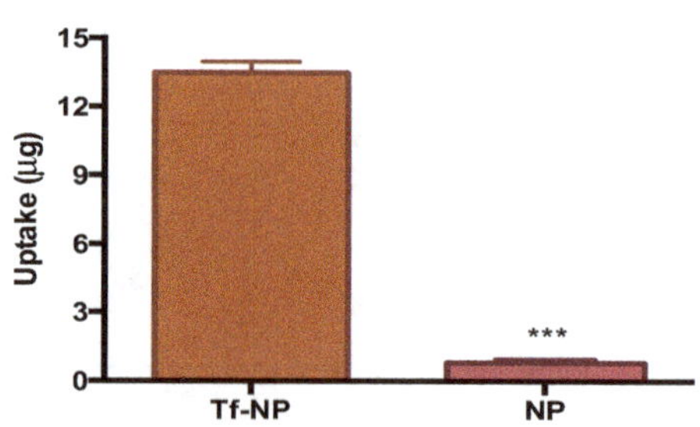

Figure 4. Uptake of transferrin-adsorbed nanoparticles ('Tf-NP') and bare nanoparticles (NP) by Caco-2 cells cultured as differentiated monolayers. Tf-NP were applied to the apical side of Caco-2 monolayers at 40 µg/mL in Hank's Balanced Salt Solution (HBSS) as biological buffer. Cells were incubated with the samples at 37 °C for two hours. Cells were permeabilised via the application of 100 µL of Triton X-100 (1% *v/v* in HBSS). Nanoparticles were quantified by fluorescence. Data presented as the mean ± SD ($n = 3$). *** denotes $p < 0.001$

Following the demonstration of Tf-NP uptake by intestinal Caco-2 cells, the final set of experiments looked into the transepithelial transport. In this regard, Figure 5 shows that Tf-NP traversed differentiated Caco-2 monolayers remarkably more efficiently; specifically a 23-fold higher rate of NP translocation was observed with Tf-NP compared to bare counterparts.

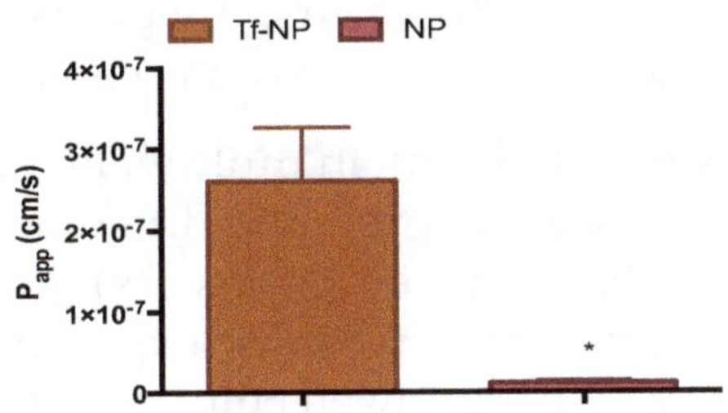

Figure 5. Transport of transferrin-adsorbed nanoparticles ('Tf-NP') and bare nanoparticles (NP) across differentiated Caco-2 cells (cultured on inserts for three weeks). Tf-NP were applied to the apical side of Caco-2 monolayers at 40 μg/mL in Hank's Balanced Salt Solution (HBSS) as biological buffer. Cells were incubated with the samples at 37 °C for two hours, during which sampling from the basolateral compartment was carried out periodically. Data presented as the mean ± SD ($n = 3$). * denotes $p < 0.05$.

4. Discussion

The intestinal mucosa acts as a selective barrier to systemic absorption of material present in the lumen. Large and complex biologics are usually not capable of crossing the intestinal epithelium, therefore displaying very low bioavailabilities following oral administration. One way to improve the oral bioavailability of such drugs is to enhance epithelial absorption by targeting the transcytosis pathways as physiological routes of transport in the intestinal epithelium. This strategy has been made possible by advances in biotechnology and nanotechnology, which have facilitated the production of fusion proteins and drug nanocarriers, respectively. We and other groups have demonstrated that a number of physiological transcytosis processes functioning in the intestinal epithelium can potentially be used to shuttle material (nanoparticles and macromolecules) across the intestinal epithelium, including the transport system for IgG [20,21], neurotensin [22] and albumin [23,24]. This study provides further progress in this arena, by demonstrating that the biological machinery for Tf transport can also be considered as a potential pathway for intestinal delivery of nanomedicines.

Tf is an abundant human plasma glycoprotein responsible for transport of iron, binding to TfR when bound to iron, activating receptor mediated endocytosis [25]. As tumour cells generally overexpress the TfR because of high demand for iron, Tf-mediated drug delivery strategy has been predominantly used for its potential to target cancer cells, usually as a ligand to guide NP to these cells.

Transferrin receptor (TfR)-mediated endocytosis and transcytosis in intestinal Caco-2 cells was previously investigated using Tf-fusion proteins. It was shown that apically-endocytosed Tf in Caco-2 cells is transported to a Rab11-positive compartment, which may control its release to follow either slow recycling to apical membrane or progress to transcytotic compartments [26]. Shah and Shen studied the transport of Tf-conjugated insulin across Caco-2 cell monolayers and reported that transport of the complex, which was mediated via the TfR, was increased by 5- to 15-fold compared to free insulin [16]. In another study, Tf recombinant fusion protein approach was explored for oral delivery for human growth hormone (hGH) [15]. Fusion proteins of 100 kDa, which retained bioactivity of both hGH and Tf, were tested in hGH-deficient hypophysectomised rats for in vivo biological activity. It was shown that one of the tested fusion proteins—containing a helical linker as spacer between hGH and Tf domain—induced a statistically significant weight gain after oral dosing.

We utilised fluorescently-labelled model polystyrene NP systems and achieved ligand (Tf) presentation on NP via physical adsorption. This produced Tf-NP of approximately 180 nm (Figure 2), which fall within the optimal size range for intestinal epithelial transport [6,20,27,28]. Furthermore, it was previously shown that following presentation as coating on the surface of NP via physical adsorption, Tf retains the ability to target and interact with TfR [29].

We first probed the internalisation of Tf by Caco-2 cells, demonstrating that the extent of Tf uptake by Caco-2 cells (0.18 μg/1.9 cm^2) is likely to be comparable with a previous study [16] showing that cell internalization of insulin-Tf conjugate was around 1.9 pmoles per 3.5 cm^2 monolayer (Caco-2), equivalent to around 0.15 μg (the final insulin:Tf ratio in the conjugate was 3:1).

Cell internalisation of Tf-NP was tested both in multiwell-cultured cells and differentiated cell monolayers. This was done to determine any potential difference in cell uptake capacity between undifferentiated and differentiated cells (cultured on inserts), given the difference in surface area available for uptake and potential differential receptor expression between undifferentiated and differentiated cells. In undifferentiated cells (multiwell culture) cell uptake of Tf-NP was over five-fold higher relative to bare NP. Furthermore, excess free Tf reduced cell uptake of Tf-NP by more than three-fold (Figure 3). With regards to cell uptake of Tf-NP in differentiated cells, data revealed more than 16-fold higher cell uptake of Tf-NP compared to bare NP (Figure 4), with the latter displaying a similar uptake level to that previously reported by us (around 2 μg here versus 5 μg in previously published work [30]), confirming the pattern observed in undifferentiated cells. The notably larger magnitude of effect (enhanced cell uptake following Tf presentation on NP) may be related to differential TfR expression in undifferentiated *versus* differentiated cells. The implications of these findings are important, pointing to significant enhancement of cell uptake of NP following presentation of Tf on their surface.

It is noted that the definitive biological pathway of Tf-NP uptake in Caco-2 cells cannot be ascertained from this work. However, suppression of internalisation by excess free Tf does point to a TfR-dependent uptake, similarly to the study by Shah and Shen [16] who demonstrated that the binding and uptake of the radiolabelled insulin-Tf conjugate in Caco-2 cells were inhibited by 70% and 80%, respectively, with excess unlabeled Tf.

We finally considered the transport of Tf-NP across differentiated Caco-2 monolayers. The data concerning this showed remarkably higher (23-fold) transport of Tf-NP across cells compared to bare NP (Figure 5). It must be pointed out that this remarkable enhancement in the permeation of NP across intestinal epithelium in vitro is much higher than that previously seen with other transcytosis receptor systems exploited in a similar manner (i.e., for intestinal NP delivery). This includes the neonatal Fc receptor (FcRn), whereby the uptake into Caco-2 cells of polyethylene glycol-poly(lactic-*co*-glycolic acid) (PEG-PLGA) NP modified with Fc was improved (compared to non Fc-modified NP) by a maximum three-fold [20]. Similarly, a different study showed that the translocation of 63 nm Fc-targeted poly(lactic acid)-*b*-poly(ethylene glycol) (PLA-PEG) across Caco-2 monolayers was increased by approximately a factor of two (compared to non-modified NP) [21].

Overall, this work highlights that the TfR transport system shows potential as a pathway for cell entry and transepithelial permeation of NP in the intestinal epithelium. Therefore, this system should be given consideration as a potential pathway for intestinal delivery of nanomedicines intended for systemic effect or local action. The latter is particularly applicable to colon cancer and IBD, given TfR overexpression in the intestinal mucosa in these diseases [12,13]. Therefore, TfR-mediated delivery should be probed further for its potential usefulness in the area of oral or intestinal delivery of nanomedicines.

Author Contributions: Conceptualization, D.V.; Methodology, D.V., J.M. and J.M.Y.; Software, D.V., J.M.Y.; Validation, J.M.Y. and J.M.; Formal Analysis, D.V., J.M.Y. and J.M.; Investigation, J.M.Y., Y.C. and J.M.; Resources, D.V.; Data Curation, J.M.Y., Y.C. and J.M.; Writing-Original Draft Preparation, D.V. and J.M.Y.; Writing-Review & Editing, D.V.; Supervision, D.V.

References

1. Nordisk, N. Available online: https://www.novonordisk.com/content/Denmark/HQ/www-novonordisk-com/en_gb/home/media/news-details.2226662.html (accessed on 17 December 2018).
2. Vllasaliu, D.; Shubber, S.; Fowler, R.; Garnett, M.; Alexander, C.; Stolnik, S. Epithelial toxicity of alkylglycoside surfactants. *J. Pharm. Sci.* **2013**, *102*, 114–125. [CrossRef] [PubMed]
3. Anselmo, A.C.; Gokarn, Y.; Mitragotri, S. Non-invasive delivery strategies for biologics. *Nat. Rev. Drug Discov.* **2018**, *18*, 19–40. [CrossRef] [PubMed]
4. Therapeutics, R. Available online: https://www.ranitherapeutics.com (accessed on 17 December 2018).
5. Vllasaliu, D.; Alexander, C.; Garnett, M.; Eaton, M.; Stolnik, S. Fc-mediated transport of nanoparticles across airway epithelial cell layers. *J. Control. Release* **2012**, *158*, 479–486. [CrossRef] [PubMed]
6. Kim, K.S.; Suzuki, K.; Cho, H.; Youn, Y.S.; Bae, Y.H. Oral Nanoparticles Exhibit Specific High-Efficiency Intestinal Uptake and Lymphatic Transport. *ACS Nano* **2018**, *12*, 8893–8900. [CrossRef] [PubMed]
7. Pridgen, E.M.; Alexis, F.; Farokhzad, O.C. Polymeric nanoparticle drug delivery technologies for oral delivery applications. *Expert. Opin. Drug Deliv.* **2015**, *12*, 1459–1473. [CrossRef] [PubMed]
8. Lajoie, J.M.; Shusta, E.V. Targeting receptor-mediated transport for delivery of biologics across the blood-brain barrier. *Annu. Rev. Pharmacol. Toxicol.* **2015**, *55*, 613–631. [CrossRef]
9. Lam, F.C.; Morton, S.W.; Wyckoff, J.; Han, T.L.; Hwang, M.K.; Maffa, A.; Balkanska-Sinclair, E.; Yaffe, M.B.; Floyd, S.R.; Hammond, R.T. Enhanced efficacy of combined temozolomide and bromodomain inhibitor therapy for gliomas using targeted nanoparticles. *Nat. Commun.* **2018**, *9*, 1991. [CrossRef]
10. Uchida, Y.; Ohtsuki, S.; Katsukura, Y.; Ikeda, C.; Suzuki, T.; Kamiie, J.; Terasaki, T. Quantitative targeted absolute proteomics of human blood-brain barrier transporters and receptors. *J. Neurochem.* **2011**, *117*, 333–345. [CrossRef]
11. Banerjee, D.; Flanagan, P.R.; Cluett, J.; Valberg, L.S. Transferrin receptors in the human gastrointestinal tract. Relationship to body iron stores. *Gastroenterology* **1986**, *91*, 861–869. [CrossRef]
12. Shen, Y.; Li, X.; Dong, D.; Zhang, B.; Xue, Y.; Shang, P. Transferrin receptor 1 in cancer: A new sight for cancer therapy. *Am. J. Cancer Res.* **2018**, *8*, 916–931.
13. Tirosh, B.; Khatib, N.; Barenholz, Y.; Nissan, A.; Rubinstein, A. Transferrin as a luminal target for negatively charged liposomes in the inflamed colonic mucosa. *Mol. Pharm.* **2009**, *6*, 1083–1091. [CrossRef] [PubMed]
14. Du, W.; Fan, Y.; Zheng, N.; He, B.; Yuan, L.; Zhang, H.; Wang, X.; Wang, J.; Zhang, X.; Zhang, Q. Transferrin receptor specific nanocarriers conjugated with functional 7peptide for oral drug delivery. *Biomaterials* **2013**, *34*, 794–806. [CrossRef] [PubMed]
15. Amet, N.; Wang, W.; Shen, W.C. Human growth hormone-transferrin fusion protein for oral delivery in hypophysectomized rats. *J. Control. Release* **2010**, *141*, 177–182. [CrossRef] [PubMed]
16. Shah, D.; Shen, W.C. Transcellular delivery of an insulin-transferrin conjugate in enterocyte-like Caco-2 cells. *J. Pharm. Sci.* **1996**, *85*, 1306–1311. [CrossRef] [PubMed]
17. Yang, D.; Liu, D.; Deng, H.; Zhang, J.; Qin, M.; Yuan, L.; Zou, X.; Shao, B.; Li, H.; Dai, W.; et al. Transferrin Functionization Elevates Transcytosis of Nanogranules across Epithelium by Triggering Polarity-Associated Transport Flow and Positive Cellular Feedback Loop. *ACS Nano* **2019**, *13*, 5058–5076. [CrossRef] [PubMed]
18. Ganugula, R.; Arora, M.; Guada, M.; Saini, P.; Kumar, M.N.R. Noncompetitive Active Transport Exploiting Intestinal Transferrin Receptors for Oral Delivery of Proteins by Tunable Nanoplatform. *ACS Macro Lett.* **2017**, *6*, 161–164. [CrossRef]
19. Pitek, A.S.; O'Connell, D.; Mahon, E.; Monopoli, M.P.; Bombelli, F.B.; Dawson, K.A. Transferrin coated nanoparticles: Study of the bionano interface in human plasma. *PLoS ONE* **2012**, *7*, e40685. [CrossRef]
20. Shi, Y.; Sun, X.; Zhang, L.; Sun, K.; Li, K.; Li, Y.; Zhang, Q. Fc-modified exenatide-loaded nanoparticles for oral delivery to improve hypoglycemic effects in mice. *Sci. Rep.* **2018**, *8*, 726. [CrossRef]
21. Pridgen, E.M.; Alexis, F.; Kuo, T.T.; Levy-Nissenbaum, E.; Karnik, R.; Blumberg, R.S.; Langer, L.; Farokhzad, O.C. Transepithelial transport of Fc-targeted nanoparticles by the neonatal fc receptor for oral delivery. *Sci. Transl. Med.* **2013**, *5*, 213ra167. [CrossRef]
22. Bird, J.L.; Simpson, R.; Vllasaliu, D.; Goddard, A.D. Neurotensin receptor 1 facilitates intracellular and transepithelial delivery of macromolecules. *Eur. J. Pharm. Biopharm.* **2017**, *119*, 300–309. [CrossRef]
23. Hashem, L.; Swedrowska, M.; Vllasaliu, D. Intestinal uptake and transport of albumin nanoparticles: Potential for oral delivery. *Nanomedicine (Lond.)* **2018**, *13*, 1255–1265. [CrossRef] [PubMed]

24. Martins, J.P.; D'Auria, R.; Liu, D.; Fontana, F.; Ferreira, M.P.; Correia, A.; Kemell, M.; Moslova, K.; Makila, K.; Salonen, J.; et al. Engineered Multifunctional Albumin-Decorated Porous Silicon Nanoparticles for FcRn Translocation of Insulin. *Small* **2018**, *14*, e1800462. [CrossRef] [PubMed]
25. Qian, Z.M.; Li, H.; Sun, H.; Ho, K. Targeted drug delivery via the transferrin receptor-mediated endocytosis pathway. *Pharmacol. Rev.* **2002**, *54*, 561–587. [CrossRef] [PubMed]
26. Lim, C.J.; Norouziyan, F.; Shen, W.C. Accumulation of transferrin in Caco-2 cells: A possible mechanism of intestinal transferrin absorption. *J. Control. Release* **2007**, *122*, 393–398. [CrossRef] [PubMed]
27. Fowler, R.; Vllasaliu, D.; Falcone, F.H.; Garnett, M.; Smith, B.; Horsley, H.; Alexander, C.; Stolnik, S. Uptake and transport of B12-conjugated nanoparticles in airway epithelium. *J. Control. Release* **2013**, *172*, 374–381. [CrossRef]
28. Song, Y.; Shi, Y.; Zhang, L.; Hu, H.; Zhang, C.; Yin, M.; Chu, L.; Yan, X.; Zhao, M.; Zhang, X.; et al. Synthesis of CSK-DEX-PLGA Nanoparticles for the Oral Delivery of Exenatide to Improve Its Mucus Penetration and Intestinal Absorption. *Mol. Pharm.* **2019**, *16*, 518–532. [CrossRef] [PubMed]
29. Chang, J.; Paillard, A.; Passirani, C.; Morille, M.; Benoit, J.P.; Betbeder, D.; Garcion, E. Transferrin adsorption onto PLGA nanoparticles governs their interaction with biological systems from blood circulation to brain cancer cells. *Pharm. Res.* **2012**, *29*, 1495–1505. [CrossRef]
30. Bannunah, A.M.; Vllasaliu, D.; Lord, J.; Stolnik, S. Mechanisms of nanoparticle internalization and transport across an intestinal epithelial cell model: Effect of size and surface charge. *Mol. Pharm.* **2014**, *11*, 4363–4373. [CrossRef]

12

Preparation and Characterization of Oxidized Inulin Hydrogel for Controlled Drug Delivery

Franklin Afinjuomo, Paris Fouladian, Ankit Parikh, Thomas G. Barclay, Yunmei Song and Sanjay Garg *

School of Pharmacy and Medical Sciences, University of South Australia, Adelaide, South Australia 5001, Australia

* Correspondence: sanjay.garg@unisa.edu.au

Abstract: Inulin-based hydrogels are useful carriers for the delivery of drugs in the colon-targeted system and in other biomedical applications. In this project, inulin hydrogels were fabricated by crosslinking oxidized inulin with adipic acid dihydrazide (AAD) without the use of a catalyst or initiator. The physicochemical properties of the obtained hydrogels were further characterized using different techniques, such as swelling experiments, in vitro drug release, degradation, and biocompatibility tests. The crosslinking was confirmed with Fourier transform infrared spectroscopy (FTIR), thermal gravimetric analysis (TGA), and differential scanning calorimetry (DSC). In vitro releases of 5-fluorouracil (5FU) from the various inulin hydrogels was enhanced in acidic conditions (pH 5) compared with physiological pH (pH 7.4). In addition, blank gels did not show any appreciable cytotoxicity, whereas 5FU-loaded hydrogels demonstrated efficacy against HCT116 colon cancer cells, which further confirms the potential use of these delivery platforms for direct targeting of 5-FU to the colon.

Keywords: hydrogels; oxidized inulin; periodate oxidation; colon targeting

---

1. Introduction

Inulin is an important fructan found in plants and vegetables, such as garlic, leeks, bananas, and Jerusalem artichokes [1]. Inulin belongs to the fructan class of polysaccharides typically containing about 2–60 fructose units in linear chains with $\beta(2\rightarrow1)$ glycosidic linkages and typically linked to a terminal glucose unit [2]. There is a growing interest in inulin because of the key role that fructans play in both food and the pharmaceutical industry. Inulin is only digested by colon bacteria and not in the small intestine, promoting its health benefits as a prebiotic and in food [3–5]. Inulin also serves as a replacement for fat and sugar in the food industry [6,7]. Inulin is Food and Drug Administration (FDA) approved Generally Recognized As Safe (GRAS) polysaccharide with excellent biodegradability, biocompatibility, water solubility, renewability, and non-toxicity, making it very attractive as a drug delivery carrier targeting colon delivery and pulmonary delivery [8–13]. Other important applications include use as a flocculant for wastewater treatment [14] and in tissue engineering scaffolds [15]. The modification of inulin hydroxyl groups allows the introduction of new functional groups into the polymer. In addition to the multiple hydroxyl groups, the flexible furanose backbone, as well as its increased solubility compared with other polysaccharides, means that it can be readily modified chemically. This allows the use of inulin derivatives as carriers for a variety of pharmaceutical applications. Inulin is considered to be a very attractive polysaccharide for colon targeting, because it is only degraded by specific inulinase enzymes found in the colon [9].

For this reason, we hope to exploit the variation in the microflora concentration of various segments of the gastrointestinal tract for site-specific delivery of drugs to the colon. The chemical modification or derivatization of hydrophilic inulin results in new materials with hydrophobic characters making them suitable for drug delivery systems (DDSs), including hydrogels [16–19], micelles [20–22], liposomes [23], nanoparticles [24–26], vaccine adjuvants [27–29], solid dispersion [30,31], microparticles [8,12,32], and macromolecular bioconjugates/prodrugs [33,34]. To develop hydrogel drug delivery systems, different chemical strategies and techniques have been utilized for hydrogel synthesis. Reported methods of preparation include radical polymerization of inulin derivatives [10,11], Michael-addition crosslinking [35], condensation reaction [36], chemical crosslinking using crosslinkers [5,16,37], or chemical crosslinking followed by UV radiation [19] with subsequent formation of pH-sensitive inulin hydrogels. The limitations with the methods reported above include the use of a toxic catalyst [10,16], initiators [36,38], several reaction steps during synthesis, and long gelation period [37]. The use of modified polysaccharides with aldehyde functionality crosslinked with adipic acid hydrazide has been reported for biodegradable polysaccharides, such as pectin [39,40], dextran [41], chitosan [42], alginate [43,44], xanthan, hyaluronic acid [45–48], and gum with potential application as injectable hydrogel. Periodate oxidation of inulin is a well-known method of functionalizing inulin with an aldehyde group [33,49]. This enables the use of oxidized inulin as a macromolecular bioconjugate to couple a cardiac depressant and antiarrhythmic agent procainamide [33], as well as an enzyme immobilizing agent [49].

However, the use of oxidized inulin for hydrogel fabrication by crosslinking the polyaldehyde inulin with adipic acid hydrazide (AAD) has yet to be reported. To the best of our knowledge, there are no prior studies on the use of oxidized inulin in the formation of a hydrogel via crosslinking with non-toxic AAD. In this work, sodium periodate was used as an oxidizing agent to attack the hydroxyl group of inulin between C_3–C_4, breaking the C–C bond and producing two aldehyde groups (Scheme 1A,B). The resulting intermediate obtained from periodate oxidation is highly reactive toward nucleophilic compounds, such as carbazates, amines, and hydrazines. This oxidized inulin reacts with AAD to form a crosslink without the use of a catalyst. It is worth mentioning that this inulin hydrogel was fabricated in physiologic pH conditions (pH 7.4) in phosphate-buffered saline (PBS) as compared with the organic solvents used in most reported inulin hydrogels. Other clear advantages include (1) the fact that the oxidized inulin/AAD hydrogels were formed within 2–4 min and (2) the potential to control their mechanical and degradation properties with the amount of crosslinker used.

We hypothesized that the chemical crosslinking of oxidized inulin with different ratios of AAD would result in hydrogels with different degrees of crosslinking density, which can allow the controlled release of 5-fluorouracil (5FU). The aim of this study was to crosslink oxidized inulin with AAD to obtain a hydrogel with a hydrazone bond. The oxidized inulin was characterized using ^{1}H NMR and FTIR, as well as colorimetric titration. The three hydrogels formed were evaluated using different techniques, such as swelling experiments, rheological measurement, FTIR, TGA, differential scanning calorimetry (DSC), SEM, and degradation as well as biocompatibility and cytotoxicity studies using 33-(4,5-dimethylthiazol-2-yl)-2,5-diphenyl-tetrazolium bromide blue-indicator dye (MTT) assay.

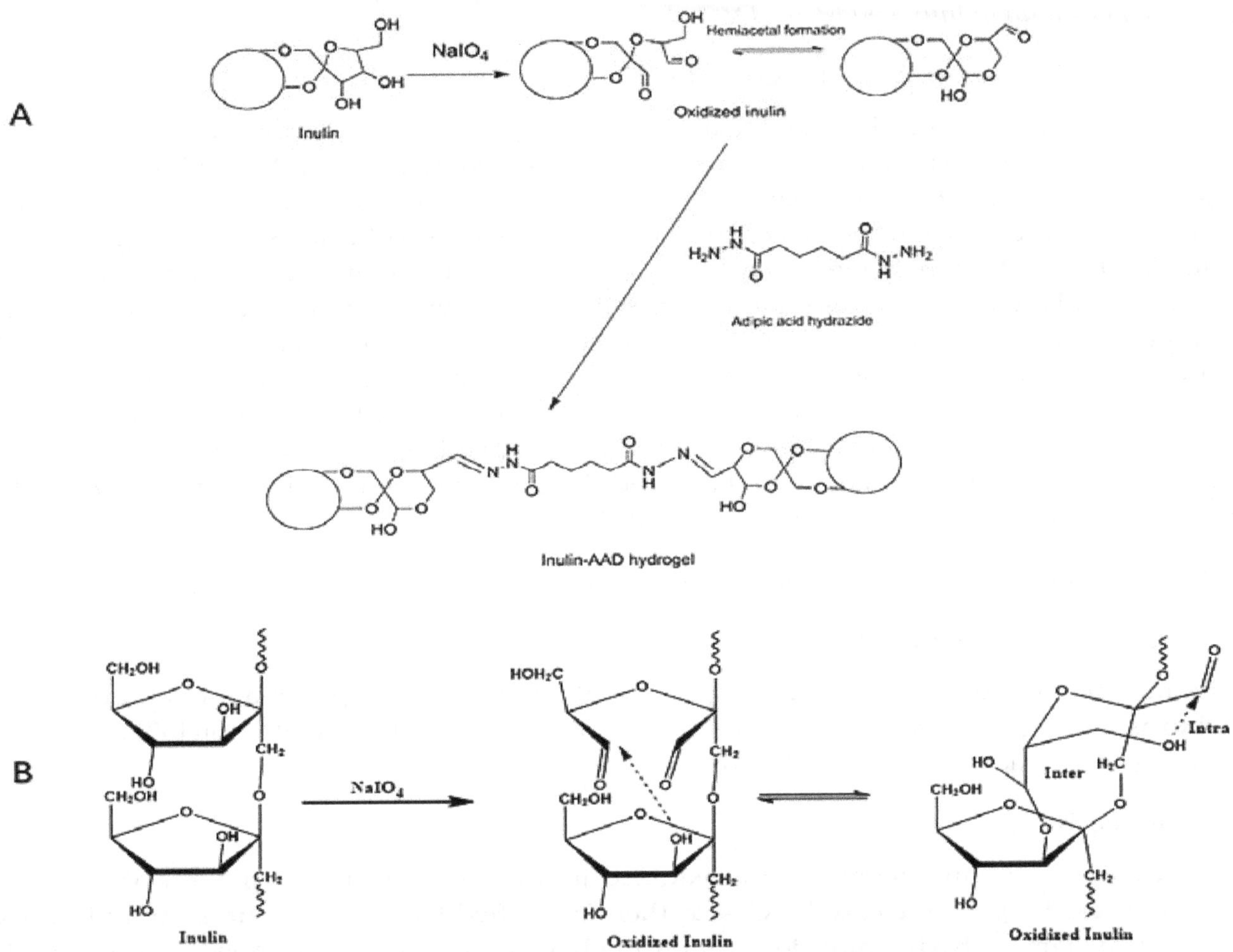

Scheme 1. (**A**) Periodate oxidation of inulin and subsequent crosslinking with adipic acid dihydrazide (AAD) and (**B**) periodate oxidation of inulin with cleavage at C_3–C_4.

2. Materials and Methods

2.1. Materials

Inulin polysaccharide from a Dahlia plant was purchased from Sigma-Aldrich (Castle Hill, New South Wales, Australia), and the average chain length (DPn) 39.2 and MWn = 6381.7 was determined by using end-group analysis via an 1H NMR spectroscopy method previously reported by Barclay et al. [50]. Adipic acid dihydrazide, phosphate-buffered saline tablets, 5-fluorouracil, hydrochloride acid 32%, trichloroacetic acid, sodium metaperiodate, tert-butyl carbazate (tBC), ethylene glycol, hydroxylamine hydrochloride, trinitrobenzenosulfonic acid, methyl orange, McCoy's 5A (Modified) Medium, L-glutamine, potassium bromide (KBr), inulinase and sodium bicarbonate were all acquired from Sigma–Aldrich. Sodium hydroxide was obtained from Ajax FineChem (Taren Point, New South Wale, Australia). CelluSep T4 25-mm flat width 12,000 MWCO Dialysis membranes were purchased from Fisher Biotec Australia (Wembley, Western Australia, Australia). Acetonitrile from Merck Pty Ltd. (Baywaters, Victoria, Australia). Deuterated water (D_2O) and DMSO (DMSO-d_6) for 1H NMR were obtained from Cambridge Isotope Laboratories (Tewksbury, MA, USA). For the MTT assay, 3-(4,5-dimethylthiazol-2-yl)-5-(3-carboxymethoxyphenyl)-2-(4-sulfophenyl)-2H-tetrazolium; 96-well plates; media ingredients including penicillin, streptomycin, and trypsin; and fetal bovine serum (FBS) were purchased from Thermo Fisher Scientific (Thebarton, Adelaide, Australia). All chemicals were of analytic grade and used as received without any further modification or purification.

2.2. Oxidation of Inulin to Inulin Aldehyde Derivative

Preparation and Characterization of Oxidized Inulin

Inulin was modified to obtain an aldehyde derivative by using the method previously reported [51]. Briefly, 1.2 g of inulin (12.3 mmol fructose units) was dissolved in 25 mL of distilled water, and a half equimolar amount of $NaIO_4$ sodium periodate (0.6 g, 6 mmol) to fructose-repeating unit of inulin was added to the inulin suspension and stirred at 25 °C. The molar ratio of fructose-repeating units of raw inulin to $NaIO_4$ was 2:1, which was expected to give a theoretical degree of oxidation (DO) of 50%. The periodate oxidation reaction was protected from light by carrying out the reaction in the dark and at room temperature. The reaction was allowed to proceed for different times (2 h, 3 h, 4 h, 15 h, and 20 h) in order to investigate the effect of reaction time on the oxidation process. The reaction was terminated by adding an excess quantity of ethylene glycol (molar ratio of 3:1 to $NaIO_4$). Then, the reaction mixture was purified using a simple dialysis membrane bag in milliQ water for 3 days [52]. During the dialysis process, the water was changed daily, and the final oxidized inulin product (a white fluffy product) was obtained after freeze-drying the resulting solution.

2.3. Determination of the Degree of Oxidation (Aldehyde Content Analysis)

2.3.1. Determination of Degree of Oxidation

The number of aldehyde functional groups obtained from the periodate oxidation reaction, referred to as the degree of oxidation, was quantified using hydroxylamine titration [53] and ^{1}H NMR spectroscopy after reaction with tBC [41,54].

Hydroxylamine Titration

The reaction of hydroxylamine with oxidized inulin results in the formation of oximes and hydrochloric acid [53]. The released HCl was then quantified by titration with sodium hydroxide. For the hydroxylamine hydrochloride titration method, an accurately weighed amount of about 50.0 mg of each freeze-dried oxidized inulin sample was dissolved in 20 mL of 0.25 N hydroxylamine hydrochloride solution–methyl orange solution, and the pH was adjusted to 4.5 before use. The resulting mixture was allowed to react for 24 h with continuous stirring, resulting in the formation of oximes and hydrochloric acid. The released hydrochloric acid was then titrated with a standardized 0.5 mol/L NaOH solution, while the progress of the titration was monitored with a pH meter and visual observation of the color change until a red-to-yellow endpoint was achieved. The change in pH and the volume of sodium hydroxide consumed was recorded. Inulin oxidation using periodate produces two equivalent aldehyde groups for each mole of periodate consumed [51]. The related reactions and calculation formulas are as follows:

$$\text{INU-(CHO)n} + \text{NH}_2\text{OH}\cdot\text{HCL} \rightarrow \text{INU-(CH=N-OH)n} + \text{nH}_2\text{O} + \text{nHCL}$$

$$\text{HCL} + \text{NaOH} \rightarrow \text{NaCL} + \text{H}_2\text{O}.$$

The degree of oxidation can be calculated from the formula below:

$$\frac{\text{The volume of NaOH consumed } \times \text{Concentration (NaOH) } \times 10^{-3}}{\text{Weight of the sample (g) } \times \text{ Molecular Weight of inulin}} = \frac{\text{Mol of aldehyde}}{\text{Mol of inulin}} \quad (1)$$

^{1}H NMR Spectroscopy after Titration with tBC

The degree of oxidation was also characterized using the ^{1}H NMR spectroscopy method previously reported by Maia et al. [41]. In this method, a mixture of about 20 mg of oxidized inulin samples dissolved in about 3 mL of sodium acetate buffer with pH 5.0 (acidic condition) was reacted with excess tBC (81.278 mg) at room temperature for 24 h. Thereafter, the unreacted tBC was removed using dialysis. The resulting solution was then freeze-dried, and the ^{1}H NMR spectroscopy spectrum was obtained using DMSO-d_6 solvent. The ^{1}H NMR spectroscopy method used in this experiment enables the quantification of the degree of oxidation (aldehyde content of the oxidized inulin) by comparing the ratio of the integral peak (δ) at 7.2 ppm belonging to the proton of the carbazone group to the glucose anomeric proton from inulin at δ 5.2 ppm. This method provides a similar result to that of colorimetric titration in the case of oxidized dextran. However, the formation of precipitates with highly oxidized sugar may limit the application of this method [41]. Using ^{1}H NMR, the degree of oxidation of inulin can be determined using the equation below:

$$\text{The degree of oxidation} = \frac{A \times 100}{B} \quad (2)$$

where A represents the integral peak (δ) at 7.2 ppm from the carbazone proton and B is the integral of the glucose anomeric proton at 5.2 ppm.

2.4. *Preparation and Characterization of Hydrogels (Wissembourg, France)*

The oxidized inulin (Oxi-4h) was dissolved in PBS (pH 7.4) to obtain a 6% (*w*/*v*) polysaccharide concentration [47]. AAD was also dissolved in PBS solution (pH 7.4) in order to obtain 2.5%, 5%, and 10% concentration. Finally, 800 µL of oxidized inulin solution was mixed with 200 µL of each different concentration of the AAD solution to form hydrogels [47]. The crosslinking of the hydrogels was allowed to proceed at 37 °C. Three hydrogels were formed using a different amount of crosslinker, namely INUAAD2.5, INUAAD5, and INUAAD10, corresponding to the gel obtained with 2.5%, 5% and 10% of crosslinker, respectively. The synthesized hydrogels were soaked in de-ionized water for 1 day in order to remove any unbound crosslinker and other unreacted reagents before freeze-drying.

2.5. *Characterization of Oxidized Polymer and Hydrogels: FTIR and ^{1}H NMR*

The modification of the vicinal hydroxyl groups in inulin into aldehyde functional groups was confirmed by ^{1}H NMR (Bruker Avance III 500 NMR, Wissembourg, France) and FTIR spectrophotometer (Shimadzu IRPrestige-21 FTIR 8400 spectrophotometer, Kyoto, Japan). The FTIR spectra of all the oxidized samples and hydrogels were acquired using a Schimadzu FTIR spectrophotometer in the region of 4000–400 cm^{-1} by recording 128 scans with a resolution of 4 cm^{-1}. Briefly, about 2 mg of the freeze-dried samples and hydrogels were ground into powder before being mixed with about 100 mg of KBr and pressed into pellets using a hydraulic press. The ^{1}H NMR spectra were acquired with a Brucker NMR spectrometer using a 5-mm broadband NMR probe, and DMSO was used as the solvent for all the samples except where stated otherwise.

2.6. *Characterization of Hydrogels: TGA*

Based on preliminary characterization, oxidized inulin obtained after 4 h of oxidation time was selected for further characterization and for hydrogel fabrication. About 6 ± 0.1 mg of each freeze-dried sample of oxidized inulin, crosslinker (AAD), and the hydrogels (INUAAD2.5, INUAAD5, and INUAAD10) were accurately weighed, and thermal gravimetric analysis was carried out in a TA Instrument (Thermogravimetric Analyzer Discovery TGA 550, New Castle, DE, USA) by heating the sample from 25 to 500 °C at a heating rate of 10 °C/min under a nitrogen atmosphere (10 mL min^{-1}).

2.7. *Characterization of Hydrogels: DSC*

Differential scanning (DSC) of the synthesized inulin hydrogels (INUAAD2.5, INUAAD5, and INUAAD10), AAD, and the modified inulin was investigated using a Discovery DSC TA Instrument (model Discovery DSC 2920, New Castle, DE, USA). Briefly, ~2 ± 0.1 mg of each freeze-dried sample was weighed accurately in a platinum cup before being heated from 25 to 250 °C in a nitrogen atmosphere at a rate of 10 °C/min.

2.8. Rheological Evaluation

The rheological measurement of the synthesized inulin hydrogel was carried out using a rheometer (Malvern Kinexus pro+ Rotational, Worcestershire, UK) with parallel plates (diameter, 25-mm steel). In order to investigate the viscoelastic behavior of the hydrogels, the procured hydrogel was placed between the parallel plates with a gap of 1 mm in oscillatory mode while maintaining the temperature at 37 °C. Prior to rheological analysis, the inulin hydrogel was procured at 37 °C and allowed to stand for 30 min before testing. In order to ensure that all measurement was within the viscoelastic region, prior to the start of the frequency sweep experiments, a strain sweep was conducted using 1.0-Hz frequency and 0.1% strain. Thereafter, storage modulus (G′) and loss modulus (G′′) of the inulin hydrogels were determined using a frequency sweep test from 0.1 to 10 Hz and controlled strain ($\gamma = 0.01$).

2.9. Scanning Electron Microscope (SEM) Analysis

SEM imaging was conducted using FEI Quanta 450 FEG Environmental SEM (FEI, Hillsboro, OR, USA). Before the imaging process, the fully swollen hydrogels in sodium acetate buffer (pH 5.0) and PBS buffer (pH 7.4) were frozen using liquid nitrogen before freeze-drying to ensure that the morphology of the hydrogels was preserved. The freeze-dried hydrogels (INUAAD2.5, INUAAD5, and INUAAD10) were then transferred to double-sided tape before being sputter-coated with 10 mm of palladium, and the morphology was viewed using FEI Quanta 450 FEG Environmental SEM at an accelerated voltage of 10 KV. Furthermore, the pore size was determined from the SEM micrographs using image J software 1.49 v from the National Institutes of Health, Bethesda, MD, USA.

2.10. Dynamic Swelling Experiments: Swelling Analysis

The swelling properties of the hydrogels (INUAAD2.5, INUAAD5, and INUAAD10) were determined by the gravimetry method. Briefly, dry inulin hydrogel was weighed (Wd) before being immersed in deionized water and PBS buffer solution (pH 7.4) until the equilibrium swelling was reached, after which the hydrogels were removed. Excess surface water on the hydrogels was then blotted with the use of tissue paper before the swollen hydrogel was finally weighed. All the swelling experiments were performed in triplicate and at 37 °C. Finally, the equilibrium swelling ratio and percentage of swelling were calculated from Equations (3) and (4), respectively:

$$\text{Equilibrium swelling ratio of the hydrogel} = \frac{(\text{Ws} - \text{Wd})}{\text{Wd}} \tag{3}$$

$$\%\text{S} = \frac{(\text{Ws} - \text{Wd}) \times 100}{\text{Wd}} \tag{4}$$

where Ws represents the final weight of the fully swollen hydrogel and Wd is the dry weight of the hydrogel before swelling.

2.11. Release Kinetics of 5FU from Crosslinked Hydrogels

The encapsulation of 5FU to the hydrogels was accomplished during the crosslinking of the hydrogels. Briefly, 0.8 mL of oxidized inulin solution was mixed with 1 mg of 5FU before crosslinking this mixture with 0.2 mL of AAD, and subsequently, the mixture was incubated at 37 °C. The 5FU in the hydrogels was fixed at 1 mg/mL, and subsequently, the hydrogels were freeze-dried to obtain dried powder. Furthermore, the in vitro release experiment was carried out using the obtained freeze-dried powder. The release experiment was performed at physiological body temperature 37 °C in a 50-mL falcon tube. Then, 10 mL of release medium (phosphate buffer at pH 7.4 or sodium acetate buffer at pH 5.0) was added with constant stirring at 50 RPM. At scheduled time intervals, about 500 µL of the release aliquot was collected from the release medium, and the 5FU concentration in this aliquot was assayed using the HPLC method previously reported [55]. The HPLC system (Shimadzu Corporation, Kyoto, Japan) consisted of a pump (LC-20ADXR), an autosampler, a photodiode array (PDA) detector set to 268 nm, and a column for separation (Agilent Zorbax 300–SCX C18, 250 mm × 4.6 mm, 5 μm, Agilent Technologies Australia, Mulgrave, Victoria, Australia). The mobile phase for the HPLC assay was 10% acetonitrile and 90% water, and the flow rate was maintained at 0.9 mL/min in isocratic mode [55]. The injection volume of 5FU into the HPLC was 20 μL, the run time was 6 min, and the retention time for the 5FU peak was 3.061 min. The concentration of analytes was diluted to ensure that they fall within the standard calibration curve concentration range. A linear calibration curve of 5FU was plotted in the concentration range of 0.1–10 μg/mL ($R^2 > 0.999$). All measurements were conducted in triplicate.

2.12. Degradation Studies

The degradation studies of the fabricated inulin hydrogels (INUAAD2.5, INUAAD5, and INUAAD10) were conducted in PBS (pH 7.4) without inulinase enzyme [49]. In addition, the in vitro degradation of the inulin hydrogels in the presence of inulinase was also investigated by immersing the three different hydrogels (INUAAD2.5, INUAAD5, and INUAAD10) into sodium acetate buffer (pH 5.0) containing 10 units inulinase/mL [36]. Inulinase was chosen because this enzyme is specifically expressed by the colon and is capable of degrading inulin polysaccharide [56–58]. In brief, dry inulin hydrogels (0.050 g) were added into 5 mL of the medium (PBS or acetate), followed by incubation at 37 °C with and without inulinase enzyme. At a predetermined time interval, the hydrogels were removed from the falcon tube and washed with water to remove any remnant of the enzyme. Finally, the remaining hydrogels were dried and weighed, and the weight was recorded as Wdt. All the experiments were performed in triplicate.

The degradation of the hydrogels was determined using Equation (5) below:

$$\% \text{ Degradation} = \frac{(\text{Wd} - \text{Wdt}) \times 100}{\text{Wd}} \quad (5)$$

where Wd and Wdt are the initial starting weights before and after degradation, respectively.

2.13. MTT Assay

The cytotoxicity of the synthesized inulin hydrogels and drug-loaded hydrogels were investigated against HCT116 human colorectal carcinoma cell lines (a gift from Professor Shudong of Wang Laboratory) using 3-(4,5-dimethylthiazol-2-yl)-2,5-diphenyl-tetrazolium bromide blue-indicator dye (MTT assay). First, HCT116 cancer cell lines were seeded in 96-well plates at 3×10^3 cells per well, maintained under the expected standard growth condition (37 °C, 5% CO_2, 10% FBS containing McCoy's 5A (Modified) Medium), and incubated for 24 h to allow for proper cell attachment. Subsequently, the drug-loaded hydrogels and blank inulin hydrogels were sterilized for 15 min using an ultraviolet ray. This was followed by rinsing with sterile PBS. Then, 5 mL of McCoy's 5A (Modified) Medium was added into the sterile hydrogel, and it was shaken for 24 h. Thereafter, the hydrogel was removed, and the resulting extracts were filtered using a 0.22-mm syringe. For the MTT assay, cells were incubated for 24 h with a free 5FU solution and the sterilized extracts from the hydrogels after diluting with McCoy's 5A (Modified) Medium to obtain concentrations of 10, 50, and 100 μg/mL [59–61]. This incubation process was followed by washing with PBS, and then, the cells were further treated with 5 mg/mL of MTT solution at 37 °C for 4 h. The culture medium containing MTT reagent was removed, and 0.1 mL of DMSO was added. Finally, the absorbance of the resulting solution was measured at 570 nm using a microplate reader.

3. Results and Discussion

The vicinal hydroxyl groups on inulin were oxidized using sodium periodate, resulting in a highly reactive hemiacetal aldehyde derivative that subsequently reacted with adipic acid dihydrazide to form an inulin hydrogel via a hydrazone bond. Scheme 1 shows the oxidation of inulin by $NaIO_4$ to create two aldehyde functional groups. Note that there is a chance of double oxidation from the glucose end group with the subsequent release of formic acid. However, this would likely represent a small portion of the polyaldehyde formed. This periodate oxidation occurred in an aqueous medium without utilizing any catalyst or any chemical initiator. The oxidation involved breaking the C3–C4 bond, resulting in two aldehyde groups [51], which then crosslinked with AAD to form a hydrogel. Prior studies suggest that one of the reactive aldehyde functional groups at C_3 can undergo a reaction with the neighboring C_6 hydroxyl group, which ultimately leads to the formation of stable intra-residue and inter-residue hemiacetals [62,63]. The stable hemiacetal could restrict the aldehyde functional groups available for nucleophilic reaction to one per fructose residue [51].

During the early stages of the reaction (the first 10 min), an aldehyde functional group peak with very low intensity was observed around 9.5 ppm (Supplementary Materials Figure S1). This peak was not observed at the end of the reaction, possibly suggesting that a masked aldehyde group was involved in the formation of hemiacetals as the reaction progressed. The formation of hemiacetals was further supported by the appearance of a new peak in the ^{1}H NMR spectra of the oxidized samples, with several distinctive peaks in the region of 3.5–5.0 ppm that were not present in the original raw inulin sample (Figure 1A,B). This result helps confirm that raw inulin was modified. (Supplementary Materials Figures S2 and S3A–E). The ^{1}H NMR spectra of the oxidized inulin samples show visible change with the increase in time of the reaction from 2 to 20 h. (Supplementary Materials Figure S3A–E). The formation of hemiacetals, as shown in Figure 1B, is consistent with reports in the literature regarding some oxidized polysaccharides, such as dextran [41,64], cellulose [65], hyaluronic acid [48], alginate [66], starch, pectin, and chitosan [67]. There was rapid release of formic acid, possibly from the oxidation of the reducing end glucose as the reaction proceeded, resulting in a pH drop from 4.15 to 3.88; however, as the reaction proceeded the pH of the reaction medium remained stable at 3.88 for the remaining part of the reaction process (Figure 1D and Supplementary Materials Figure S1). The hemiacetals are behind the disappearance of the aldehyde functional group formed during oxidation.

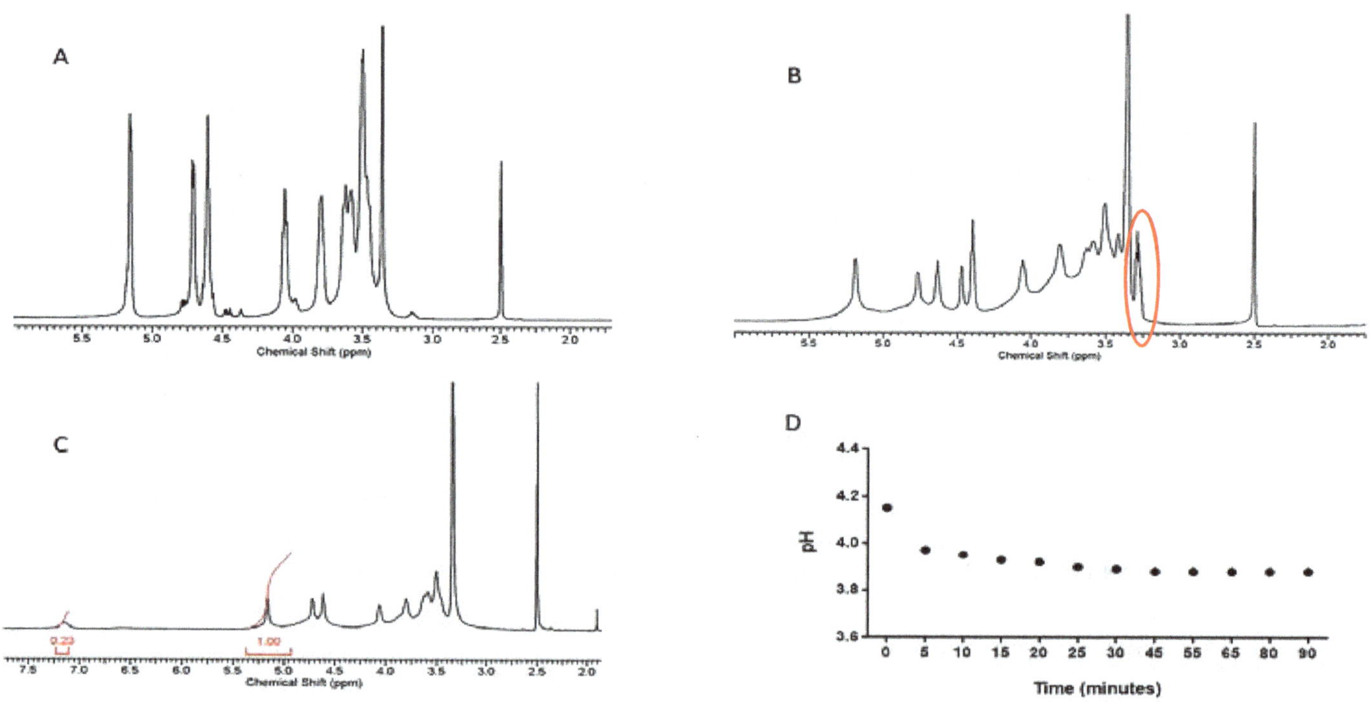

Figure 1. The ^{1}H NMR spectra of (**A**) raw inulin, (**B**) oxidized inulin 2 h (Oxi-2h), and (**C**) oxidized inulin after titration with tert-butyl carbazate (tBC) using DMSO solvent; (**D**) the variation of pH during the oxidation of inulin with periodate. (Red circle show appearance of new peaks after oxidation).

3.1. Oxidized Inulin Characterization

The oxidized inulin derivative was also characterized using ^{1}H NMR spectroscopy. From Figure 1C showing the ^{1}H NMR spectrum of raw inulin, peaks between δ 3.0–4.80 ppm were assigned to fructose and glucose carbon-attached protons except for the anomeric proton from glucose that occurs at 5.2 ppm. The quantification of aldehyde groups, i.e., degree of oxidation (DO), was evaluated using tBC. The aldehyde content of the modified inulin was also investigated using ^{1}H NMR spectroscopy by taking advantage of the reaction of the aldehydes with carbazate to form stable carbazones in same way as in hydrazone formation [41].

As shown in Figure 1C, the formation of carbazone shows that the reactive aldehyde portion of the oxidized inulin reacted with the amine portion of the tBC with evidence of a peak around 7.2 ppm. It is suggested that this peak resulted from the proton attached to the carbon atom modified by reacting the oxidized sample with tBC. Furthermore, there was evidence of the disappearance of peaks attributed to some of the hemiacetals after the formation of the final product. Comparing the carbazone integral's peak δ at 7.2 ppm to that of the glucose anomeric proton at δ 5.2 ppm allowed DO quantification using ^{1}H NMR spectroscopy (Figure 1A and Supplementary Materials Figure S5A–C). The DO of oxidized inulin (oxi-inu) 15 h and 20 h was not assayed by ^{1}H NMR because of the slight oxidation of the anomeric glucose after the long oxidation period, making quantification difficult and inaccurate. Hydroxylamine titration converted the aldehydes into oximes with the release of acid quantified via a titrimetric method. The volume of sodium hydroxide at the endpoint was determined using the first derivative curve of the titration between sodium hydroxide and hydrochloric acid. The result of the ^{1}H NMR spectroscopy for the oxidized inulin samples was lower than the result obtained from the hydroxylamine titration. The slight difference in the DO for the oxidized inulin samples (Table 1) can possibly be attributed to precipitation of the samples by the bulky tBC, as well as the pH of the reaction medium [51,68].

Table 1. The aldehyde content determination using ^{1}H NMR spectroscopy and hydroxylamine titration.

Oxidized Inulin	The Degree of Oxidation by Hydroxylamine (%) ^{a}	The Degree of Oxidation by NMR (%) ^{b}
Oxi-2h	25.6 ± 0.6	23 ± 0.9
Oxi-3h	31 ± 0.8	26 ± 0.7
Oxi-4h	34 ± 0.3	31 ± 1.2
Oxi-15h	38 ± 0.4	n
Oxi-20h	43.6 ± 0.5	n

^{a} The results of all titration experiments were the average of three titrations; ^{b} ^{1}H NMR results calculated from four independent integrations with Advanced Chemistry Development (ACD) software; ^{n} not estimated.

3.2. FTIR

In order to investigate the changes and alterations to the inulin structure as a result of the periodate oxidation, both the raw inulin and modified samples were analyzed using FTIR. Despite the oxidation reaction, the inulin structure was partly preserved. Figure 2A shows the FTIR spectra of the raw inulin and modified inulin samples with different degrees of oxidation based on the reaction time. In Figure 2A, it is difficult to see any difference between the oxidized and raw inulin. However, for the highly oxidized inulin samples (oxi-15h and oxi-20h) there was a low-intensity signal at 1730 cm^{-1} ascribed to the stretching of the carbonyl group from an aldehyde [69]. In addition, there were several changes in the position of the bands, especially in the region of 1300–800 cm^{-1} for the oxidized inulin compared with the raw inulin (Supplementary Materials Figure S6A). The formation of hemiacetals made it difficult to notice any aldehyde groups in the oxidized sample [41], and this is consistent with the reported FTIR of oxidized polysaccharides, such as dextran [41] and alginates [52,70].

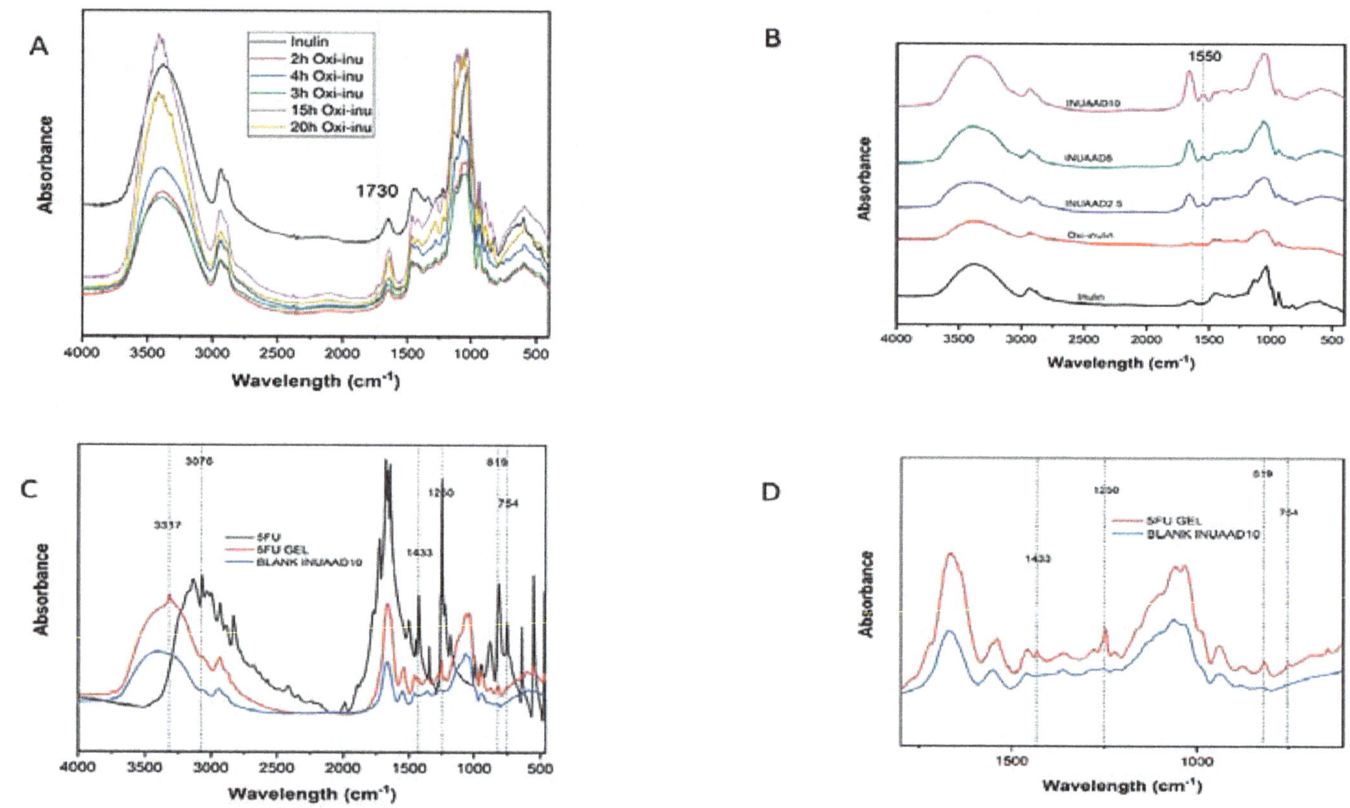

Figure 2. (**A**) The spectra of all the oxi-inulin and raw inulin samples. (**B**) The spectra of inulin, oxidized inulin (oxi-inulin), and the hydrogels. (**C**) Spectra of pure 5-fluorouracil (5FU), blank INUAAD10 gel, and 5FU-loaded hydrogel. (**D**) spectra of blank INUAAD10 and 5FU-loaded hydrogel.

The formation of the hydrogels by crosslinking oxidized inulin with AAD was confirmed by FTIR spectroscopy (Figure 2B). The spectra of the hydrogels show the appearance of the new band at 1550 cm^{-1}, which can be attributed to the NH bending from the crosslinker (AAD). The 5FU-loaded inulin hydrogels were also characterized using FTIR (Figure 2C,D). The FTIR spectra of the 5FU-loaded inulin hydrogels reveal small changes compared with the blank inulin hydrogels, including new bands at 3076, 1433, 1246, 819, and 754 cm^{-1} [71], which were attributed to the incorporation of 5FU. Furthermore, the change in the broad peak of the blank gels compared with that of the 5FU-loaded gels was presumably due to the hydrogen bonding interaction between the OH of the hydrogel and the NH stretching of 5FU, resulting in the formation of a sharp peak around 3317 cm^{-1} [71,72] (Figure 2C). The disappearance of some typical 5FU peaks can also be attributed to the strong hydrogen bond interactions between the blank gels and 5FU (Figure 2C,D and Supplementary Materials Figure S6B,C).

3.3. SEM

The interior morphologies of the fabricated inulin hydrogels, as well as their porous structures, were evaluated by SEM. Figure 3A,B clearly shows that the freeze-dried hydrogels (INUAAD2.5, INUAAD5, and INUAAD10) had irregular, interconnecting inner pores. It is evident that the pore size of the hydrogels decreased with the increase in AAD, as higher concentrations of AAD resulted in higher crosslink density, producing gels with smaller pore size. SEM was also able to show the pore size variation and hydrolysis of the hydrazone bond when the gels were immersed in acetate buffer (pH 5.0) as compared with PBS (pH 7.4) for 2 days. The SEM images confirm the slight degradation of the hydrogels in acetate buffer due to the hydrolysis of the bonds, as well as the increase in pore size (Figure 3A). The formation of porous materials has also been reported for other oxidized polysaccharides crosslinked with AAD in the literature [41,50], and pore formation with controllable pore size is important for drug encapsulation and delivery of drugs such as 5FU.

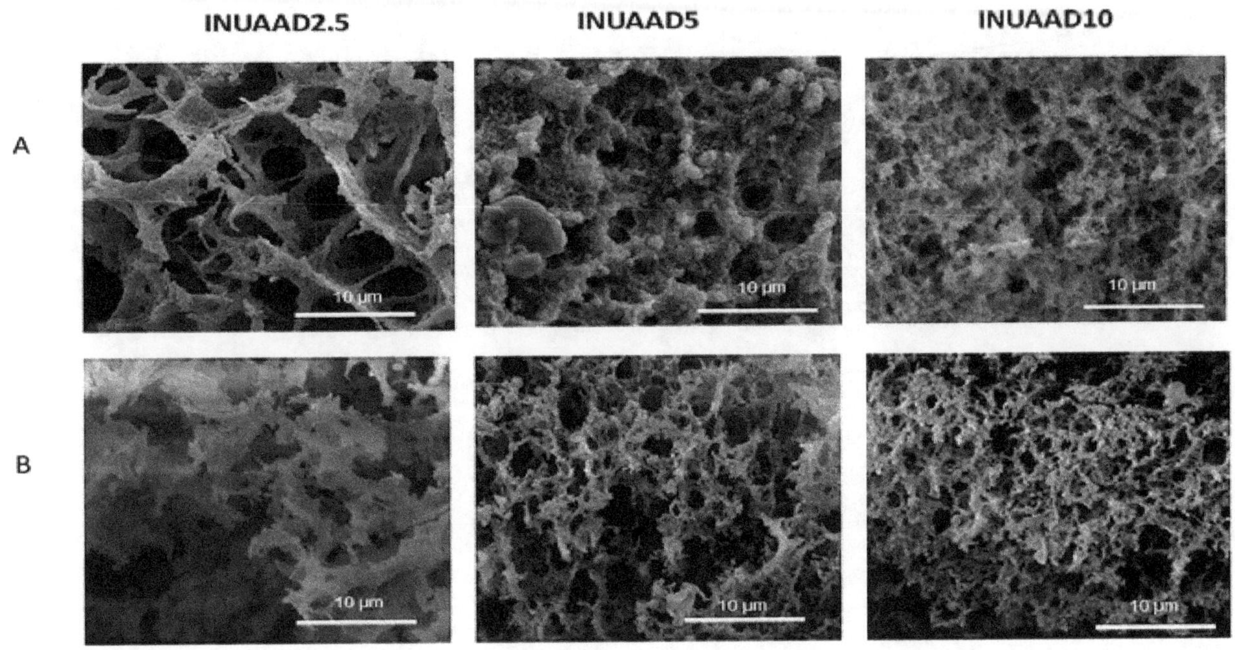

Figure 3. (**A**) SEM images of hydrogels (INUAAD2.5, INUAAD5, and INUAAD10) after immersion in acetate buffer for 2 days. (**B**) SEM images of hydrogels (INUAAD2.5, INUAAD5, and INUAAD10) after immersion in phosphate-buffered saline (PBS) for 2 days.

3.4. TGA/First derivative of the TGA Curve (DTG)

The thermal stability of the raw inulin, oxidized inulin, AAD, and hydrogels was assessed using TGA/DTG. As shown in Figure 4A,B, the crosslinker showed higher thermal stability compared with oxidized inulin. The TGA curve for AAD shows an onset of degradation at 282 °C, and raw inulin showed slight weight loss due to the elimination of water at a temperature below 100 °C and major weight loss occurring between 225 and 325 °C, which was attributed to inulin backbone degradation [73]. There was a clear shift in the onset temperature for degradation from 215 °C for raw inulin to 192 °C for oxidized inulin (reduced by 25 °C), and there was a different character of the thermogram that can be attributed to the damage to the raw inulin chain caused by its oxidation [74–77]. After crosslinking the oxidized inulin with AAD, the thermal stability of the synthesized hydrogels was enhanced and improved compared with the oxidized inulin, as seen in the TGA and DTG curve (Figure 4C). This was due to formation of a stable hydrazone bond and strong hydrogen bonding interactions introduced onto the molecular chain [78–80]. As expected, the hydrogels exhibited three stage mass loss. Below 100 °C, there was the removal of bound and free water in the hydrogels (about 7% weight loss). The second weight loss was due to the decomposition of the inulin backbone, and finally, the third stage was due to the degradation of the AAD. Increasing the AAD concentration during crosslinking resulted in hydrogels with higher decomposition temperature. The maximum thermal decomposition temperature for the hydrogels was found to be 218.4, 225.9, and 227.5 °C for the three hydrogel samples, INUAAD2.5, INUAAD5, and INUAAD10, respectively. The corresponding residual weight at 600 °C for the INUAAD2.5, INUAAD5, and INUAAD10 hydrogels was 17.2%, 3.02%, and 1.55% respectively. It is important to mention that all the oxi-inu hydrogels showed a similar degradation profile (Figure 4D). Proof of crosslinking between the modified oxidized inulin and AAD was confirmed by the change in the maximum temperature of degradation of the hydrogels when compared with that of the oxidized inulin.

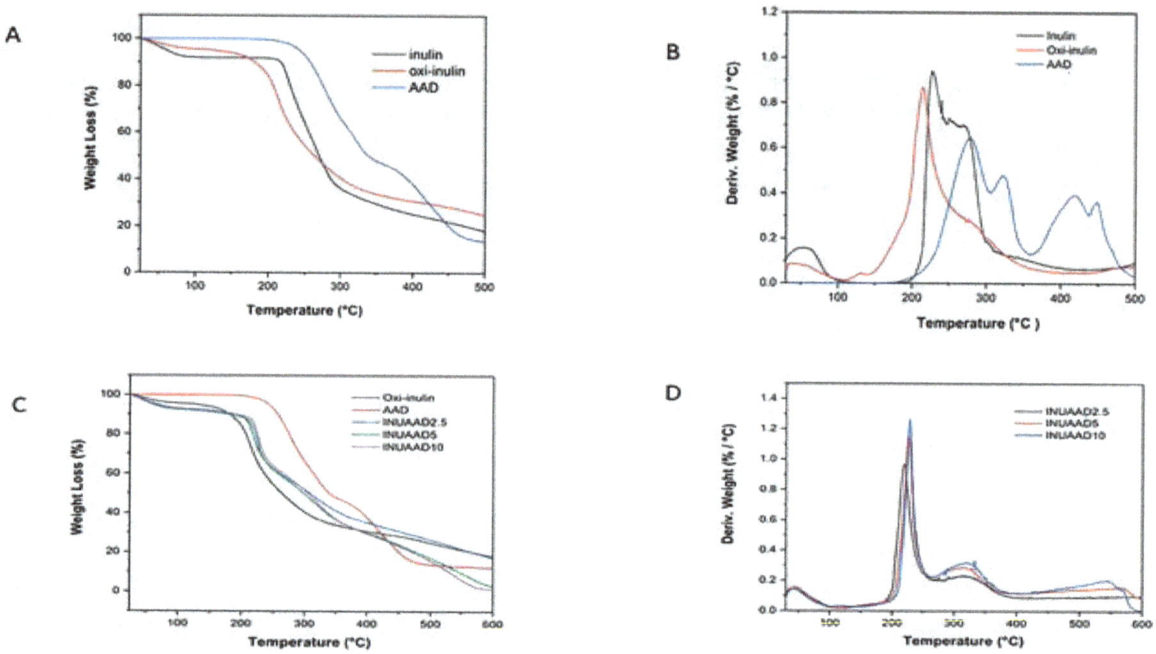

Figure 4. (**A**) Thermograms of the raw inulin, oxidized inulin, and AAD. (**B**) DTG thermograms of the raw inulin, oxidized inulin, and AAD. (**C**) Thermograms of the raw inulin, oxidized inulin, AAD, and hydrogels. (**D**) DTG thermograms of the hydrogels.

3.5. DSC

The DSC of the oxidized inulin, AAD, and hydrogels was also investigated (Figure 5A,B). As shown in the DSC thermogram, the melting point peak of the oxidized inulin was 161.3 °C, and the melting point of AAD was 183.22 °C. However, these peaks were absent in the final hydrogels, indicating the formation of new crosslinked polymeric material. In Figure 5B, the hydrogels exhibited endothermic peaks at 166, 164, and 160 °C for INUAAD2.5, INUAAD5.0, and INUAAD10 respectively, due to degradation of the hydrazone bond [16,81]. Interestingly, as the amount of AAD increased, the temperature of the endothermic peak decreased. In addition, there was a broad exothermic transition for all the hydrogels after the degradation of the hydrazone bond. Another endothermic peak at 196.96, 199.42, and 200.26 °C for INUAAD2.5, INUAAD5.0, and INUAAD10, respectively, can be seen in Figure 5B, which was attributed to the start of the hydrogel degradation. It is very clear that the degradation temperature was dependent on the crosslinking density.

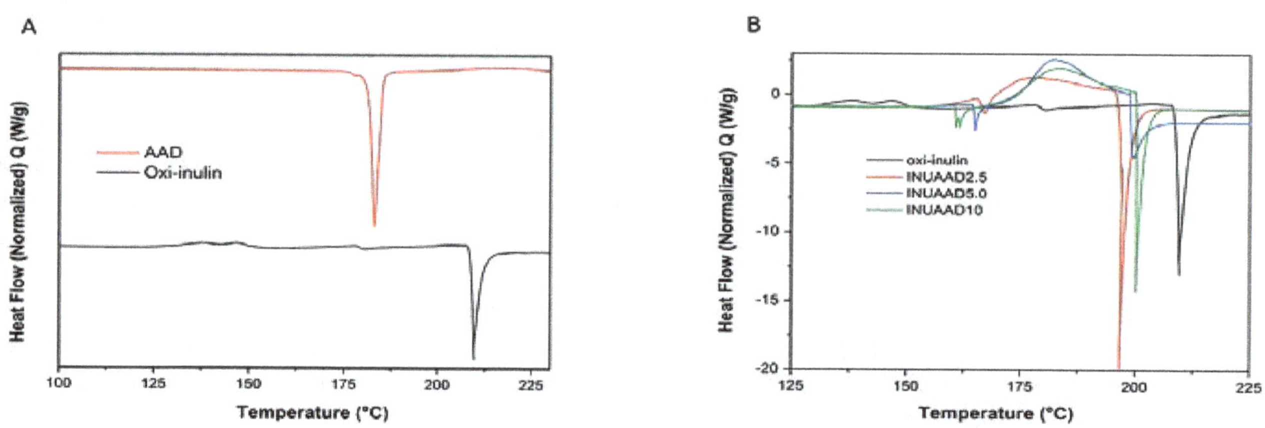

Figure 5. (**A**) Differential scanning calorimetry (DSC) thermograms of the oxidized inulin and AAD; (**B**) thermograms of the oxidized inulin and hydrogels.

3.6. Rheological Properties

As shown in Figure 6A,B, all three fabricated inulin hydrogels, INUAAD2.5, INUAAD5, and INUAAD10, showed higher G′ compared with the G′′ for all the frequencies tested using the frequency sweep mode. As shown in Figure 5A, it is obvious that the G′ increased with the increase in the concentration of the crosslinker from 2.5% to 10%, whereas there was little change with respect to G′′. By increasing the crosslinker from 2.5% to 10%, the G′ increased from ca. 711 to 3015 (Pa) at a frequency of 1 Hz (Supplementary Materials Table S1). This increase in G′ indicates that a stiff and highly crosslinked gel was formed at high AAD concentration [48]. These results indicate that the fabricated hydrogels possessed viscoelastic properties [52,82]. All the hydrogels exhibited high G′ value, which was independent of the frequency that is indicative of a gel with stable viscoelastic solid-like behavior [52]. In addition, all the synthesized inulin hydrogels had similar loss moduli. The difference in elastic moduli also shows that the crosslinking density for the gels differed. This result corroborates the finding that, by varying crosslinker concentration, we can synthesize hydrogels with different degrees of crosslinking. The rheology measurements, particularly the elastic moduli of all the hydrogels, as well as the crosslink density, had a direct correlation to the content of AAD used during crosslinking.

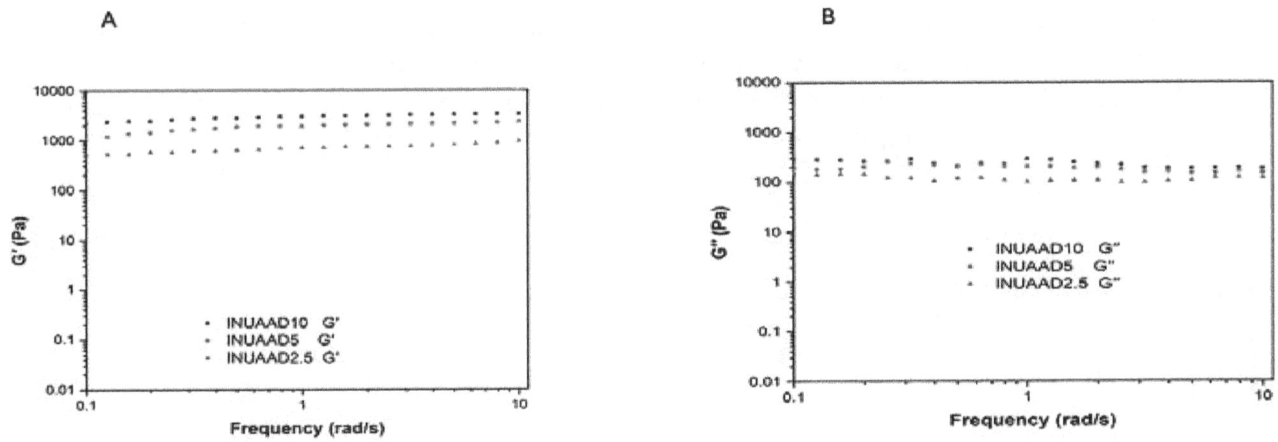

Figure 6. (**A**) Rheological properties of the INUAAD hydrogels showing the storage moduli (G′) and (**B**) the loss moduli (G″) of the different crosslinked inulin hydrogels.

3.7. Gelation and Swelling Studies

The swelling ratio of the fabricated inulin hydrogels in de-ionized water and PBS (pH 7.4) (Supplementary Materials Figure S7) shows a higher swelling ratio (SR) in de-ionized water compared with PBS, as expected. The gels showed moderate swelling in water, with a swelling ratio of 6.95, 5.61, and 3.8 for INUAAD2.5, INUAAD5, and INUAAD10, respectively. The result demonstrates that the swelling ratio of the hydrogels was inversely related to the degree of crosslinking. Furthermore, all the hydrogels reached equilibrium before 24 h, which can help facilitate the diffusion and release of drug molecules from such hydrogels. The SR obtained was comparable to pH-sensitive inulin hydrogels with reported values from 3.5 to 6.5 [19,37] but lower than inulin hydrogels made from pyromellitic dianhydride crosslinker [16]. The SR was also lower than the values reported for oxidized dextran crosslinked with AAD (4.3–8.7) [41] and polyaldehyde guluronate (12.6–15.3) [69]. The gelation time for the fabricated hydrogels obtained by the tube inversion method was directly related to the concentration of AAD used during hydrogel synthesis. The gelation time was reduced from 178 to 128 s with an increase in AAD concentration, which was very close to those reported for oxidized hyaluronic acid/ adipic acid dihydrazide hydrogels (143–175 s) [48] and oxidized dextran/AAD gels (117–230 s) [41]. By controlling the amount of AAD used, we can easily tune the gelation time. As the concentration of AAD used during the hydrogel fabrication increases, the time required for the formation of the hydrogel decreases, which is attributed to the higher percentage of hydrazide available for effective crosslinking.

3.8. Release Kinetics of 5FU from Crosslinked Hydrogels

The drug delivery capability of the fabricated inulin hydrogels was further evaluated using 5FU as the model drug for in vitro release. The in vitro release results show that the amount of 5FU released can be tuned by varying the crosslinker ratio. The release of 5FU was initially characterized by burst release, which was subsequently followed by sustained release, as expected. In this study, the hydrogels with hydrazone linkages allowed faster cleavage at low acidic pH. The inulin hydrogel system exploited acidic pH around colon cancer tissues to achieve better drug release properties. Overall the release profile of 5FU from the crosslinked hydrogels was governed by both the pH of the release medium and the crosslinking density. As shown in Figure 7A,B, as expected, all the hydrogels demonstrated faster drug release in pH 5.0 than in pH 7.4. The hydrazone bond of the inulin hydrogels was relatively stable in physiological pH but was cleaved in acidic pH. As shown in Figure 7A,B, there was a burst release in both pH 5 and 7.4 on the first day, which was followed by a very slow release of 5FU. In the release study, 50%, 38%, and 35% of 5FU was released from INUAAD2.5, INUAAD5.0, and INUAAD10, respectively, in pH 7.4 after 24 h. In contrast, in the acidic media with pH 5.0, after 24 h, 68%, 47%, and 38% of 5FU was released from INUAAD2.5, INUAAD5.0, and INUAAD10, respectively. Moreover, after the initial burst release in pH 5.0, there was a continuous release of 5FU, with about 85% of 5FU released within 2 days for INUAAD2.5. The gels showed higher release in pH 5.0 compared with physiological pH 7.4.

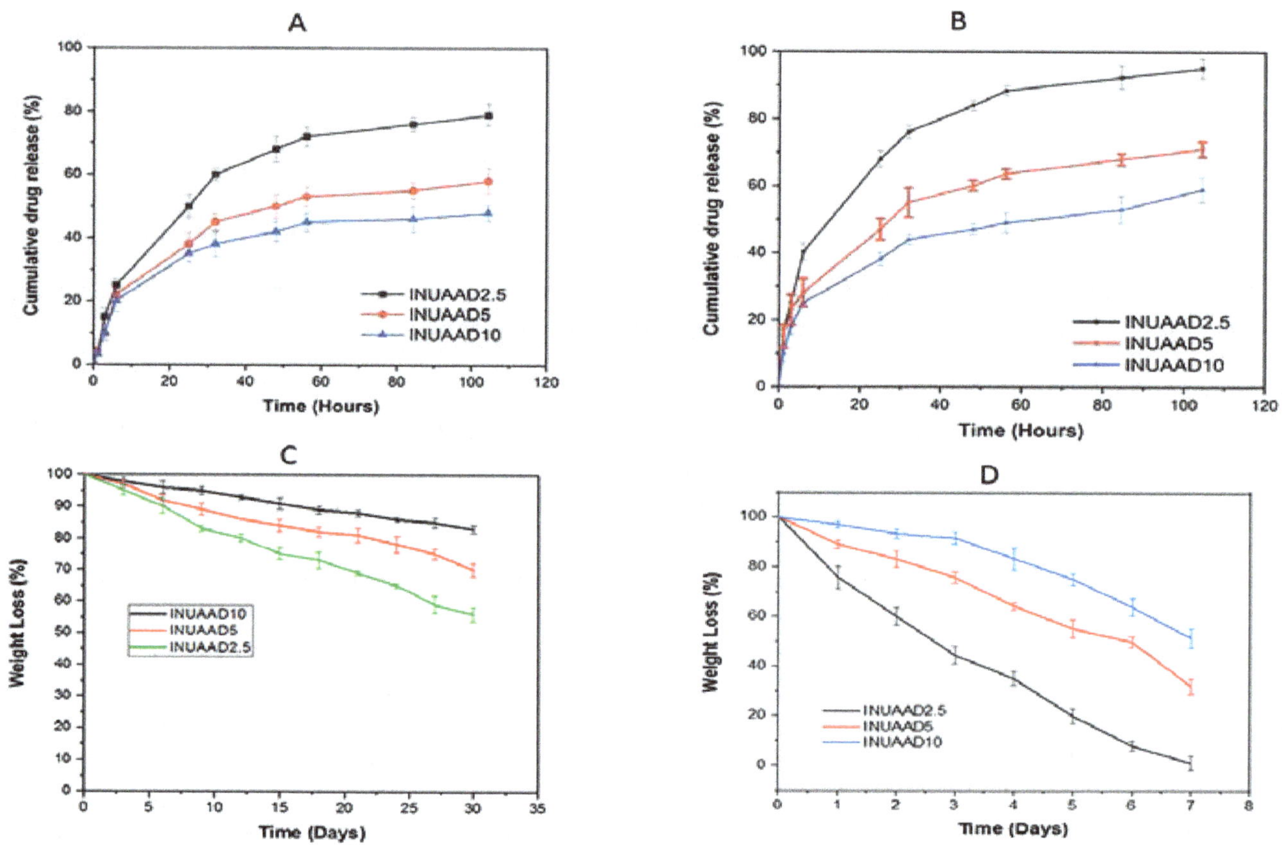

Figure 7. (**A**) The in vitro release rate of 5FU from the hydrogel batches in pH 7.4; (**B**) the in vitro release rate of 5FU from the hydrogel batches in pH 5.0; (**C**) the degradation of the hydrogels in pH 7.4; (**D**) the degradation of the hydrogels in pH 5.0 with the addition of inulinase.

The release of 5FU from the hydrogels was dependent on the crosslinking density and pH of the release media. The FTIR result for the 5FU-loaded hydrogels show that the 5FU amine group and inulin polymer hydroxyl may have formed a hydrogen bond interaction [71,83,84]. This polymer–drug interaction may have resulted in slow drug release from the hydrogel due to entrapment of the remaining drug in the gel network (Figure 2C,D). The smaller pore size allowed the encapsulation of structurally smaller drug moieties, such as 5FU, into the hydrogels [71]. The difference in the stability of the hydrazone bond in pH 7.4 compared with pH 5.0 was exploited for selective and localized targeting of 5FU between colon normal and cancers cells. The difference performance with respect to pH enables the use of this hydrogel as a useful strategy for delivering 5FU to the colon. This result clearly suggests that the acidic environment within colon cancer cells would trigger the degradation of the crosslinked hydrogel, which would result in a higher drug release from the hydrogel. This hydrogel system can potentially maintain a higher concentration of drugs around cancer cells and can possibly reduce adverse side effects on healthy tissue. In order to achieve successful colon targeting, the inulin drug delivery system will require enteric coating to prevent gastric degradation and premature release of drugs as the hydrogel passes through the stomach and small intestine.

3.9. *Degradation*

The degradation rate of the hydrogels was investigated by examining the weight loss in both PBS and acetate buffer, as shown in Figure 7C,D. INUAAD10, INUAAD5.0, and INUAAD2.5 experienced weight loss of 17%, 30%, and 44%, respectively, in PBS after 30 days of incubating, implying that a higher concentration of the crosslinker results in higher resistance to biodegradability. In addition, the in vitro degradation of the inulin hydrogels in the presence of inulinase incubated in sodium acetate buffer (pH 5.0) after one week was 49%, 68%, and 95% degradation for INUAAD10, INUAAD5, and INUAAD2.5, respectively (Figure 7D). Inulinase is known to degrade inulin in the colon and function better around pH 4.7, which is close to pH 5.0 [56]. As shown in Figure 7C,D, the degradation rate decreased with the increase in AAD concentration. This finding could be attributed to the increase in degree of crosslinking, making it harder for the inulinase to attack the hydrogel, as well as the higher hydrazone bond, which tends to be resistant to hydrolytic cleavage. The degradation behavior in acetate buffer was related to the cleavage of the hydrazone bond due to the acidic pH of the medium, as well as partial activity from the enzyme. The hydrogels' degradation was pronounced in acetate buffer with inulinase but slow in physiologic pH conditions. The in vitro degradation data clearly show that it is possible to tune the degradation rate by varying the ratio of the crosslinker. The prolonged degradation profile of these hydrogels make them useful for controlled delivery of drugs to the colon.

3.10. *Cytotoxicity*

The blank crosslinked inulin hydrogels were assayed against the HCT116 cancer cell line using MTT assay, because the application of the synthesized inulin hydrogel as a drug delivery carrier requires the biomaterials to be non-toxic and the 5FU-loaded inulin hydrogels were expected to cause high cytotoxicity to tumor cells. The cell cytotoxicity of different concentrations of extracts from the crosslinked inulin hydrogels, oxidized inulin, and crosslinker was evaluated. As shown in Figure 8A, the viabilities of HCT116 with different extracts of empty inulin hydrogel samples were all above 85% after 24 h of incubation, which clearly demonstrates that these hydrogels were biocompatible with negligible cytotoxicity at concentrations between 10 and 100 μg/mL and that they can be utilized as a delivery platform to deliver drugs to the colon.

In Figure 8A, we can clearly observe, as expected, a dose-dependent decrease in the cell viability as the concentration of the sample increased from 10 to 100 μg/mL with respect to the hydrogel extracts. The blank crosslink hydrogels did not have any appreciable cytotoxicity towards the HCT116 cancer cells. As expected, after 24 h of incubation, both the modified inulin with the aldehyde functional group and AAD showed reduced cell viability with a viability of 77.1% and 88%, respectively (Supplementary Materials Figure S8). This can be attributed to the reactive aldehyde group in the oxidized inulin, which tends to react to the nucleophilic portion of the cells. In addition, the 5FU-loaded hydrogels were assayed for its antitumor activity against the HCT116 cancer cells via MTT assay, and the free 5FU solution was employed as a control. After 24 h of incubation, the 5FU-loaded hydrogels showed a dose-dependent antitumor effect. Furthermore, the gel with the lowest concentration of crosslinker swelled better in the medium, causing a greater release of 5FU and more activity. As shown in Figure 8B, the cell viability of the 5FU-loaded gels against the HCT116 cell line was 65.2%, 71.1%, and 75.2%, respectively, compared with free 5FU, which was 35.9% at 100 μg/mL concentration. The difference in cell viability between the pure and loaded hydrogels was due to the slow release of 5FU from the hydrogel structure. The free 5FU exhibited more antitumor activity compared with the 5FU-loaded hydrogels. This was expected, because the fabricated hydrogel releases 5FU slowly as and a pH of 7.0 does not break the hydrazone bond of the gel. These results support the finding that inulin hydrogel could be utilized as a delivery platform. Based on these results, we can conclude that extracts obtained from the blank inulin hydrogels did not show any significantly difference from the control in terms of cell viability.

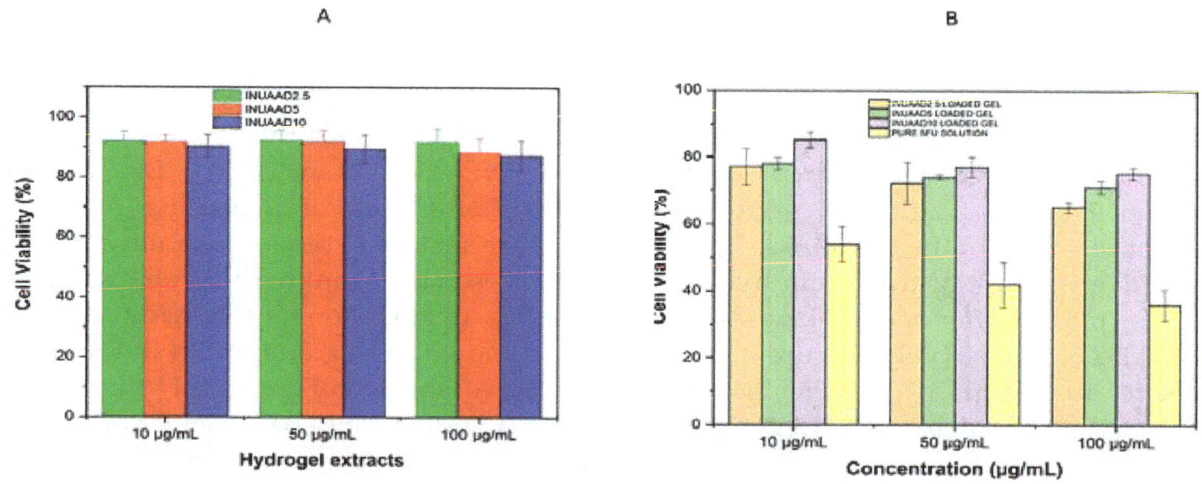

Figure 8. (**A**) Cell viability of the HCT116 cancer cells after treatment with the blank hydrogel extracts, and (**B**) cell viability of HCT116 cancer cells after treatment with the 5FU-loaded hydrogel extracts.

4. Conclusions

New injectable inulin hydrogels based on hydrazone crosslinking for potential use as drug delivery vehicles were fabricated by reacting oxidized inulin with AAD without the use of a catalyst. The novel hydrogels were formed within 2–3 min at 37 °C. The initial degree of oxidation was determined by hydroxylamine titration and ^{1}H NMR spectroscopy, whereas FTIR spectroscopy was used to confirm the covalent crosslinking by AAD with a new band at 1550 cm^{-1}. Changes in thermal properties was detected using DSC and TGA. By varying, the amount of AAD crosslinker used during hydrogel synthesis, the swelling, rheological properties, pore size, degradation, and 5FU release of the hydrogels can be tuned. The in vitro release rate of 5FU from all the hydrogels tested exhibited initial burst release followed by a controlled release pattern. The hydrogels are degradable both hydrolytically in physiologic conditions and by inulinase. In addition, the MTT results confirm that, at a concentration of 10–100 μg/mL, the INUAAD hydrogels showed no appreciable cytotoxicity. These findings demonstrate that these novel hydrogels could serve as delivery systems for anticancer drugs in the treatment of colon cancer.

Author Contributions: Conceptualization—S.G., T.G.B., and F.A.; method—F.A., T.G.B., S.G., A.P., and Y.S.; investigation–synthesis, characterization, release, and in vitro work—F.A. and P.F.; writing original draft—F.A., P.F., and S.G.; Review and editing and result interpretation—F.A., T.G.B., A.P., Y.S., and S.G.; supervision—Y.S., T.G.B., and S.G., and project administration—S.G.

Acknowledgments: The authors would like to thank Ken Neubauer for help with SEM imaging and Karen Teague for assistance with laboratory set-up.

References

1. Mensink, M.A.; Frijlink, H.W.; Maarschalk, K.V.; Hinrichs, W.L. Inulin, a flexible oligosaccharide I: Review of its physicochemical characteristics. *Carbohydr. Polym.* **2015**, *130*, 405–419. [CrossRef] [PubMed]
2. Barclay, T.; Ginic-Markovic, M.; Cooper, P.; Petrovsky, N. Inulin—A versatile polysaccharide with multiple pharmaceutical and food chemical uses. *J. Excip. Food Chem.* **2010**, *1*, 27–50.
3. Flamm, G.; Glinsmann, W.; Kritchevsky, D.; Prosky, L.; Roberfroid, M. Inulin and oligofructose as dietary fiber: A review of the evidence. *Crit. Rev. Food Sci. Nutr.* **2001**, *41*, 353–362. [CrossRef] [PubMed]
4. Roberfroid, M.B.; Delzenne, N.M. Dietary fructans. *Annu. Rev. Nutr.* **1998**, *18*, 117–143. [CrossRef] [PubMed]
5. Maris, B.; Verheyden, L.; van Reeth, K.; Samyn, C.; Augustijns, P.; Kinget, R.; van den Mooter, G. Synthesis and characterisation of inulin-azo hydrogels designed for colon targeting. *Int. J. Pharm.* **2001**, *213*, 143–152. [CrossRef]
6. Keenan, D.F.; Resconi, V.C.; Kerry, J.P.; Hamill, R.M. Modelling the influence of inulin as a fat substitute in comminuted meat products on their physico-chemical characteristics and eating quality using a mixture design approach. *Meat Sci.* **2014**, *96*, 1384–1394. [CrossRef] [PubMed]
7. Furlan, L.T.R.; Padilla, A.P.; Campderros, M.E. Development of reduced fat minced meats using inulin and bovine plasma proteins as fat replacers. *Meat Sci.* **2014**, *96*, 762–768. [CrossRef] [PubMed]
8. Poulain, N.; Dez, I.; Perrio, C.; Lasne, M.C.; Prud'homme, M.P.; Nakache, E. Microspheres based on inulin for the controlled release of serine protease inhibitors: Preparation, characterization and in vitro release. *J. Control Release* **2003**, *92*, 27–38. [CrossRef]
9. Lopez-Molina, D.; Chazarra, S.; How, C.W.; Pruidze, N.; Navarro-Peran, E.; Garcia-Canovas, F.; Garcia-Ruiz, P.A.; Rojas-Melgarejo, F.; Rodriguez-Lopez, J.N. Cinnamate of inulin as a vehicle for delivery of colonic drugs. *Int. J. Pharm.* **2015**, *479*, 96–102. [CrossRef]
10. Vervoort, L.; van den Mooter, G.; Augustijns, P.; Busson, R.; Toppet, S.; Kinget, R. Inulin hydrogels as carriers for colonic drug targeting: I. Synthesis and characterization of methacrylated inulin and hydrogen formation. *Pharm. Res.* **1997**, *14*, 1730–1737. [CrossRef]
11. Vervoort, L.; Vinckier, I.; Moldenaers, P.; van den Mooter, G.; Augustijns, P.; Kinget, R. Inulin hydrogels as carriers for colonic drug targeting. Rheological characterization of the hydrogel formation and the hydrogel network. *J. Pharm. Sci.* **1999**, *8*, 209–214. [CrossRef] [PubMed]
12. Jain, A.K.; Sood, V.; Bora, M.; Vasita, R.; Katti, D.S. Electrosprayed inulin microparticles for microbiota triggered targeting of colon. *Carbohydr. Polym.* **2014**, *112*, 225–234. [CrossRef] [PubMed]
13. Zijlstra, G.S.; Ponsioen, B.J.; Hummel, S.A.; Sanders, N.; Hinrichs, W.L.; De Boer, A.H.; Frijlink, H.W. Formulation and process development of (recombinant human) deoxyribonuclease I as a powder for inhalation. *Pharm. Dev. Technol.* **2009**, *14*, 358–368. [CrossRef] [PubMed]
14. Rahul, R.; Jha, U.; Sen, G.; Mishra, S. Carboxymethyl inulin: A novel flocculant for wastewater treatment. *Int. J. Biol. Macromol.* **2014**, *63*, 1–7. [CrossRef] [PubMed]
15. Palumbo, F.S.; Fiorica, C.; Di Stefano, M.; Pitarresi, G.; Gulino, A.; Agnello, S.; Giammona, G. In situ forming hydrogels of hyaluronic acid and inulin derivatives for cartilage regeneration. *Carbohydr. Polym.* **2015**, *122*, 408–416. [CrossRef] [PubMed]
16. Afinjuomo, F.; Barclay, T.G.; Song, Y.; Parikh, A.; Petrovsky, N.; Garg, S.; Parikh, A. Synthesis and characterization of a novel inulin hydrogel crosslinked with pyromellitic dianhydride. *React. Funct. Polym.* **2019**, *134*, 104–111. [CrossRef]
17. Mooter, G.V.D.; Vervoort, L.; Kinget, R. Characterization of methacrylated inulin hydrogels designed for colon targeting: In vitro release of BSA. *Pharm. Res.* **2003**, *20*, 303–307. [CrossRef]
18. Tripodo, G.; Pitarresi, G.; Cavallaro, G.; Palumbo, F.S.; Giammona, G. Controlled release of IgG by novel UV induced polysaccharide/poly(amino acid) hydrogels. *Macromol. Biosci.* **2009**, *9*, 393–401. [CrossRef]
19. Castelli, F.; Sarpietro, M.G.; Micieli, D.; Ottimo, S.; Pitarresi, G.; Tripodo, G.; Carlisi, B.; Giammona, G. Differential scanning calorimetry study on drug release from an inulin-based hydrogel and its interaction with a biomembrane model: pH and loading effect. *Eur. J. Pharm. Sci.* **2008**, *35*, 76–85. [CrossRef]
20. Licciardi, M.; Scialabba, C.; Sardo, C.; Cavallaro, G.; Giammona, G. Amphiphilic inulin graft co-polymers as self-assembling micelles for doxorubicin delivery. *J. Mater. Chem. B* **2014**, *2*, 4262–4271. [CrossRef]

21. Muley, P.; Kumar, S.; El Kourati, F.; Kesharwani, S.S.; Tummala, H. Hydrophobically modified inulin as an amphiphilic carbohydrate polymer for micellar delivery of paclitaxel for intravenous route. *Int. J. Pharm.* **2016**, *500*, 32–41. [CrossRef] [PubMed]
22. Mandracchia, D.; Rosato, A.; Trapani, A.; Chlapanidas, T.; Montagner, I.M.; Perteghella, S.; Di Franco, C.; Torre, M.L.; Trapani, G.; Tripodo, G. Design, synthesis and evaluation of biotin decorated inulin-based polymeric micelles as long-circulating nanocarriers for targeted drug delivery. *Nanomed. Nanotechnol. Biol. Med.* **2017**, *13*, 1245–1254. [CrossRef] [PubMed]
23. Essien, H.; Lai, J.Y.; Hwang, K.J. Synthesis of diethylenetriaminepentaacetic acid conjugated inulin and utility for cellular uptake of liposomes. *J. Med. Chem.* **1988**, *31*, 898–901. [CrossRef] [PubMed]
24. Volsi, A.L.; de Aberasturi, D.J.; Henriksen-Lacey, M.; Giammona, G.; Licciardi, M.; Liz-Marzan, L.M.Y. Inulin coated plasmonic gold nanoparticles as a tumor-selective tool for cancer therapy. *J. Mater. Chem. B* **2016**, *4*, 1150–1155. [CrossRef] [PubMed]
25. Zhang, L.; Li, Y.; Wang, C.; Li, G.; Zhao, Y.; Yang, Y. Synthesis of methylprednisolone loaded ibuprofen modified inulin based nanoparticles and their application for drug delivery. *Mater. Sci. Eng. C* **2014**, *42*, 111–115. [CrossRef] [PubMed]
26. Licciardi, M.; Volsi, A.L.; Mauro, N.; Scialabba, C.; Cavallaro, G.; Giammona, G. Preparation and characterization of inulin coated gold nanoparticles for selective delivery of doxorubicin to breast cancer cells. *J. Nanomater.* **2016**, *2016*, 1–12. [CrossRef]
27. Silva, D.G.; Cooper, P.D.; Petrovsky, N. Inulin-derived adjuvants efficiently promote both Th1 and Th2 immune responses. *Immunol. Cell Biol.* **2004**, *82*, 611–616. [CrossRef] [PubMed]
28. Cooper, P.D.; Petrovsky, N. Delta inulin: A novel, immunologically active, stable packing structure comprising beta-D-[2 -> 1] poly(fructo-furanosyl) alpha-D-glucose polymers. *Glycobiology* **2011**, *21*, 595–606. [CrossRef] [PubMed]
29. Kumar, S.; Tummala, H. Development of soluble inulin microparticles as a potent and safe vaccine adjuvant and delivery system. *Mol. Pharm.* **2013**, *10*, 1845–1853. [CrossRef] [PubMed]
30. Srinarong, P.; Hamalainen, S.; Visser, M.R.; Hinrichs, W.L.; Ketolainen, J.; Frijlink, H.W. Surface-active derivative of inulin (Inutec(R) SP1) is a superior carrier for solid dispersions with a high drug load. *J. Pharm. Sci.* **2011**, *100*, 2333–2342. [CrossRef] [PubMed]
31. Fares, M.M.; Salem, M.S.; Khanfar, M. Inulin and poly(acrylic acid) grafted inulin for dissolution enhancement and preliminary controlled release of poorly water-soluble Irbesartan drug. *Int. J. Pharm.* **2011**, *410*, 206–211. [CrossRef] [PubMed]
32. Robert, P.; Garcia, P.; Reyes, N.; Chávez, J.; Santos, J. Acetylated starch and inulin as encapsulating agents of gallic acid and their release behaviour in a hydrophilic system. *Food Chem.* **2012**, *134*, 1–8. [CrossRef]
33. Schacht, E.; Ruys, L.; Vermeersch, J.; Remon, J.P.; Duncan, R. Use of polysaccharides as drug carriers. Dextran and inulin derivatives of procainamide. *Ann. N. Y. Acad. Sci.* **1985**, *446*, 199–212. [CrossRef] [PubMed]
34. Hartzell, A.L.; Maldonado-Gómez, M.X.; Yang, J.; Hutkins, R.W.; Rose, D.J. In vitro digestion and fermentation of 5-formyl-aminosailcylate-inulin: A potential prodrug of 5-aminosalicylic acid. *Bioact. Carbohydr. Diet. Fibre* **2013**, *2*, 8–14. [CrossRef]
35. Sahiner, N.; Sagbas, S.; Yoshida, H.; Lyon, L.A. Synthesis and properties of inulin based microgels. *Coll. Interface Sci. Commun.* **2014**, *2*, 15–18. [CrossRef]
36. Mandracchia, D.; Denora, N.; Franco, M.; Pitarresi, G.; Giammona, G.; Trapani, G. New biodegradable hydrogels based on inulin and alpha,beta-polyaspartylhydrazide designed for colonic drug delivery: In vitro release of glutathione and oxytocin. *J. Biomater. Sci. Polym. Ed.* **2011**, *2*, 313–328. [CrossRef] [PubMed]
37. Pitarresi, G.; Tripodo, G.; Calabrese, R.; Craparo, E.F.; Licciardi, M.; Giammona, G. Hydrogels for potential colon drug release by thiol-ene conjugate addition of a new inulin derivative. *Macromol. Biosci.* **2008**, *8*, 891–902. [CrossRef]
38. Chiu, H.; Hsu, Y.; Lin, P. Synthesis of pH-sensitive inulin hydrogels and characterization of their swelling properties. *J. Biomed. Mater. Res.* **2002**, *61*, 146–152. [CrossRef]
39. Chen, S.; Cui, S.; Zhang, H.; Pei, X.; Hu, J.; Zhou, Y.Z.; Liu, Y. Cross-linked pectin nanofibers with enhanced cell adhesion. *Biomacromolecules* **2018**, *19*, 490–498. [CrossRef]
40. Gupta, B.; Tummalapalli, M.; Deopura, B.; Alam, M.S. Functionalization of pectin by periodate oxidation. *Carbohydr. Polym.* **2013**, *98*, 1160–1165. [CrossRef]
41. Maia, J.; Ferreira, L.; Carvalho, R.; Ramos, M.A.; Gil, M.H. Synthesis and characterization of new injectable and degradable dextran-based hydrogels. *Polymer* **2005**, *46*, 9604–9614. [CrossRef]

42. Cai, M.; Gong, J.; Cao, J.; Chen, Y.; Luo, X. In situ chemically crosslinked chitosan membrane by adipic acid. *J. Appl. Polym. Sci.* **2013**, *128*, 3308–3314. [CrossRef]
43. Maiti, S.; Singha, K.; Ray, S.; Dey, P.; Sa, B. Adipic acid dihydrazide treated partially oxidized alginate beads for sustained oral delivery of flurbiprofen. *Pharm. Dev. Technol.* **2009**, *14*, 461–470. [CrossRef] [PubMed]
44. Paşcalău, V.; Popescu, V.; Popescu, G.L.; Dudescu, M.C.; Borodi, G.; Dinescu, A.M.; Moldovan, M. Obtaining and characterizing alginate/k-carrageenan hydrogel cross-linked with adipic dihydrazide. *Adv. Mater. Sci. Eng.* **2013**, *2013*, 1–12. [CrossRef]
45. Hu, M.H.; Yang, K.C.; Sun, Y.H.; Chen, Y.C.; Yang, S.H.; Lin, F.H. In situ forming oxidised hyaluronic acid/adipic acid dihydrazide hydrogel for prevention of epidural fibrosis after laminectomy. *Eur. Cells Mater.* **2017**, *34*, 307–320. [CrossRef] [PubMed]
46. Shoham, N.; Sasson, A.L.; Lin, F.-H.; Benayahu, D.; Haj-Ali, R.; Gefen, A. The mechanics of hyaluronic acid/adipic acid dihydrazide hydrogel: Towards developing a vessel for delivery of preadipocytes to native tissues. *J. Mech. Behav. Biomed. Mater.* **2013**, *28*, 320–331. [CrossRef]
47. Su, W.-Y.; Chen, K.-H.; Chen, Y.-C.; Lee, Y.-H.; Tseng, C.-L.; Lin, F.-H. An injectable oxidated hyaluronic acid/adipic acid dihydrazide hydrogel as a vitreous substitute. *J. Biomater. Sci. Polym. Ed.* **2011**, *22*, 1777–1797. [CrossRef]
48. Su, W.-Y.; Chen, Y.-C.; Lin, F.-H. Injectable oxidized hyaluronic acid/adipic acid dihydrazide hydrogel for nucleus pulposus regeneration. *Acta Biomater.* **2010**, *6*, 3044–3055. [CrossRef]
49. Tabandeh, M.R.; Aminlari, M. Synthesis, physicochemical and immunological properties of oxidized inulin–l-asparaginase bioconjugate. *J. Biotechnol.* **2009**, *141*, 189–195. [CrossRef]
50. Barclay, T.; Ginic-Markovic, M.; Johnston, M.R.; Cooper, P.D.; Petrovsky, N. Analysis of the hydrolysis of inulin using real time 1H NMR spectroscopy. *Carbohydr. Res.* **2012**, *352*, 117–125. [CrossRef]
51. Schacht, E.; Vermeersch, J.; Vandoorne, F.; Vercauteren, R.; Remon, J. Synthesis and characterization of some modified polysaccharides containing drug moieties. *J. Control. Release* **1985**, *2*, 245–256. [CrossRef]
52. Zhang, K.; Yan, S.; Wang, T.; Feng, L.; Zhu, J.; Chen, X.; Cui, L.; Yin, J. Injectable in situ self-cross-linking hydrogels based on poly(l -glutamic acid) and alginate for cartilage tissue engineering. *Biomacromolecules* **2014**, *15*, 4495–4508.
53. Zhao, H.; Heindel, N.D. Determination of degree of substitution of formyl groups in polyaldehyde dextran by the hydroxylamine hydrochloride method. *Pharm. Res.* **1991**, *8*, 400–402. [CrossRef] [PubMed]
54. Jia, X.; Burdick, J.A.; Kobler, J.; Clifton, R.J.; Rosowski, J.J.; Zeitels, S.M.; Langer, R. Synthesis and characterization of in situ cross-linkable hyaluronic acid-based hydrogels with potential application for vocal fold regeneration. *Macromolecules* **2004**, *37*, 3239–3248. [CrossRef]
55. De Mattos, A.C.; Khalil, N.M.; Mainardes, R. Development and validation of an HPLC method for the determination of fluorouracil in polymeric nanoparticles. *Braz. J. Pharm. Sci.* **2013**, *49*, 117–126. [CrossRef]
56. Vervoort, L.; Rombaut, P.; van den Mooter, G.; Augustijns, P.; Kinget, R. Inulin hydrogels. II. In vitro degradation study. *Int. J. Pharm.* **1998**, *172*, 137–145. [CrossRef]
57. Damian, F.; Mooter, G.V.D.; Samyn, C.; Kinget, R. In vitro biodegradation study of acetyl and methyl inulins by Bifidobacteria and inulinase. *Eur. J. Pharm. Biopharm.* **1999**, *47*, 275–282. [CrossRef]
58. Pitarresi, G.; Tripodo, G.; Cavallaro, G.; Palumbo, F.S.; Giammona, G. Inulin–iron complexes: A potential treatment of iron deficiency anaemia. *Eur. J. Pharm. Biopharm.* **2008**, *68*, 267–276. [CrossRef]
59. Prabaharan, M.; Grailer, J.J.; Pilla, S.; Steeber, D.A.; Gong, S. Amphiphilic multi-arm block copolymer based on hyperbranched polyester, poly(L-lactide) and poly(ethylene glycol) as a drug delivery carrier. *Macromol. Biosci.* **2009**, *9*, 515–524. [CrossRef]
60. Seeli, D.S.; Prabaharan, M. Guar gum oleate-graft-poly(methacrylic acid) hydrogel as a colon-specific controlled drug delivery carrier. *Carbohydr. Polym.* **2017**, *158*, 51–57. [CrossRef]
61. Parikh, A.; Kathawala, K.; Li, J.; Chen, C.; Shan, Z.; Cao, X.; Zhou, X.-F.; Garg, S. Curcumin-loaded self-nanomicellizing solid dispersion system: Part II: In vivo safety and efficacy assessment against behavior deficit in Alzheimer disease. *Drug Deliv. Transl. Res.* **2018**, *8*, 1406–1420. [CrossRef] [PubMed]
62. Stevens, C.V.; Meriggi, A.; Booten, K. Chemical modification of inulin, a valuable renewable resource, and its industrial applications. *Biomacromolecules* **2001**, *2*, 1–16. [CrossRef] [PubMed]

63. Ishak, M.F.; Painter, T. Kinetic evidence for hemiacetal formation during the oxidation of dextran in aqueous periodate. *Carbohydr. Res.* **1978**, *64*, 189–197.
64. Pan, J.-F.; Yuan, L.; Guo, C.-A.; Geng, X.-H.; Fei, T.; Fan, W.-S.; Li, S.; Yuan, H.-F.; Yan, Z.-Q.; Mo, X.-M. Fabrication of modified dextran–gelatin in situ forming hydrogel and application in cartilage tissue engineering. *J. Mater. Chem. B* **2014**, *2*, 8346–8360. [CrossRef]
65. Kim, U.-J.; Kuga, S.; Wada, M.; Okano, T.; Kondo, T. Periodate oxidation of crystalline cellulose. *Biomacromolecules* **2000**, *1*, 488–492. [CrossRef] [PubMed]
66. Gomez, C.; Rinaudo, M.; Villar, M.; Gomez, C. Oxidation of sodium alginate and characterization of the oxidized derivatives. *Carbohydr. Polym.* **2007**, *67*, 296–304. [CrossRef]
67. Kristiansen, K.A.; Potthast, A.; Christensen, B.E. Periodate oxidation of polysaccharides for modification of chemical and physical properties. *Carbohydr. Res.* **2010**, *345*, 1264–1271. [CrossRef] [PubMed]
68. Maia, J.; Ribeiro, M.P.; Ventura, C.; Carvalho, R.A.; Correia, I.J.; Gil, M.H. Ocular injectable formulation assessment for oxidized dextran-based hydrogels. *Acta Biomater.* **2009**, *5*, 1948–1955. [CrossRef]
69. Bouhadir, K.H.; Hausman, D.S.; Mooney, D.J. Synthesis of cross-linked poly(aldehyde guluronate) hydrogels. *Polymer* **1999**, *40*, 3575–3584. [CrossRef]
70. Li, X.; Xu, A.; Xie, H.; Yu, W.; Xie, W.; Ma, X. Preparation of low molecular weight alginate by hydrogen peroxide depolymerization for tissue engineering. *Carbohydr. Polym.* **2010**, *79*, 660–664. [CrossRef]
71. Villanueva-Carcia, D.N.; Rangel-Vazquez, N.A.; Kalla, J. Structural analysis of adsorption processes of 5FU and imiquimod on hydrogels using AMBER/PM3 hybrid model. *Rev. Colomb. Quím.* **2018**, *47*, 28–35.
72. Miralinaghi, P.; Kashani, P.; Moniri, E.; Miralinaghi, M.; Monir, E.; Miralinaghi, M. Non-linear kinetic, equilibrium, and thermodynamic studies of 5-fluorouracil adsorption onto chitosan–functionalized graphene oxide. *Mater. Res. Express* **2019**, *6*, 65305. [CrossRef]
73. Dan, A.; Ghosh, S.; Moulik, S.P. Physicochemical studies on the biopolymer inulin: A critical evaluation of its self-aggregation, aggregate-morphology, interaction with water, and thermal stability. *Biopolymers* **2009**, *91*, 687–699. [CrossRef] [PubMed]
74. Bouhadir, K.; Lee, K.; Alsberg, E.; Damm, K.; Anderson, K.; Mooney, D. Degradation of partially oxidized alginate and its potential application for tissue engineering. *Biotechnol. Prog.* **2001**, *17*, 945–950. [CrossRef] [PubMed]
75. Maia, J.; Carvalho, R.A.; Coelho, J.F.; Simões, P.N.N.; Gil, M.H. Insight on the periodate oxidation of dextran and its structural vicissitudes. *Polymer* **2011**, *52*, 258–265. [CrossRef]
76. Balakrishnan, B.; Jayakrishnan, A. Self-cross-linking biopolymers as injectable in situ forming biodegradable scaffolds. *Biomaterials* **2005**, *26*, 3941–3951. [CrossRef] [PubMed]
77. Rinaudo, M. Periodate oxidation of methylcellulose: Characterization and properties of oxidized derivatives. *Polymer* **2010**, *2*, 505–521. [CrossRef]
78. Mitra, T.; Sailakshmi, G.; Gnanamani, A.; Mandal, A.B. Adipic acid interaction enhances the mechanical and thermal stability of natural polymers. *J. Appl. Polym. Sci.* **2012**, *125*. [CrossRef]
79. Chen, Y.-C.; Su, W.-Y.; Yang, S.-H.; Gefen, A.; Lin, F.-H. In situ forming hydrogels composed of oxidized high molecular weight hyaluronic acid and gelatin for nucleus pulposus regeneration. *Acta Biomater.* **2013**, *9*, 5181–5193. [CrossRef]
80. Zhu, R.; Chen, R.; Duo, Y.; Zhang, S.; Xie, D.; Mei, Y. An industrial scale synthesis of adipicdihydrazide (ADH)/polyacrylate hybrid with excellent formaldehyde degradation performance. *Polymer* **2019**, *11*, 86. [CrossRef]
81. Larrañeta, E.; Henry, M.; Irwin, N.J.; Trotter, J.; Perminova, A.A.; Donnelly, R.F. Synthesis and characterization of hyaluronic acid hydrogels crosslinked using a solvent-free process for potential biomedical applications. *Carbohydr. Polym.* **2018**, *181*, 1194–1205. [CrossRef] [PubMed]
82. Song, F.; Zhang, L.-M.; Li, N.-N.; Shi, J.-F. In situ crosslinkable hydrogel formed from a polysaccharide-based hydrogelator. *Biomacromolecules* **2009**, *10*, 959–965. [CrossRef] [PubMed]
83. Mohana, M.; Muthiah, P.; McMillen, C. Supramolecular hydrogen-bonding patterns in 1:1 cocrystals of 5-fluorouracil with 4-methylbenzoic acid and 3-nitrobenzoic acid. *Acta Crystallogr. Sect. C Struct. Chem.* **2017**, *73*, 259–263. [CrossRef] [PubMed]
84. Anirudhan, T.S.; Nima, J.; Divya, P.L. Synthesis, characterization and in vitro cytotoxicity analysis of a novel cellulose based drug carrier for the controlled delivery of 5-fluorouracil, an anticancer drug. *Appl. Surf. Sci.* **2015**, *355*, 64–73. [CrossRef]

13

N-(2-Hydroxy)-propyl-3-trimethylammonium, *O*-Myristoyl Chitosan Enhances the Solubility and Intestinal Permeability of Anticancer Curcumin

Daniella S. Silva [1], Danilo M. dos Santos [2], Andreia Almeida [3,4,5], Leonardo Marchiori [1], Sérgio P. Campana-Filho [6], Sidney J. L. Ribeiro [1] and Bruno Sarmento [3,4,5,*]

1 Institute of Chemistry, São Paulo State University—UNESP, Araraquara 4800-900, Brazil; danyss8@hotmail.com (D.S.S.); leonardo.marchiori.lm@gmail.com (L.M.); sidney.jl.ribeiro@unesp.br (S.J.L.R.)
2 Embrapa Instrumentação, Rua XV de Novembro 1452, São Carlos 13560-970, Brazil; danilomartins_1@hotmail.com
3 Institute for Research and Innovation in Health (i3S), Rua Alfredo Allen, 208, 4200-393 Porto, Portugal; andreia.almeida@ineb.up.pt
4 ICBAS—Institute of Biomedical Sciences Abel Salazar, University of Porto, Rua de Jorge Viterbo Ferreira, 228, 4050-313 Porto, Portugal
5 CESPU—Institute for Research and Advanced Training in Health Sciences and Technologies, Rua Central de Gandra, 1317, 4585-116 Gandra, Portugal
6 Sao Carlos Institute of Chemistry, University of Sao Paulo—USP, Av. Trabalhador São-Carlense, 400, São Carlos 13566-590, Brazil; scampana@iqsc.usp.br
* Correspondence: bruno.sarmento@ineb.up.pt

Abstract: An amphiphilic derivative of chitosan containing quaternary ammonium and myristoyl groups, herein named as ammonium myristoyl chitosan (DMCat), was synthesized by reacting glycidyltrimethylammonium chloride (GTMAC) and myristoyl chitosan (DMCh). The success of the modification was confirmed using Fourier-transform infrared spectroscopy (FTIR) and ^{1}H nuclear magnetic resonance (NMR) spectroscopy. The average degrees of alkylation and quaternization ($\overline{DQ}$) were determined by using ^{1}H NMR and conductometric titration. The zeta potential of the micelles was higher than 28 mV while its average size and encapsulation efficiency ranged from 280 nm to 375 nm and 68% to 100%, respectively. The in vitro cytotoxicity of the unloaded and curcumin (CUR)-loaded micelles was tested against Caco-2 and HT29-MTX intestinal epithelial cell lines. The results showed no cytotoxic effect from loaded and unloaded micelles as compared to free CUR. In the permeability test, it was observed that both types of micelles, i.e., DMCh and DMCat, improved CUR permeability. Additionally, higher permeability was verified for both systems in Caco-2/HT29-MTX:Raji B because of the mucoadhesive character of chitosan and its ability to open tight junctions. The results indicated that DMCat micelles, due to the physico-chemical, improved characteristics may be a promising carrier to encapsulate CUR aiming cancer therapy.

Keywords: chitosan derivatives; amphiphilic polymers; polymeric micelles; quaternization; curcumin; intestinal delivery

---

1. Introduction

Polymeric micelles have attracted considerable interest for controlled drug delivery over the last few years, due to their unique properties and behaviors resulting from their small size and high load capacity [1]. These nanostructured materials show potential to deliver chemotherapeutics to tumor cells maintaining their concentration at the desired site for a sufficient time to have a therapeutic effect, increasing the efficacy of treatment and reducing the toxicity [2].

Curcumin (CUR) is a naturally occurring phytochemical that has been widely used as a therapeutic agent against a variety of cancers [3–8]. In particular, CUR is a cheap compound (especially when compared with popular anticancer agents like paclitaxel and camptothecin) and has properties in antioxidant, anti-inflammatory, antimicrobial, anticancer, anticarcinogenic, chemopreventive, chemotherapeutic, and chemosensitizing activities [9,10]. Although CUR possesses remarkable medicinal properties, its bioavailability during cancer treatments is limited due to its low solubility and poor stability in aqueous solution. Other than its rapid degradation in physiological conditions, however, there is a wide interest in the development of systems to solve problems related to the limitations of the applicability of CUR as a therapeutic agent [4–7,11]. To enhance solubility, stability, pharmacokinetics profile of curcumin and thus its therapeutic efficiency, various drug delivery systems have been investigated, including nanoemulsions, nanosuspensions, and polymeric micelles [11,12].

In recent years, drug delivery systems based on polymeric micelles have been the subject of research. Several formulations are undergoing clinical trials due to the ability of the micelles to encapsulate hydrophobic and hydrophilic drugs [13–15]. In addition, these systems have shown greater physical stability and encapsulation efficiency, when compared to liposomes [16–20]. Shell/core polymeric micelles, in particular, exhibit advantages regarding encapsulation and controlled release of drugs since their hydrophobic nuclei promote the solubilization of hydrophobic actives, avoiding drug degradation. On the other hand, hydrophilic outer shells avoid recognition by the immune system, prolonging the circulation time of the drug in the body [21,22].

Lately, micelles formulations based on chitosan have presented promising results in the drug delivery field [23–28]. This cationic biopolymer exhibits biological activities, such as biocompatibility, biodegradability, mucoadhesiveness, and antimicrobial activity, in addition to presenting antioxidant properties [29–31]. Chitosan has present in its backbone reactive groups (–OH and $–NH_2$) that make it susceptible to chemical modifications. Various derivatives of chitosan are obtained via the addition of hydrophobic groups with different degrees of substitution (DS). In particular, chitosan modified with stearic acid (DS = 4.96%) [32] and linoleic acid (DS = 1.8%) [33] exhibit self-assembly and loading abilities, which improve the solubility of hydrophobic drugs [34,35]. However, the addition of a small portion of hydrophobic units makes chitosan extremely insoluble in neutral medium, leading to a low loading capacity of the micelles for non-ionic hydrophobic drugs [34,36].

Previous studies with the structural modification of chitosan via an *O*-acylation reaction with myristoyl chloride showed excellent capacity for encapsulation and solubilization of hydrophobic drugs, such as paclitaxel [37]. This is due to the affinity of the acyl chains within the drug. However, because such a derivative exhibited a low degree of substitution (DS = 6.8%), the characteristics of the starting chitosan have been maintained, and its limited solubility at a neutral pH has hindered its application. Thus, the limitations resulting from the modification of chitosan with myristoyl chloride via an *O*-substitution reaction can be solved by carrying out a further chemical modification.

The introduction of hydrophilic and hydrophobic groups has shown excellent results in the encapsulation of hydrophobic drugs, such as paclitaxel and doxorubicin. In this sense, different amphiphilic derivatives of chitosan have been synthesized, such as *N*-octyl-*N*, *O*-carboxymethylchitosan [18], colic acid grafted *N*-(2,3-(dihydroxypropyl) chitosan [38], chitosan-*g*-polylactic [39], *N*-octyl-*N*-trimethylchitosan [40], *N*-propyl-*N*-methylenephosphonic chitosan [41], *N*-naphthyl-*N*, *O*-succinylchitosan [42]. In all of these studies, amphiphilic derivatives of chitosan are suggested to be promising efficient carriers for hydrophobic drugs, especially when compared to hydrophobically modified chitosan.

This work aims to develop a new amphiphilic derivative of chitosan via *O*-acylation and quaternization reactions in chitosan (Scheme 1), since the first step (*O*-acylation) has already been conducted with excellent results for anticancer drug delivery [37]. Studies showed that the synthesis of quaternized chitosan via *N*-substitution by reacting it with *N*-(2-hydroxyl) propyl-3-trimethyl ammonium chloride presented properties of interest, such as water solubility, antibacterial activity, mucoadhesiveness, increased permeability to hydration, and strong stereochemical hindrance of quaternary amine groups [43–45].

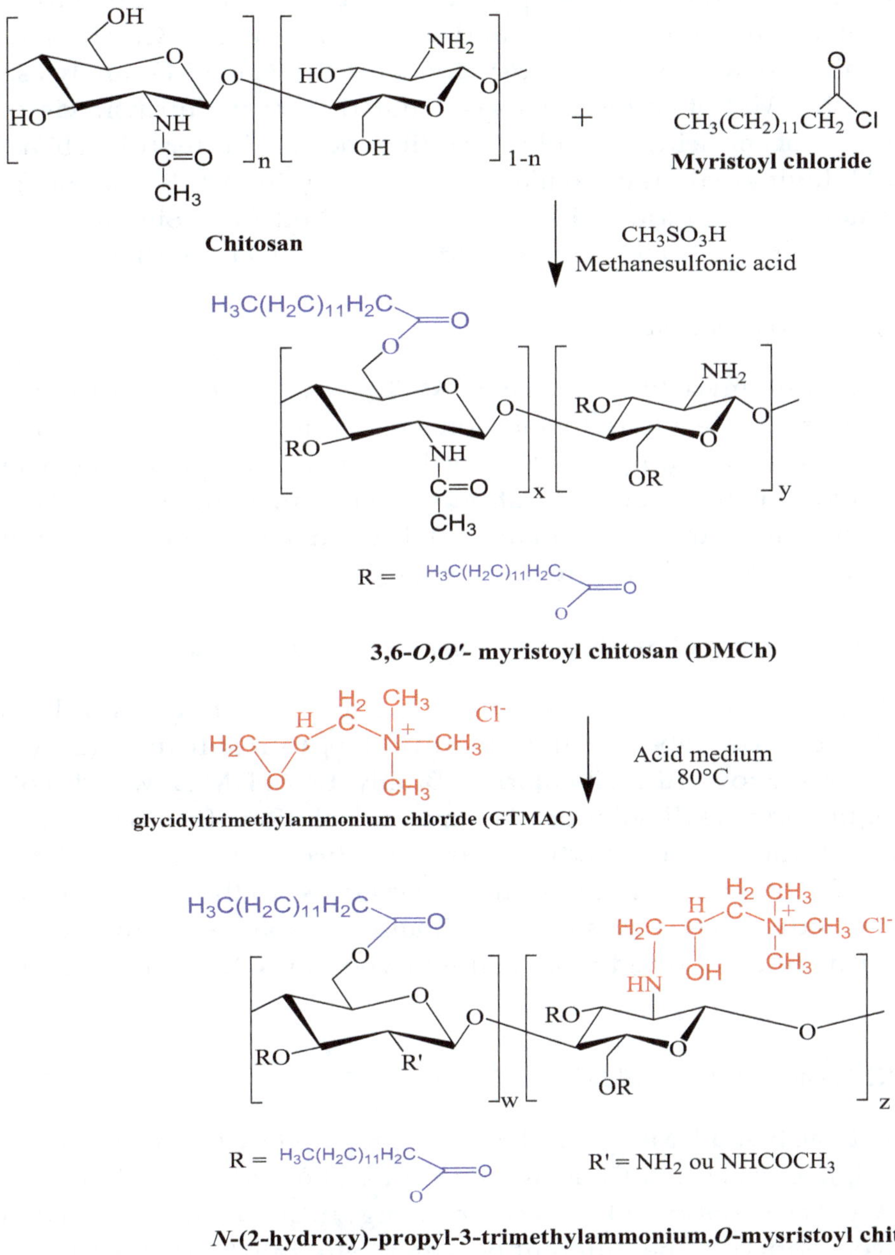

Scheme 1. The synthesis of *N*-(2-hydroxy)-propyl-3-trimethylammonium,*O*-myristoyl chitosan.

In this study, an amphiphilic derivative of chitosan containing quaternary ammonium and myristoyl goups was prepared and its ability to form self-assembled micelles with ability to encapsulate curcumin was explored. The efficiency of the structural modification was evaluated by FTIR and ^1H nuclear magnetic resonance (NMR) spectroscopy and conductometric titration. The physical-chemical characteristics such as average size, zeta potential, drug loading efficiency, and critical aggregation concentration (CAC) were determined. The in vitro cytotoxicity was evaluated using Caco-2 (clone C2BBe1) and HT29-MTX cell lines, as well as the in vitro intestinal permeability.

2. Materials and Methods

2.1. Materials

Chitosan acquired from a commercial supplier (Cheng Yue Plating Co. Ltd.; Pequim, China) was purified according to Santos et al. [46], and then dried at 30 °C. The average degree of acetylation ($\overline{DA}$) of chitosan was 5%, as determined by the ^{1}H NMR analysis. The viscosity average molecular weight ($\overline{Mv}$) of chitosan was calculated from its intrinsic viscosity, which was determined in 0.3 mol L^{-1} acetic acid/0.2 mol L^{-1} sodium acetate buffer (pH 4.5) at 25.00 $\pm$ 0.01 °C, by using the Mark-Houwink-Sakurada equation, resulting in $\overline{Mv} \approx$ 87.000 g mol^{-1} [46,47]. Glycidyltrimethylammonium chloride (GTMAC) was acquired from Sigma-Aldrich (Saint Louis, MO, USA). All other reagents and solvents were used as acquired, i.e., without any purification.

2.2. Synthesis of 3,6-O,O′-Myristoyl Chitosan

The synthesis of 3,6-*O*,*O*′-myristoyl chitosan (DMCh) was realized by adding 1 g of chitosan in 25 mL of methanesulfonic acid ($MeSO_3H$). In addition, an amount of myristoyl chloride was added in order to generate an excess of chitosan ($\approx$13.3). After 1 h of reaction, the product was (i) neutralized with 5% (*w*/*v*) aqueous sodium bicarbonate solution, (ii) centrifugated, (iii) extensively washed with distilled water, (iv) purified in Soxhlet, and finally, (v) dried in a vacuum oven at room temperature. This procedure can be found in detail in a previous work [37].

2.3. Synthesis of N-(2-Hydroxy)-Propyl-3-Trimethylammonium Chitosan Chloride

The reaction of glycidyltrimethylammonium chloride (GTMAC) and DMCh in an acid medium was carried out as described in the literature [46] to result in *N*-(2-hydroxy)-propyl-3-trimethylammonium, *O*-myristoyl chitosan chloride. Briefly, 1 g of DMCh was dissolved in 60 mL of acetic acid 1% (*v*/*v*), until complete dissolution. An aqueous solution of GTMAC was added dropwise to the DMCh solubilized; the reaction mixture was then stirred in a glycerin bath for 8 h, under constant stirring at 80 °C. Following, excess acetone was added to the reaction medium to result in the precipitation of the product, which was filtered. Finally, the solid was purified by extraction with acetone in Soxhlet during 6 h and dried in a vacuum oven (30 °C), obtaining as final product the DMCat polymer.

2.4. Preparation of CUR-Loaded DMCh and DMCat Micelles

Both CUR-loaded DMCh and DMCat micelles were prepared by following the steps described in earlier works [37,48,49]. In essence, DMCh is dissolved in acetic acid 0.1% while DMCat is dissolved in deionized water. CUR was dissolved in acetone (1 mg/mL). Next, aliquots containing 50, 100 and 150 μg of CUR were added in the different polymer solutions (DMCh and DMCat). Then, the solutions are magnetically stirred at 300 rpm for 2 h (room temperature) and freeze-dried. Finally, the CUR-loaded micelles are resuspended and separated by centrifugation at 5000 rpm for 10 min.

2.5. Characterization

2.5.1. Fourier-Transform Infrared Spectroscopy (FTIR)

FTIR was performed on an IRAffinity Shimadzu spectrometer (Shimadzu Scientific Instruments, Columbia, MD, USA) in a 4000–400 cm^{-1} wavelength range, with an accumulation of 32 scans and resolution of 4 cm^{-1}. In order to prepare the pellets, the sample and KBr were dried at 60 °C for 8 h and mixed in a ratio of 1:100 (sample:KBr).

2.5.2. ^{1}H NMR Spectroscopy

A Bruker AVANCE III spectrophotometer 400 MHz (Bruker, Billerica, MA, EUA) was used to obtain ^{1}H NMR spectra, aiming the samples' characterization. Basically, the Equations (1)–(3) are used to determine the average degree of acetylation of chitosan ($\overline{DA}$) ([50,51]), degree of substitution ($\overline{DS}$) of the derivative 3,6-*O*,*O'*-myristoyl chitosan ([37]) and degree of quaternization ($\overline{DQ}$) of the derivative *N*-(2-hydroxy)-propyl-3-trimethylammonium, *O*-myristoyl chitosan ([46]), respectively. In other words, $\overline{DA}$, $\overline{DS}$, and $\overline{DQ}$ refers to the amount of acetylated units present in chitosan, as well as both the myristoyl groups added to chitosan and the quaternary groups present in derivative *N*-(2-hydroxy)-propyl-3-trimethylammonium,*O*-myristoyl chitosan.

$$\overline{DA}(\%) = \left(\frac{A_{CH_3}/3}{A_{H_2-H_6}/6}\right) * 100 \quad (1)$$

A_{CH3} = area of the methyl hydrogens of the acetamido group (of GlcNAc units);
$A_{H2\text{–}H6}$ = area of hydrogens bonded to the C (2–6) carbon of the glycopyranose ring.

$$\overline{DS}(\%) = \left(\frac{A_{Me}/3}{A_{H_2-H_6}/6}\right) * 100 \quad (2)$$

A_{Me} = area of the methyl hydrogens of the myristoyl group;
$A_{H2\text{–}H6}$ = area of hydrogens bonded to the C (2–6) carbon of the glycopyranose ring.

$$\overline{DQ}(\%) = \frac{IH1'}{IH1' + IH1} \cdot 100 \quad (3)$$

$I_{H1'}$= the integral of the signal due to the anomeric hydrogen bonded to *N*-substituted GlcN (units);
I_{H1} = is the integral of the signal due to the anomeric units hydrogen bonded to unsubstituted GlcN (units).

2.5.3. Conductometric Titration

The $\overline{DQ}$ of DMcat samples were also determined by dosing the counter-ions Cl^- through titration with standardized 0.017 mol L^{-1} aqueous $AgNO_3$ solution. Thus, the quaternized derivative (0.1 g) was dissolved in deionized water (100 mL) and the conductivity of the solution was measured at 25.00 ± 0.01 °C as a function of the added volume of aqueous $AgNO_3$ by using a Handylab LF1 conductivimeter (SI Analytics, Mainz, Germany). The value of $\overline{DQ}$ of samples was calculated from the titration curves according to [46].

2.5.4. Critical Aggregation Concentration (CAC)

The conductivity method was performed to determine the CAC by using a Consort C863 conductivity meter. In order to prepare the samples, different polymer concentrations were utilized (1×10^{-6} mg/mL $\leq$ Cp $\leq$ 1 mg/mL). The DMCh sample was solubilized in acid medium due to its limited solubility in neutral medium, while deionized water was used to dissolve DMCat.

2.5.5. Particle Size and Surface Charge

The average size, polydispersity, and zeta potential of DMCh (in acid medium) and DMCat (in water) micelles were determined using dynamic light scattering (DLS) measurements (ZetaSizer Nano ZS, Malvern, UK). Three replicates of each formulation were produced and analyzed.

2.5.6. Drug Encapsulation Efficiency

The drug encapsulation efficiency (EE%) was quantified by measuring the absorbance of the CUR solution at 340 nm using a UV-Vis spectrophotometer [3,7]. The measurements were performed by an indirect method in triplicate, in which the unencapsulated drug was solubilized in acetone and quantified. The amount of CUR loaded into the DMCh and DMCat micelles was determined according to Equation (4):

$$EE\% = \frac{(CUR_{total} - CUR_{free})}{CUR_{total}} \times 100 \quad (4)$$

2.6. *In Vitro Studies*

2.6.1. Cell Culturing Reagents

Caco-2 cells (clone C2BBe1) were obtained from American Type Culture Collection (ATCC, Manassas, VA, USA) and HT29-MTX cell line was kindly provided by Dr. T. Lesuffleur (INSERMU178, Villejuif, France). Dulbecco's Modified Eagle Medium (DMEM, Lonza, Basel, Switzerland), supplemented with 10% (*v*/*v*) fetal bovine serum (FBS, Merck Millipore, USA), 1% (*v*/*v*) penicillin (100 UI/mL, Merck Millipore), streptomycin (100 µg/mL, Merck Millipore), and 1% (*v*/*v*) nonessential amino acids (NEAA, Merck Millipore). 3-(4,5-dimethylthiazol-2-yl)-2,5-diphenyltetrazolium bromide (MTT), dimethyl sulfoxide (DMSO) and Triton X-100 were obtained from Sigma Aldrich.

2.6.2. Cytotoxicity Assay

The cytotoxicity of CUR-loaded micelles and free CUR was assessed in Caco-2 and HT29-MTX cell lines, using the MTT reagent. Cells were seeded (200 µL) into 96-well plates at a density of 1×10^4 cells/well for HT29-MTX cell line and 2×10^4 cells/well for Caco-2 and then incubated during 24 h in a Binder® incubator at 37 °C with a humidified atmosphere and 5% CO_2 to reach exponential growth prior to the assay test. On the following day, the medium was removed and the cells were washed twice with 200 µL of phosphate buffered saline (PBS). Next, the cells were treated with free CUR and CUR-loaded and unloaded micelles at the concentrations of 5, 10, 20, and 50 µg/mL. The negative control, which were cells treated with cell culture medium and positive control and treated with 1% (*w*/*v*) Triton X-100 in DMEM [52]. The cultured cells were incubated for 4 h in the presence of different concentrations of the referred samples. After this period, the wells were washed twice with PBS at 37 °C and 200 µL of the MTT reagent (0.5 mg/mL in cell culture medium) was added to each well, followed by an incubation period of 4 h. After, the MTT was removed and 200 µL of DMSO was added to each well to dissolve the formazan crystals. The plates were shaken for 10 min inside the microplate reader before the relative color intensity has been measured at 570 nm and taking the absorbance at 630 nm as a reference, by using a microplate reader (Synergy 2, Biotek Instruments Ltd., Winooski, VT, USA). The percentage of cell viability was calculated according to the Equation (5):

$$\text{Cell viability (\%)} = \frac{\text{experimental value} - \text{negative control}}{\text{positive control} - \text{negative control}} \times 100 \quad (5)$$

2.6.3. Permeability Studies

Monoculture model of Caco-2 cells and triple co-culture model of Caco-2/HT29-MTX:Raji B cells were seeded on 6-well Transwell™ cell culture inserts (transparent PET, 3 µm pore size, 4.67 cm^2, Corning Life Sciences, New York, NY, USA), according to Araújo. F [53,54]. The cell lines were seeded on the apical compartment at a density of 1×10^5 cells/cm^2. In the case of the triple co-culture model, Caco-2 and HT29-MTX were seeded at the proportion 90:10 and at the 14th day of culture, Raji B cells were added to the basolateral compartment in a density of 1×10^5 cells/cm^2. Cells were grown for 21 days until reaching confluency and the medium was changed every 2 days.

Before permeability experiments, cells were washed twice with pre-warmed Hank's buffered salt solution (HBSS) and then replaced with new HBSS and allowed to equilibrate for 30 min at 37 °C at 100 rpm. Permeability studies of CUR-loaded micelles and free CUR (20 µg/mL) were run at similar conditions during 3 h and samples were collected at different time (15, 30, 60, 90, 120, and

180 min). Each sample was taken from the basolateral side of the Transwell™ cell culture insert, which contained 1% (*v*/*v*) DMSO in HBSS in order to maintain the sink conditions. The same volume of pre-warmed 1% (*v*/*v*) DMSO in HBSS was added to replace the withdrawn volume. The cell monolayers integrity was measured at the during 21 days of growth and during the experiment, using an epithelial voltohmmeter EVOM2® with chopstick electrodes (World Precision Instruments, Sarasota, FL, USA). The transepithelial electrical resistance (TEER) values, expressed in percentage, were normalized in function of the TEER value after equilibrium. All experiments were performed in triplicate and the CUR was quantified by measuring the absorbance at 340 nm as referred previously.

2.7. Statistical Analysis

The experiments were performed in triplicate and are represented as mean ± standard deviation (SD). A two-way ANOVA with Bonferroni multiple/post hoc group comparisons was used to analyze the cytotoxicity and permeability data. GraphPadPrism software (GraphPad Software, San Diego, CA, USA) was used and the level of significance was set at probabilities of * $p < 0.05$, ** $p < 0.01$, *** $p < 0.001$ and **** $p < 0.0001$.

3. Results and Discussion

3.1. Spectroscopic Characterizatio

The infrared spectra of chitosan, DMCh, and DMCat derivatives (Figure 1) were characterized by an intense and broad band centered at 3434 cm^{-1}, associated to the axial stretching of hydroxyl and amine groups; a band at 2915 cm^{-1} corresponding to stretching vibration of CH; the bands at 1654 and 1600 cm^{-1} assigned to the C=O stretching and N–H bending, respectively [55]. The spectrum of DMCh (Figure 1B) also exhibits a weak band centered at 1732 cm^{-1}, due to axial deformation of carbonyl ester that is related to the *O*-acylation of chitosan [37]. In the spectrum of DMCat, a new band is observed at 1483 cm^{-1}, which is attributed to the CH bending of $^{+}N(CH_3)_3$ group [56]. Additionally, the band corresponding to the primary amine observed at 1600 cm^{-1} in the spectrum of chitosan and DMCh is less intense in the spectrum of DMCat and it is shifted to lower wavenumber while that band observed at 1654 cm^{-1} is more intense in the spectra of DMCat, which confirms that the primary amine group of GlcN units of DMCh has been modified to secondary amine group as a consequence of the reaction with GTMAC [46,57].

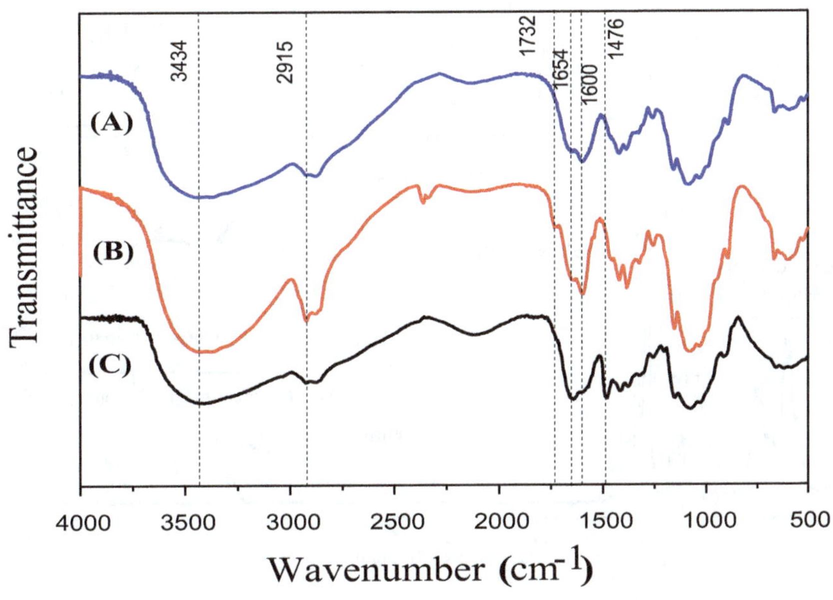

Figure 1. (**A**) Infrared spectra of chitosan, (**B**) DMCh, and (**C**) DMCat.

The comparison of the ^{1}H NMR of chitosan (Figure 2A), DMCh (Figure 2B), and DMCat (Figure 2C) provide additional evidences for the structural modifications resulting of *O*-acylation of chitosan and the quaternization of DMCh. The ^{1}H NMR spectrum of chitosan exhibited singlets at 2.0 ppm and 3.2 ppm characteristics of methyl hydrogens of GlcNAc units and to the hydrogen bonded to C2 of GlcN units, respectively. The set of signals in the range of 3.3–4.0 ppm is attributed to the hydrogens H3–H6 from GlcN unit and the hydrogen bonded to C2 of GlcNAc unit, while that signal occurring at 4.80 ppm is due to the hydrogen (H1) bonded to the anomeric carbon (C1) [46]. The average degree of deacetylation of chitosan was calculated from its ^{1}H NMR spectrum by taking into account the intensity of the signals due to methyl hydrogens from acetamido groups (2.0 ppm) and due to H2–H6 of GlcN/GlcNAc units (3.3–4.0 ppm) and resulted in $\overline{DA} = 5\%$.

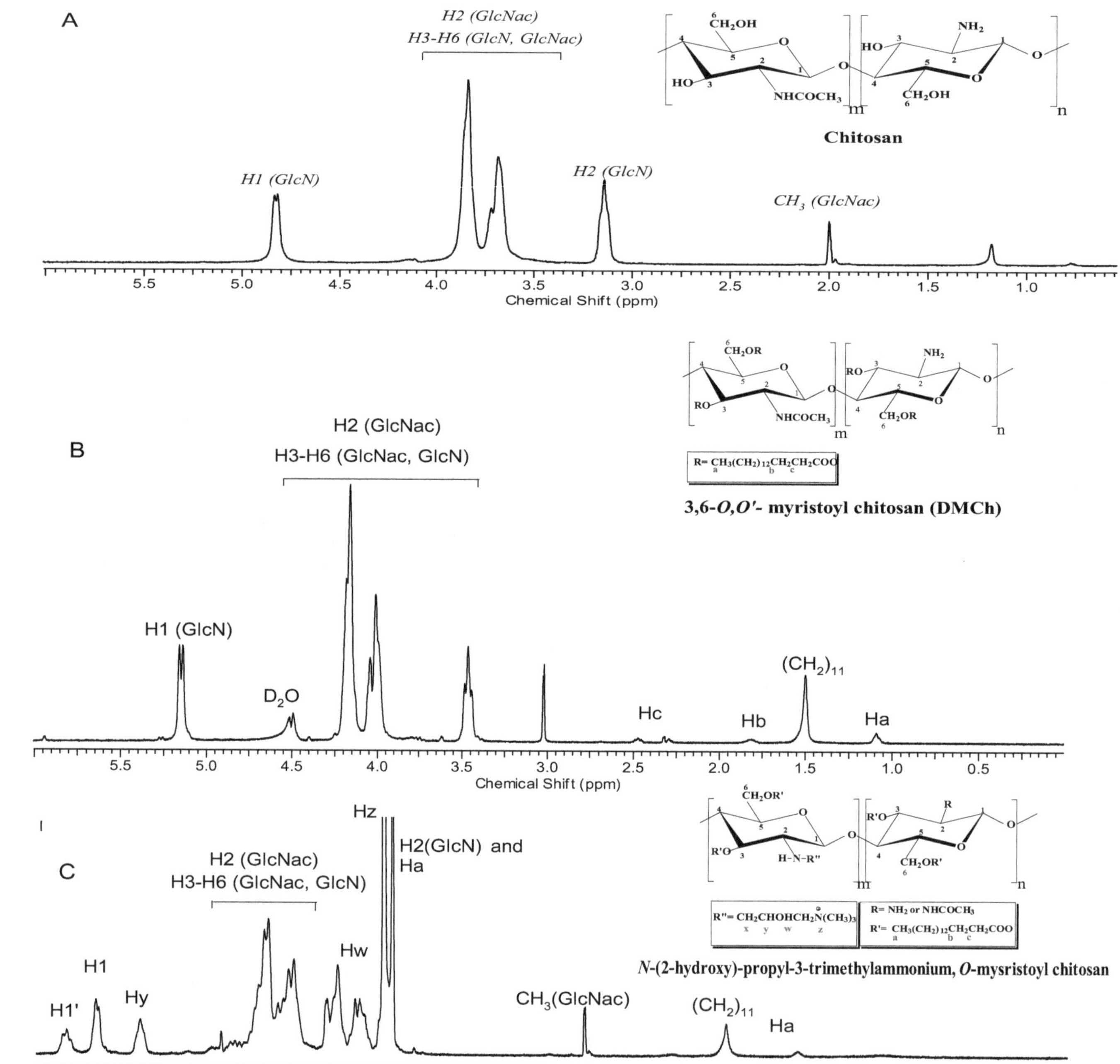

Figure 2. (**A**) ^{1}H nuclear magnetic resonance (NMR) spectra of chitosan, (**B**) DMCh, and (**C**) DMCat in solution D_2O/HCl 1% (*v*/*v*) acquired at 80 °C.

The ^{1}H NMR spectrum of DMCh (Figure 2B) exhibits additional signals at 1.1, 1.5, 1.8, 2.5, and 3.1 ppm corresponding to the hydrogen atoms of CH3, CH2, CH2 (β), and CH2 (α) moieties of myristoyl group. The peaks at 3.2–4.2 ppm refer to the hydrogens H3–H6 from the GlcN unit and the hydrogen bonded to C2 of the GlcNAc unit [37]. The $\overline{DS}$ of DMCh was calculated from ^{1}H NMR spectrum, as described in the Section 2.5.2, and resulted in $\overline{DS}$ = 6%. As a consequence of quaternization of DMCh, the ^{1}H NMR spectrum of DMCat (Figure 2B) showed signals at 4.0 ppm and 4.2 ppm assigned to the methyl hydrogens of $N^+(CH_3)_3$ and methylene hydrogens of $NHCH_2$, respectively, which were due to the introduction of the substituent on the chitosan chains. Additionally, the signals of the hydrogens H3–H6 from GlcN unit and the hydrogen bonded to C2 of GlcNAc unit shifted from 3.2–4.2 ppm to 4.4–4.9 ppm upon the chemical modification of DMCh. The signals at 5.6 ppm and 5.7 ppm are ascribed to the hydrogen bonded to the anomeric carbon of unsubstituted and substituted GlcN units, respectively. The $\overline{DQ}$ was calculated from the corresponding ^{1}H NMR spectrum by using Equation (2) and resulted in $\overline{DQ}$ = 34.7%. The average degree of quaternization of DMcat was also determined from conductometric titration and resulted in $\overline{DQ}$ = 36%, thus demonstrating a good agreement with that calculated from the ^{1}H NMR spectra.

3.2. *Critical Aggregation Concentration*

The critical aggregation concentration (CAC) was evaluated with the conductivity measurements of sample aqueous solutions of DMCh and DMCat at different concentrations, resulting in CAC values of 8.9×10^{-3} mg/mL [37] and 9.38×10^{-6} mg/mL, respectively. The CAC result of the DMCat sample was calculated from the data shown in Figure 3; the result related to the DMCh sample is presented in a previous work [37]. It is also important to note that each polymer was solubilized in a different aqueous medium, according to its solubility, because the aggregation behavior of the polymers was evaluated depending on their solubility as a function of the polymer concentration, thus enabling quantification of the dilution limit that each system presents until its aggregation occurs. When it came to evaluating the stability of micellar systems, the CAC of the polymer was extremely important, as it was possible to know the minimum concentration required of the amphiphilic polymer to obtain stable micelles [18]. Therefore, the ability of the micelles to withstand the dilution is described in terms of their thermodynamic stability and micelles with low CAC values can be maintained in a more dilute solution, and therefore, thermodynamically more stable [58]. A previous study [37] on the physical chemical properties of DMCh evidenced its lower CAC as compared to non-polymeric surfactants, showing that the former was thermodynamically more stable as the micelles are formed and kept stable in more dilute solutions [58]. In the same sense, taking into account that the CAC value of DMCat was much lower as compared to that of DMCh, the former system was able to form micelles at more dilute solutions, evidencing its higher stability as compared to DMCh [59,60]. DMCat derivative was more stable than the DMCh, a fact that can be explained by the permanent positive charges present in the DMCat, as these charges prevent agglomeration of the micelles by the effect of electrostatic repulsion [37,49].

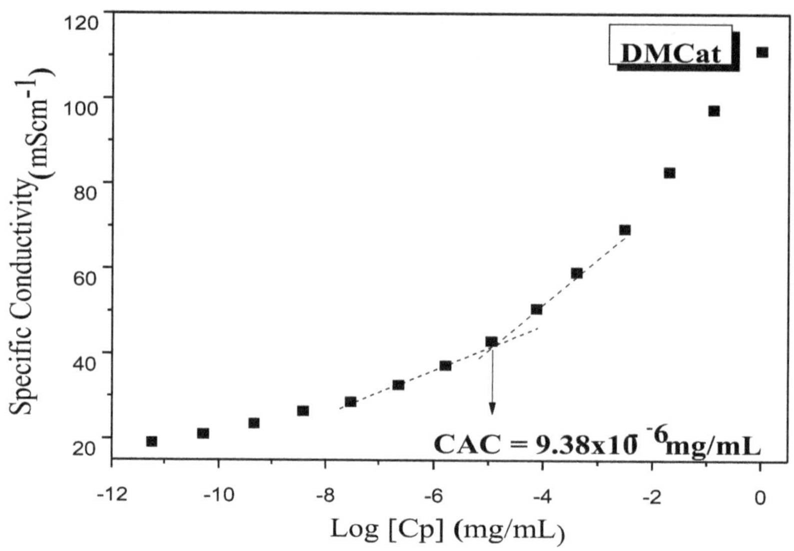

Figure 3. Graphic of specific conductivity versus function of logarithm concentration of DMCat of 1 mg/mL to 1×10^{-6} mg/mL. DMCat sample solubilized in water.

3.3. Drug Encapsulation Efficiency

The encapsulation efficiency (EE) of curcumin in the micellar systems of the DMCh and DMCat derivatives was evaluated through UV spectroscopy. The quantification was performed through the indirect method, from the no-encapsulated CUR contained in the supernatant. The EE values were calculated from the equation of the line obtained from the analytical curve and the results are presented in Table 1. According to the data in Table 1, both micellar systems presented high EE values. However, DMCh micelles had higher EE values when compared to DMCat. This difference may have occurred due to the difficulty of CUR crossing the barrier of positive charges as a consequence of the electronsteric effect. In addition, it was observed that all systems remained stable, with no formation of larger particles and/or particles precipitation.

Table 1. Size, polydispersity index, zeta potential, and encapsulation efficiency of DMCh and DMCat micelles.

Drug (µg)	Micelles–CUR							
	Sample DMCh				Sample DMCat			
	Size (nm) [1]	PDI [2]	Zeta (mV) [3]	EE (%) [4]	Size (nm) [1]	PDI [2]	Zeta (mV) [3]	EE (%) [4]
0	356 ± 21	0.53 ± 0.03	32.1 ± 4.4	-	343 ± 19	0.21 ± 0.02	34.0 ± 0.8	-
50	289 ± 17	0.49 ± 0.04	42.5 ± 2.1	92.7 ± 0.8	268 ± 43	0.62 ± 0.01	30.5 ± 1.2	100 ± 0.5
100	281 ± 38	0.44 ± 0.04	49.1 ± 0.2	81.8 ± 1.0	231 ± 15	0.66 ± 0.02	28.8 ± 1.0	73.8 ± 1.0
150	386 ± 168	0.44 ± 0.16	46.6 ± 4.12	80.9 ± 0.9	372 ± 23	0.49 ± 0.03	33.0 ± 1.5	68.6 ± 0.9

Size [1], polydispersity index [2], and zeta potential [3] were determined by carrying out dynamic light scattering measurements. Encapsulation efficiency [4] of curcumin (CUR) in percentage. Values were reported as mean ± SD ($n = 3$).

3.4. Particle Size and Surface Charge

In case of DMCh micelles, the mean diameter of the micelles varied from 281 nm to 386 nm and from 231 to 372 nm, in case of DMCat micelles (Table 1). CUR-loaded micelles presented lower values than empty micelles (Figure 4), probably due to a contraction of the micelles in the presence of the drug, caused by the greater interaction between the hydrophobic groups pertaining to the core of the micelles and the drug [37]. However, the micelles with higher CUR encapsulation reached a limit, which in turn resulted in the expansion of the volume of the micelles to accommodate a larger amount of CUR and hydrophobic groups inside. The same behavior was observed for the micelles of DMCat, showing that the hydrophobic groups present in both micellar systems have a direct influence on the size of the micelles. Therefore, from the mean diameter results it can be stated that such micelles were promising for delivery of hydrophobic drugs via oral administration.

Zeta potential of the micelles were also evaluated and according to the data presented in Table 1, loaded and empty micelles had high positive zeta potential values (> +28 mV), regardless of whether they were made up of DMCh or DMCat. In the case of DMCh micelles, the net positive charge at the micelles surface was due to the high content of amine groups pertaining to GlcN units, which were converted to ammonium groups when the polymer was dissolved in acid medium [48]. In contrast, the surface of DMCat micelles had permanent positive charges regardless of the pH of the medium because of the presence of quaternized nitrogen atoms pertaining to the substituent groups *N*-(2-hydroxy)-propyl-3-trimethylammonium.

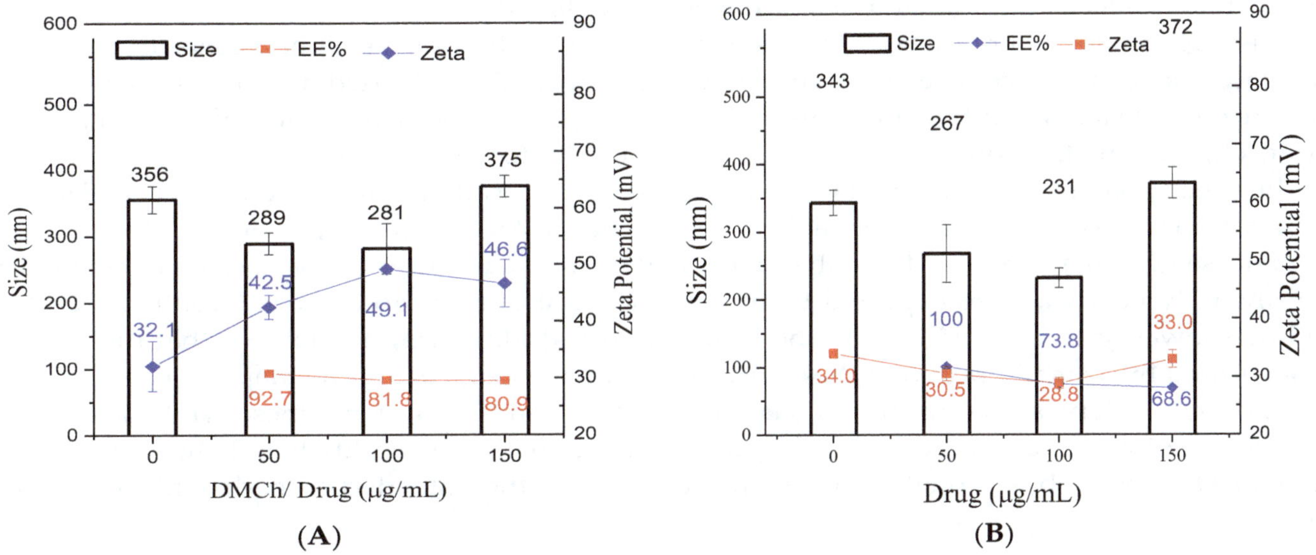

Figure 4. (**A**) the particle size, zeta potential, and encapsulation efficiency of micelles DMCh-CUR and (**B**) DMCat-CUR with different drug concentrations.

The zeta potential values of the empty and loaded micelles were slightly different. It was observed that the DMCh micelles showed an increase of the zeta potential with increase of the CUR loading. This behavior can be attributed to the fact that the formation of the micelles occurred by association of the hydrophobic moieties of the polymer chain to constitute the micelle core, while the hydrophilic portions of the positively charged polymer were exposed to the aqueous medium, i.e., the latter was predominantly located on the surface of the micelles. On the other hand, it was observed for DMCat micelles a small decrease on zeta potential values, which may be justified by the micelles surface, probably containing hydrophobic moieties, as well as a certain fraction of hydrophilic groups may be located in the micelles nuclei, varying the zeta potential in a narrow range. Thus, the high density of permanent positive charge in the hydrophilic shell of the micelles contributes strongly to stabilize them and also favors the interactions of the micelles with the negatively charged cell wall, resulting in the greater absorption and penetration of CUR.

According to the literature, formulations with PdI values $\leq$0.3 are representative of monodisperse systems [61,62]. From the PdI results of both micelles, it was possible to observe values ranging from 0.21 to 0.66 (Table 1), indicating that the systems did not present a monodisperse distribution. This fact can be justified by the non-uniform distribution of the acyl groups added to the chitosan chains, because it was a derivative from a heterogeneous reaction, which lead to the block distribution of the substituent groups. However, the values obtained were in agreement with the results obtained in the literature for chitosan derivatives [48,63–65].

3.5. Cytotoxicity Assay

The in vitro cell viability studies were carried out with Caco-2 and HT29-MTX intestinal cell lines to evaluate the biocompatibility and safety for the oral administration of the empty micelles, DMCh and DMCat, the micelles loaded with CUR, DMCh-CUR and DMCat-CUR, and free CUR. Loaded micelles were incubated during 4 h with different concentrations of drug (5 to 50 μg/mL) and the correspondent amount of empty micelles was also incubated in the same conditions. The cell viability was assessed using an MTT assay (Figure 5). According to the results shown in the Figure 4, it was observed that all the tested samples had no cytotoxic effect on both cell lines for the concentrations 5, 10, and 20 μg/mL. However, at the concentration of 50 μg/mL, it was possible to note a slight decrease on cell viability for unloaded and loaded micelles. This was more evident in the case of HT29-MTX cell line, which dropped very close to 70%. This 70% of cell viability is a threshold that was considered as the cytotoxic level, according to the ISO 10993-5 guideline [52].

It is important to notice that CUR presented a cytotoxic effect for the highest concentration tested with statistical significance when compared with the unloaded and loaded micelles. This means that both micelles systems had the ability to maintain and protect the drug inside of the core, at least during 4 h, showing their potential to be used in the micelles for the release of the drug in the intestine, avoiding the apparent cytotoxicity of CUR. It was assumed based on our previous published studies, where similar chitosan micelles were able to retain and protect the drug, providing a hydrophobic drug release less than 20% after 4 h in the gastric and intestinal fluids [49]. The absence of cytotoxicity from the polymers was also expected taking into account our previous work [37,49]. HT29-MTX cell line showed greater sensitivity to the tested samples. However, it is known that the intestine is constituted by a small portion of these mucus-producing cells, being the majority constituted by Caco-2 cells, which presented higher cell viability levels. Taking into account these cytotoxicity results, the concentration chosen to proceed for the in vitro intestinal permeability was 20 μg/mL, since no cytotoxic effect was observed either for the free drug or for the unloaded or loaded micelles in both cell lines.

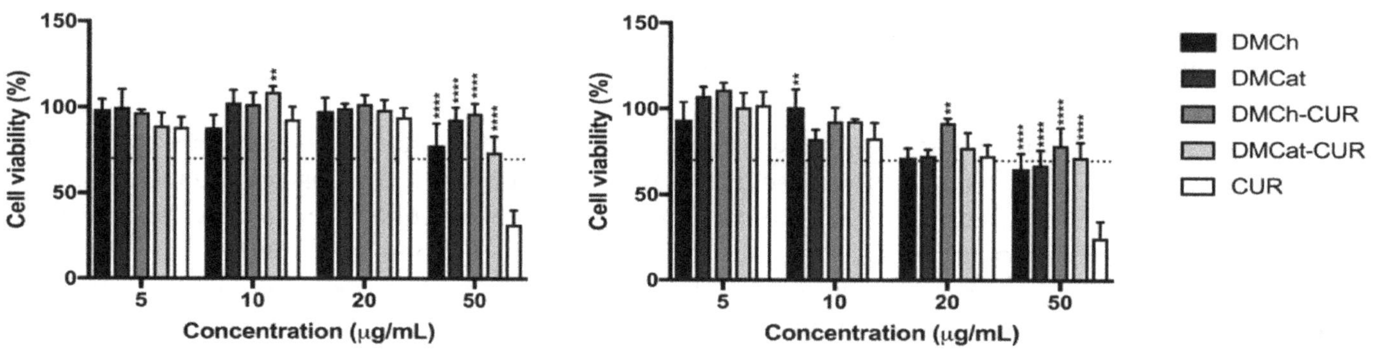

Figure 5. Cell viability of DMCh, DMCat, DMCh-CUR, DMCat-CUR, and free CUR against Caco-2 (**left**) and HT29-MTX (**right**) cell lines, respectively, at CUR concentrations between 5 and 50 μg/mL after 4 h of incubation. Values were reported as mean ± SD (n = 4). ** $p < 0.01$ and **** $p < 0.0001$ denotes a significant difference when compared with free CUR.

3.6. Permeability Studies

In order to evaluate the in vitro permeability estudies, non-toxic concentrations of free CUR and DMCh/DMCat loaded with CUR were selected based on cell viability results. Tests were carried out uni-directionally from the apical to the basolateral compartment. Therefore, a monoculture model consisting of Caco-2 cells was used, which represents the standard model that mimics human enterocytes. In addition, the triple co-culture model, Caco-2/HT29-MTX:Raji B was used due to be a model that better mimic the human intestine when compared to isolated Caco-2 cells, since HT29-MTX are secretory cells of mucus and Raji B cells can induce differentiation of the Caco-2 cell phenotype into M cells.

The monolayer's integrity and growth were carefully verified before the day of the experiment by measuring the TEER regularly during 21 days in order to make sure that a confluent monolayer was formed (Figure 6). As can be seen in Figure 6, Caco-2 model presented much higher TEER values compared to the triple model. These higher values were expected due to the tight junctions presented in Caco-2 cells [66]. On the other hand, the triple model presented lower TEER values due to the presence of HT29-MTX. Both models presented TEER values after 21 days that supported those monolayers to be used in the permeability experiment.

TEER values before starting the experiment were about 1600 Ω/cm^2 in the case of Caco-2 model and up to 450 Ω/cm^2 in the case of the triple model (Figure 6). The TEER values were normalized in percentage by the value at the beginning of the experiment (time zero). The permeability profile of CUR permeated through both models was plotted as a function of time expressed in percentage and is shown in Figure 7. It is possible to observe the permeability of CUR across Caco-2 monoculture model ranged from around 15% in the case of free CUR to around 18% and 24% for DMCh-CUR and DMCat-CUR, respectively, showing that both polymers are capable of carrying CUR. However, the micellar system constituted by DMCat-CUR presented no statistical difference in terms of permeability through monoculture compared to DMCh-CUR, as the first one appeared to have a faster CUR release over time, reaching almost the same permeability after 60 min compared to the CUR permeability at 180 min. The triple co-culture model presented a permeability value in the range of 10% in case of free CUR to 16% and 19% in the case of DMCat-CUR and DMCh-CUR, respectively.

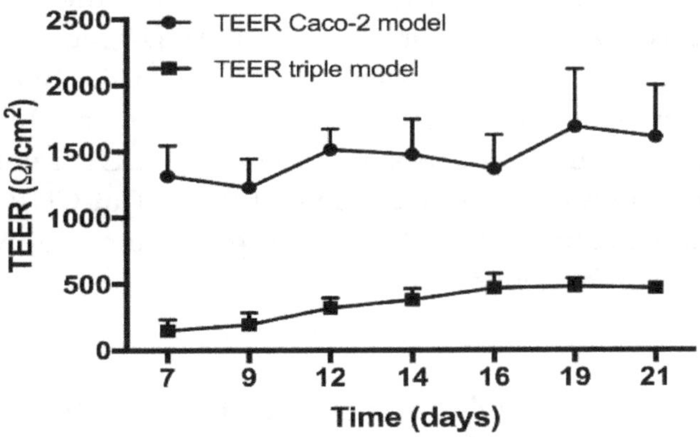

Figure 6. Transepithelial electrical resistance (TEER) values (Ω/cm^2) monitored in function of time during the 21 days of culture on Transwell™ membranes for Caco-2 monoculture model and Caco-2/HT29-MTX:Raji B triple co-culture model.

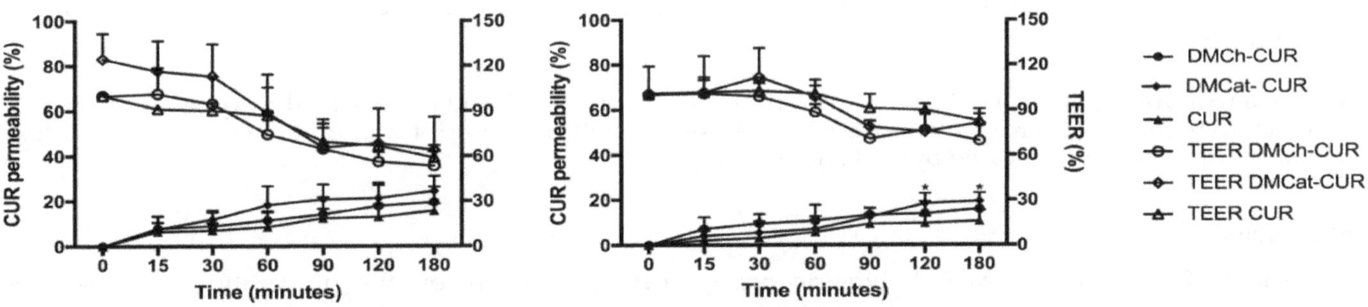

Figure 7. In vitro permeability profile of DMCh-CUR, DMCat-CUR, and free CUR across Caco-2 monoculture model (**left**) and across Caco-2/HT29-MTX:Raji B triple co-culture model (**right**) expressed in percentage. All experiments were conducted from the apical to basolateral compartment in 1% (v/v) DMSO in HBSS at 37 °C. Error bars represent mean ± SD (n = 3) and * $p < 0.05$ denotes a significant difference between DMCat-CUR and CUR.

In this model, a more controlled permeability of CUR was observed over time possibly due to the presence of mucus, which may delay the transport of CUR through the intestinal barrier. In addition, and as can be concluded, there is no significative difference in CUR permeability between both micellar systems. However, for the triple model, DMCat-CUR presented a statistical significance compared with free CUR, evidencing that this system presents a greater capacity to permeate in a more controlled way through the biological barriers and to do the release of the drug.

The decrease on TEER values in Caco-2 monoculture model were in agreement with the higher permeability observed in this mode. The triple co-culture model presented lower CUR permeability values for all the samples tested and this may be due to two important factors to consider due to the complexity of evaluating different biological systems. First, TEER values presented at the end of the 21 days for the triple model presented a lower value (below 500 Ω/cm^2) than that observed in the co-culture (above 1500 Ω/cm^2), making it impossible to compare between the two models. Second, the presence of mucus that entrapes the free CUR avoiding their passage through the monolayer. The lower ability of the micellar systems to permeate through the biological barriers is explained by the high capacity of mucoadhesion that the polymer presents. Preliminary studies show that the DMCat sample had a mucoadhesion capacity greater than the chitosan [67–69], due to the permanent charges present in the polymer chain (DMCat), emphasizing the importance of electrostatic forces for the establishment of interaction with the biological substrate. The effect of mucoadhesion is responsible for maintaining the DMCat-CUR system on the surface of the biological barrier, allowing the release of the sustained release of the drug over time, and in this case, the release of the drug occurs through degradation of the carrier or by diffusion through the polymeric wall. In the process of degradation are involved lysozyme and/or *N*-acetyl-beta-D-glucosaminidase (NAGase), which are enzymes present in the human body, capable of performing the hydrolysis of 1,4-beta-linkages between *N*-acetyl-D-glucosamine, a constituent of polymer chains of chitosan derivatives [67,70,71]. Perhaps, a longer experiment would be necessary to verify if CUR release from DMCat-CUR and subsequent CUR permeation would increase with time. Still, DMCat-CUR presented a more sustained and higher CUR intestinal permeability, which according to the previous results, demonstrate this system as a potential CUR intestinal delivery system.

4. Conclusions

Modification of the derivative 3,6-*O,O′*-dimyristoyl chitosan by the addition of quaternary groups was conducted to improve the solubility of the promising system to carry hydrophobic drugs; it was successfully performed. The presence of the permanent positive charges in the DMCat derivative allowed the solubilization of the polymer over a wide pH range. In addition, the characteristics of this polymer allowed the recognition thereof by the immunological system, thus facilitating its passage through the biological barriers, allowing the circulation of the polymer charged with a hydrophobic drug of interest.

Author Contributions: D.S.S., D.M.d.S., A.A., L.M. conceived, designed, and performed the experiments; S.P.C.-F., S.J.L.R. and B.S. contributed reagents/materials/analysis tools; the manuscript was jointly written by all authors. The manuscript has been reviewed by S.P.C.-F., S.J.L.R. and B.S.

References

1. Crucho, C.I.C.; Barros, M.T. Polymeric nanoparticles: A study on the preparation variables and characterization methods. *Mater. Sci. Eng. C* **2017**, *80*, 771–784. [CrossRef] [PubMed]
2. Lu, Z.R.; Qiao, P. Drug Delivery in Cancer Therapy, Quo Vadis? *Mol. Pharm.* **2018**, *15*, 3603–3616. [CrossRef] [PubMed]
3. Anitha, A.; Maya, S.; Deepa, N.; Chennazhi, K.P.; Nair, S.V.; Tamura, H.; Jayakumar, R. Efficient water soluble O-carboxymethyl chitosan nanocarrier for the delivery of curcumin to cancer cells. *Carbohydr. Polym.* **2011**, *83*, 452–461. [CrossRef]

4. Sajomsang, W.; Gonil, P.; Saesoo, S.; Ruktanonchai, U.R.; Srinuanchai, W.; Puttipipatkhachorn, S. Synthesis and anticervical cancer activity of novel pH responsive micelles for oral curcumin delivery. *Int. J. Pharm.* **2014**, *477*, 261–272. [CrossRef] [PubMed]
5. Ghalandarlaki, N.; Alizadeh, A.M.; Ashkani-Esfahani, S. Nanotechnology-applied curcumin for different diseases therapy. *Biomed. Res. Int.* **2014**, *2014*, 39426. [CrossRef] [PubMed]
6. Sarisozen, C.; Abouzeid, A.H.; Torchilin, V.P. The effect of co-delivery of paclitaxel and curcumin by transferrin-targeted PEG-PE-based mixed micelles on resistant ovarian cancer in 3-D spheroids and in vivo tumors. *Eur. J. Pharm. Biopharm.* **2014**, *88*, 539–550. [CrossRef] [PubMed]
7. Popat, A.; Karmaka, S.R.; Jambhrunkar, S.; Xu, C.; Yu, C. Curcumin-cyclodextrin encapsulated chitosan nanoconjugates with enhanced solubility and cell cytotoxicity. *Colloids Surf. B Biointerfaces* **2014**, *117*, 520–527. [CrossRef] [PubMed]
8. Aggarwal, B.B.; Gupta, S.C.; Sung, B. Curcumin: An orally bioavailable blocker of TNF and other pro-inflammatory biomarkers. *Br. J. Pharmacol.* **2013**, *169*, 1672–1692. [CrossRef] [PubMed]
9. Khan, S.; Imran, M.; Butt, T.T.; Ali Shah, S.W.; Sohail, M.; Malik, A.; Das, S.; Thu, H.E.; Adam, A.; Hussain, Z. Curcumin based nanomedicines as efficient Nanoplatform for treatment of cancer: New developments in reversing cancer drug resistance, rapid internalization, and improved anticancer efficacy. *Trends Food Sci. Technol.* **2018**, *80*, 8–22. [CrossRef]
10. Rauf, A.; Imran, M.; Orhan, I.E.; Bawazeer, S. Health perspectives of a bioactive compound curcumin: A review. *Trends Food Sci. Technol.* **2018**, *74*, 33–45. [CrossRef]
11. Nelson, K.M.; Dahlin, J.L.; Bisson, J.; Graham, J.; Pauli, G.F.; Walters, M.A. The Essential Medicinal Chemistry of Curcumin. *J. Med. Chem.* **2017**, *60*, 1620–1637. [CrossRef] [PubMed]
12. Anand, P.; Kunnumakkara, A.B.; Newman, R.A.; Aggarwal, B.B. Bioavailability of Curcumin: Problems and Promises. *Mol. Pharm.* **2007**, *4*, 807–818. [CrossRef] [PubMed]
13. Angeles, L.; Angeles, L.; Haven, N. Phase 1 study of PSMA-targeted docetaxel-containing nanoparticle BIND-014 in patients with advanced solid tumors. *Clin. Cancer Res.* **2016**, *22*, 3157–3163. [CrossRef]
14. Kyung, H.; Minkyu, A.; Sun, J.; Sym, J. A phase II trial of Cremorphor EL-free paclitaxel (Genexol-PM) and gemcitabine in patients with advanced non-small cell lung cancer. *Cancer Chemother. Pharmacol.* **2014**, *74*, 277–282. [CrossRef]
15. Cortez, A.J.; Tudre, P.J.; Kujawa, K.A.; Lisowska, K.M. Advances in ovarian cancer therapy. *Cancer Chemother. Pharmacol.* **2018**, *81*, 17–38. [CrossRef] [PubMed]
16. Tien, C.L.; Lacroix, M.; Ispas-Szabo, P.; Mateescu, M.A. *N*-acylated chitosan: Hydrophobic matrices for controlled drug release. *J. Control. Release* **2003**, *93*, 1–13. [CrossRef]
17. Ishihar, M.A.; Kishimoto, M.; Fujita, S.; Hattori, H.; Kanatani, Y. Biological, Chemical and Physical Compatibility of Chitosan and Biopharmaceuticals. *Chitosan-Based Syst. Biopharm. Deliv. Target. Polym. Ther.* **2012**, 93–106. [CrossRef]
18. Huo, M.; Zhang, Y.; Zhou, J.; Zou, A.; Li, J. Formation, microstructure, biodistribution and absence of toxicity of polymeric micelles formed by *N*-octyl-*N,O*-carboxymethyl chitosan. *Carbohydr. Polym.* **2011**, *83*, 1959–1969. [CrossRef]
19. Matsumura, Y.; Kataoka, K. Preclinical and clinical studies of anticancer agent-incorporating polymer micelles. *Cancer Sci.* **2009**, *100*, 572–579. [CrossRef] [PubMed]
20. Nishiyama, N.; Kataoka, K. Current state, achievements, and future prospects of polymeric micelles as nanocarriers for drug and gene delivery. *Pharmacol. Ther.* **2006**, *112*, 630–648. [CrossRef] [PubMed]
21. Gao, J.; Ming, J.; He, B.; Fan, Y.; Gu, Z.; Zhang, X. Preparation and characterization of novel polymeric micelles for 9-nitro-20(*S*)-camptothecin delivery. *Eur. J. Pharm. Sci.* **2008**, *34*, 85–93. [CrossRef] [PubMed]
22. Muley, P.; Kumar, S.; El Kourati, F.; Kesharwani, S.S.; Tummala, H. Hydrophobically modified inulin as an amphiphilic carbohydrate polymer for micellar delivery of paclitaxel for intravenous route. *Int. J. Pharm.* **2016**, *500*, 32–41. [CrossRef] [PubMed]
23. Ito, T.; Yoshida, C.; Murakami, Y. Design of novel sheet-shaped chitosan hydrogel for wound healing: A hybrid biomaterial consisting of both PEG-grafted chitosan and crosslinkable polymeric micelles acting as drug containers. *Mater. Sci. Eng. C* **2013**, *33*, 3697–3703. [CrossRef] [PubMed]
24. Du, Y.; Cai, L.; Liu, P.; You, J.; Yuan, H.; Hu, F. Biomaterials Tumor cells-speci fi c targeting delivery achieved by A54 peptide functionalized polymeric micelles. *Biomaterials* **2012**, *33*, 8858–8867. [CrossRef] [PubMed]

25. Jiao, J.; Li, X.; Zhang, S.; Liu, J.; Di, D.; Zhang, Y.; Zhao, Q.; Wang, S. Redox and pH dual-responsive PEG and chitosan-conjugated hollow mesoporous silica for controlled drug release. *Mater. Sci. Eng. C* **2016**, *67*, 26–33. [CrossRef] [PubMed]
26. Elsaid, Z.; Taylor, K.M.G.; Puri, S.; Cath, A.; Al-jamal, K.; Bai, J.; Klippstein, R.; Wang, T.; Forbes, B.; Chana, J. Mixed micelles of lipoic acid-chitosan-poly(ethylene glycol) and distearoylphosphatidylethanolamine-poly(ethylene glycol) for tumor delivery. *Eur. J. Pharm. Sci.* **2017**, *101*, 228–242. [CrossRef] [PubMed]
27. Jin, X.; Li, N.; Ju, C.; Sun, M.; Zhang, C.; Pin, Q.G. Biomaterials The mechanism of enhancement on oral absorption of paclitaxel by *N*-octyl-*O*-sulfate chitosan micelles. *Biomaterials* **2011**, *32*, 4609–4620. [CrossRef]
28. Huo, M.; Liu, Y.; Wang, L.; Yin, T.; Qin, C.; Xiao, Y.; Yin, L.; Liu, J.; Zhou, J. Redox-sensitive micelles based on *O,N*-hydroxyethyl chitosan-octylamine conjugates for triggered intracellular delivery of paclitaxel Redox-sensitive micelles based on *O,N*-hydroxyethyl chitosan-octylamine conjugates for triggered intracellular deliver. *Mol. Pharm.* **2016**, *13*, 1750–1762. [CrossRef] [PubMed]
29. Attia, E.A.B.; Ong, Z.Y.; Hedrick, J.L.; Lee, P.P.; Lee, P.L.R.; Hammond, P.T.; Yang, Y.-Y. Mixed micelles self-assembled from block copolymers for drug delivery. *Curr. Opin. Colloid Interface Sci.* **2011**, *16*, 182–194. [CrossRef]
30. Jiang, G.B.B.; Quan, D.; Liao, K.; Wang, H. Novel polymer micelles prepared from chitosan grafted hydrophobic palmitoyl groups for drug delivery. *Mol. Pharm.* **2006**, *3*, 152–160. [CrossRef] [PubMed]
31. Zhang, C.; Qu, G.; Sun, Y.; Wu, X.; Yao, Z.; Guo, Q.; Ding, Q.; Yuan, S.; Shen, Z.; Ping, Q.; et al. Pharmacokinetics, biodistribution, efficacy and safety of *N*-octyl-*O*-sulfate chitosan micelles loaded with paclitaxel. *Biomaterials* **2008**, *29*, 1233–1241. [CrossRef] [PubMed]
32. Hu, F.Q.Q.; Zhao, M.D.D.; Yuan, H.; You, J.; Du, Y.Z.Z.; Zeng, S. A novel chitosan oligosaccharide-stearic acid micelles for gene delivery: Properties and in vitro transfection studies. *Int. J. Pharm.* **2006**, *315*, 158–166. [CrossRef] [PubMed]
33. Chenguang, L.I.U.; Desai, K.G.; Xiguang, C.; Hyun-jin, P. Preparation and Charaterization of Self-assembled Nanoparticles Based on Linolenic-acid Modified Chitosan. *J. Ocean Univ. China* **2005**, *4*, 234–239. [CrossRef]
34. Hu, F.Q.; Ren, G.F.; Yuan, H.; Du, Y.Z.; Zeng, S. Shell cross-linked stearic acid grafted chitosan oligosaccharide self-aggregated micelles for controlled release of paclitaxel. *Colloids Surf. B Biointerfaces* **2006**, *50*, 97–103. [CrossRef] [PubMed]
35. Huo, M.; Zhang, Y.; Zhou, J.; Zou, A.; Yu, D.; Wu, Y.; Li, J.; Li, H. Synthesis and characterization of low-toxic amphiphilic chitosan derivatives and their application as micelle carrier for antitumor drug. *Int. J. Pharm.* **2010**, *394*, 162–173. [CrossRef] [PubMed]
36. Du, Y.Z.Z.; Wang, L.; Yuan, H.; Wei, X.H.H.; Hu, F.Q.Q. Preparation and characteristics of linoleic acid-grafted chitosan oligosaccharide micelles as a carrier for doxorubicin. *Colloids Surf. B Biointerfaces* **2009**, *69*, 257–263. [CrossRef] [PubMed]
37. Silva, D.S.; Almeida, A.; Prezotti, F.; Cury, B.; Campana-Filho, S.P.; Sarmento, B. Synthesis and characterization of 3,6-*O,O'*-dimyristoyl chitosan micelles for oral delivery of paclitaxel. *Colloids Surf. B Biointerfaces* **2017**, *152*, 220–228. [CrossRef] [PubMed]
38. Pan, Z.; Gao, Y.; Heng, L.; Liu, Y.; Yao, G.; Wang, Y.; Liu, Y. Amphiphilic *N*-(2,3-dihydroxypropyl)-chitosan-cholic acid micelles for paclitaxel delivery. *Carbohydr. Polym.* **2013**, *94*, 394–399. [CrossRef] [PubMed]
39. Di Martino, A.; Sedlarik, V. Amphiphilic chitosan-grafted-functionalized polylactic acid based nanoparticles as a delivery system for doxorubicin and temozolomide co-therapy. *Int. J. Pharm.* **2014**, *474*, 134–145. [CrossRef] [PubMed]
40. Zhang, C.; Ding, Y.; Lucy, L.; Ping, Q. Polymeric micelle systems of hydroxycamptothecin based on amphiphilic *N*-alkyl-*N*-trimethyl chitosan derivatives. *Colloids Surf. B Biointerfaces* **2007**, *55*, 192–199. [CrossRef] [PubMed]
41. Zuñiga, A.; Debbaudt, A.; Albertengo, L.; Rodríguez, M.S. Synthesis and characterization of *N*-propyl-*N*-methylene phosphonic chitosan derivative. *Carbohydr. Polym.* **2010**, *79*, 475–480. [CrossRef]
42. Woraphatphadung, T.; Sajomsang, W.; Gonil, P.; Treetong, A.; Akkaramongkolporn, P.; Ngawhirunpat, T.; Opanasopit, P. pH-Responsive polymeric micelles based on amphiphilic chitosan derivatives: Effect of hydrophobic cores on oral meloxicam delivery. *Int. J. Pharm.* **2016**, *497*, 150–160. [CrossRef] [PubMed]

43. Wu, J.; Wei, W.; Wang, L.Y.; Su, Z.G.; Ma, G.H. A thermosensitive hydrogel based on quaternized chitosan and poly(ethylene glycol) for nasal drug delivery system. *Biomaterials* **2007**, *28*, 2220–2232. [CrossRef] [PubMed]
44. Sonia, T.A.; Sharma, C.P. In vitro evaluation of *N*-(2-hydroxy) propyl-3-trimethyl ammonium chitosan for oral insulin delivery. *Carbohydr. Polym.* **2011**, *84*, 103–109. [CrossRef]
45. Ruihua, H.; Bingchao, Y.; Zheng, D.; Wang, B. Preparation and characterization of a quaternized chitosan. *J. Mater. Sci.* **2012**, *47*, 845–851. [CrossRef]
46. Santos, D.M.; Bukzem, A.L.; Campana-Filho, S.P. Response surface methodology applied to the study of the microwave-assisted synthesis of quaternized chitosan. *Carbohydr. Polym.* **2016**, *138*, 317–326. [CrossRef] [PubMed]
47. Rinaudo, M.; Milas, M.; Le Dung, P. Characterization of chitosan. Influence of ionic strength and degree of acetylation on chain expansion. *Int. J. Biol. Macromol.* **1993**, *15*, 281–285. [CrossRef]
48. Almeida, A.; Silva, D.S.; Gonçalves, V.; Sarmento, B. Synthesis and characterization of chitosan-grafted-polycaprolactone micelles for modulate intestinal paclitaxel delivery. *Drug Deliv. Transl. Res.* **2017**, *7*, 1–11. [CrossRef] [PubMed]
49. Silva, D.S.; Almeida, A.; Prezotti, F.G.; Facchinatto, W.M.; Colnago, L.A.; Campana-Filho, S.P.; Sarmento, B. Self-aggregates of 3,6-*O*,*O*′-dimyristoylchitosan derivative are effective in enhancing the solubility and intestinal permeability of camptothecin. *Carbohydr. Polym.* **2017**, *177*, 178–186. [CrossRef] [PubMed]
50. Hirai, A.; Odani, H.; Nakajim, A.A. Determination of degree of deacetylation of chitosan by ^{1}H NMR spectroscopy. *Polym. Bull.* **1991**, *94*, 87–94. [CrossRef]
51. Fiamingo, A.; Delezuk, J.A.D.M.; Trombotto, S.; David, L.; Campana-Filho, S.P. Extensively deacetylated high molecular weight chitosan from the multistep ultrasound-assisted deacetylation of beta-chitin. *Ultrason. Sonochem.* **2016**, *32*, 79–85. [CrossRef] [PubMed]
52. *ISO/EN10993-5. International Standard ISO 10993-5 Biological Evaluation of Medical Devices—Part 5: Tests for Cytotoxicity: In Vitro Methods*; International Organization for Standardization: Geneva, Switzerland, 2009; Volume 42.
53. Araújo, F.; Sarmento, B. Towards the characterization of an in vitro triple co-culture intestine cell model for permeability studies. *Int. J. Pharm.* **2013**, *458*, 128–134. [CrossRef] [PubMed]
54. Antunes, F.; Andrade, F.; Araújo, F.; Ferreira, D.; Sarmento, B. Establishment of a triple co-culture in vitro cell models to study intestinal absorption of peptide drugs. *Eur. J. Pharm. Biopharm.* **2013**, *83*, 427–435. [CrossRef] [PubMed]
55. Brugnerotto, J.; Lizardi, J.; Goycoolea, F.M.; Argüelles-Monal, W.; Desbrières, J.; Rinaudo, M. An infrared investigation in relation with chitin and chitosan characterization. *Polymer* **2001**, *42*, 3569–3580. [CrossRef]
56. Cho, J.; Grant, J.; Piquette-miller, M.; Allen, C. Synthesis and Physicochemical and Dynamic Mechanical Properties of a Water-Soluble Chitosan Derivative as a Biomaterial. *Biomacromolecules* **2006**, *10*, 2845–2855. [CrossRef] [PubMed]
57. Xiao, B.; Wan, Y.; Wang, X.; Zha, Q.; Liu, H.; Qiu, Z.; Zhang, S. Synthesis and characterization of *N*-(2-hydroxy)propyl-3-trimethyl ammonium chitosan chloride for potential application in gene delivery. *Colloids Surf. B Biointerfaces* **2012**, *91*, 168–174. [CrossRef] [PubMed]
58. Croy, S.R.; Kwon, G.S. Polymeric micelles for drug delivery. *Curr. Pharm. Des.* **2006**, *12*, 4669–4684. [CrossRef] [PubMed]
59. Li, Y.; Li, L.; Dong, H.; Cai, X.; Ren, T. Pluronic F127 nanomicelles engineered with nuclear localized functionality for targeted drug delivery. *Mater. Sci. Eng. C* **2013**, *33*, 2698–2707. [CrossRef] [PubMed]
60. Li, X.; Yu, Y.; Ji, Q.; Qiu, L. Targeted delivery of anticancer drugs by aptamer AS1411 mediated Pluronic F127/cyclodextrin-linked polymer composite micelles. *Nanomedicine* **2014**, *1*, 175–184. [CrossRef] [PubMed]
61. Rao, J.P.; Geckeler, K.E. Polymer nanoparticles: Preparation techniques and size-control parameters. *Prog. Polym. Sci.* **2011**, *36*, 887–913. [CrossRef]
62. Hickey, J.W.; Santos, J.L.; Williford, J.M.; Mao, H.Q. Control of polymeric nanoparticle size to improve therapeutic delivery. *J. Control. Release* **2015**, *219*, 535–547. [CrossRef] [PubMed]
63. Yuan, H.; Lu, L.; Du, Y.; Hu, F. Stearic acid-g-chitosan polymeric micelle for oral drug delivery: In intro transport and in vivo absorption. *Mol. Pharm.* **2010**, *8*, 225–238. [CrossRef] [PubMed]

64. Zhang, C.; Ping, Q.; Zhang, H.; Shen, J. Preparation of *N*-alkyl-*O*-sulfate chitosan derivatives and micellar solubilization of taxol. *Carbohydr. Polym.* **2003**, *54*, 137–141. [CrossRef]
65. Zhang, C.; Qineng, P.; Zhang, H. Self-assembly and characterization of paclitaxel-loaded *N*-octyl-*O*-sulfate chitosan micellar system. *Colloids Surf. B Biointerfaces* **2004**, *39*, 69–75. [CrossRef] [PubMed]
66. Lechanteur, A.; Almeida, A.; Sarmento, B. Elucidation of the impact of cell culture conditions of Caco-2 cell monolayer on barrier integrity and intestinal permeability. *Eur. J. Pharm. Biopharm.* **2017**, *119*, 137–141. [CrossRef] [PubMed]
67. Park, J.H.; Saravanakumar, G.; Kim, K.; Kwon, I.C. Targeted delivery of low molecular drugs using chitosan and its derivatives. *Adv. Drug Deliv. Rev.* **2010**, *62*, 28–41. [CrossRef] [PubMed]
68. Hejazi, R.; Amiji, M. Chitosan-based gastrointestinal delivery systems. *J. Control. Release* **2003**, *89*, 151–165. [CrossRef]
69. Tozaki, H.; Komoike, J.; Tada, C.; Maruyama, T.; Terabe, A.; Suzuki, T.; Yamamoto, A.; Muranishi, S. Chitosan capsules for colon-specific drug delivery: Improvement of insulin absorption from the rat colon. *J. Pharm. Sci.* **1997**, *86*, 1016–1021. [CrossRef] [PubMed]
70. Bernkop-Schnürch, A.; Dünnhaupt, S. Chitosan-based drug delivery systems. *Eur. J. Pharm. Biopharm.* **2012**, *81*, 463–469. [CrossRef] [PubMed]
71. Chauvierre, C.; Leclerc, L.; Labarre, D.; Appel, M.; Marden, M.C.; Couvreur, P.; Vauthier, C. Enhancing the tolerance of poly(isobutylcyanoacrylate) nanoparticles with a modular surface design. *Int. J. Pharm.* **2007**, *338*, 327–332. [CrossRef] [PubMed]

14

Probing the Action of Permeation Enhancers Sodium Cholate and N-dodecyl-β-D-maltoside in a Porcine Jejunal Mucosal Explant System

E. Michael Danielsen * and Gert H. Hansen

Department of Cellular and Molecular Medicine, The Panum Institute, Faculty of Health Sciences, University of Copenhagen, 2200 Copenhagen, Denmark; gerth@sund.ku.dk

* Correspondence: midan@sund.ku.dk

Abstract: The small intestinal epithelium constitutes a major permeability barrier for the oral administration of therapeutic drugs with poor bioavailability, and permeation enhancers (PEs) are required to increase the paracellular and/or transcellular uptake of such drugs. Many PEs act as surfactants by perturbing cell membrane integrity and causing permeabilization by leakage or endocytosis. The aim of the present work was to study the action of sodium cholate (NaC) and N-dodecyl-β-D-maltoside (DDM), using a small intestinal mucosal explant system. At 2 mM, both NaC and DDM caused leakage into the enterocyte cytosol of the fluorescent probe Lucifer Yellow, but they also blocked the constitutive endocytotic pathway from the brush border. In addition, an increased paracellular passage of 3-kDa Texas Red Dextran into the lamina propria was observed. By electron microscopy, both PEs disrupted the hexagonal organization of microvilli of the brush border and led to the apical extrusion of vesicle-like and amorphous cell debris to the lumen. In conclusion, NaC and DDM acted in a multimodal way to increase the permeability of the jejunal epithelium both by paracellular and transcellular mechanisms. However, endocytosis, commonly thought to be an uptake mechanism that may be stimulated by PEs, was not involved in the transcellular process.

Keywords: intestinal permeation enhancers; sodium cholate (NaC); N-dodecyl-β-D-maltoside (DDM); small intestine; enterocyte; brush border

---

1. Introduction

The small intestinal brush border has two equally important, but mutually conflicting bodily functions to take care of: (1) to digest and absorb dietary nutrients, and (2) to prevent harmful luminal agents from gaining access to the body. Whereas the digestive/absorptive capacity of enterocytes is optimized by the large apical surface expansion represented by numerous microvilli [1,2], the unusually high glycolipid content of the apical membrane bilayer favors the formation of "lipid raft" domains [3–5]. The ensuing membrane robustness not only renders the brush border relatively resistant to noxious luminal agents, but also proves a challenge to overcome in the pharmacological quest for permeation enhancers (PEs) suitable for oral administration of drugs with otherwise poor bioavailability [6]. Surfactants represent a large and chemically diverse group of PEs, and as amphiphilic compounds, they have a capacity to adsorb to the cell membrane bilayer, thereby rendering it more fluid and causing it to expand, leading to a loss of integrity and an increase in permeability [6,7]. At higher concentrations, PEs may cause membrane solubilization, and ultimately, buckling and lysis of the cell membrane itself [6]; ideally however, PE action should strike the optimal balance between achieving adequate drug absorption from the gut without compromising mucosal integrity [8]. Functionally, intestinal PEs may act to increase transcellular pathways and/or the paracellular permeability by the opening of tight junctions between adjacent epithelial cells. Regarding the former, permeabilization is thought to be achieved by generating pores or leaks in the cell membrane, or by engaging one of several possible endocytotic mechanisms [6,9,10].

Bile salts are a distinct group of chemically related endogenous compounds engaged in assimilation of dietary fat [11]. Their role in this process may be likened to that of other types of surfactants, and they have long attracted considerable interest as potential PEs in drug absorption, as evidenced by their listing in several patents of oral peptide delivery systems [6,12–14]. Another class of widely-used soluble surfactant PEs is alkyl maltosides, of which members like bile salts are included in some formulations currently undergoing preclinical testing for oral drug delivery [6,15].

The aim of the present work was to compare how a bile salt, sodium cholate (NaC), and an alkyl maltoside, N-dodecyl-β-D-maltoside (DDM) affect the different cellular uptake pathways of a number of fluorescent polar and lipophilic probes, using a small intestinal mucosal organ culture model. This experimental setup is simple to use and offers a more in-vivo-like alternative to commonly-used epithelial cell lines such as Caco-2 [16]. Using this model, we have previously been able to visualize directly how other types of PEs, including lauroyl-carnitine, monocaprin, the ethoxylate $C_{12}E_9$, and melittin interact with the epithelium to affect uptake of polar and lipophilic probes [17–19]. At a concentration of 2 mM (~0.1%), NaC and DDM both exhibited multimodal actions as PEs, i.e., increased paracellular, as well as transcellular, permeability, without causing excessive damage to the integrity of the epithelium. At the ultrastructural level, NaC and DDM disrupted the normally ordered hexagonal organization of microvilli of the brush border and led to the extrusion of vesicle-like and amorphous cell debris to the lumen. Otherwise, overall cell morphology, including tight junctions and basolateral cell membranes, appeared intact, implying that the brush border is the primary target of both PEs.

2. Materials and Methods

2.1. Materials

Sodium cholate hydrate (NaC, MW 409 Da) and N-dodecyl-β-D-maltoside (DDM, MW 511 Da) were supplied by Sigma-Aldrich (Copenhagen, Denmark; www.sigmaaldrich.com), Lucifer yellow CH ammonium salt (LY), a fixable analog of the FM lipophilic styryl dye FM 1-43 FX (FM), Texas Red Dextran (MW 3000 Da, lysine fixable) (TRD), ProLong antifade reagent with DAPI, and a monoclonal antibody to Na+/K+-ATPase (α-chain) by Thermo Scientific (Roskilde, Denmark; www.thermodanmark.dk), a rabbit antibody to intestinal alkaline phosphatase (IAP) was from AbD Serotec (Copenhagen, Denmark; www.bio-rad-antibodies.com), and a mouse anti-rat early endosome antigen-1 (EEA-1) antibody by BD Transduction Laboratories (Lyngby, Denmark; www.bdbiosciences.com). A rabbit antibody to pig intestinal aminopeptidase N (ApN) was prepared as previously described [20].

2.2. Animals

Animal experimentation included in this work was performed only by licensed staff at the Department of Experimental Medicine, the Panum Institute, University of Copenhagen, and was covered by license 2012-15-2934-00077 issued to the Dept. of Experimental Medicine, the Panum Institute, University of Copenhagen. A total of six animals were used in this study.

Segments of porcine jejunum, taken about 2 m from the pylorus of overnight fasted, postweaned animals, were surgically removed from the anaesthetized animals. After excision of the tissue, the animals were sacrificed by an injection with pentobarbital/lidocaine (1 mg/kg bodyweight). As this study contained no further animal experimentation, no specific approval by an ethics committee was required.

2.3. *Organ Culture of Porcine Jejunal Mucosa*

Organ culture of small intestinal mucosa was performed essentially as described previously [16,21]. Briefly, after excision from the animals, jejunal segments of ~20 cm in length were quickly opened longitudinally and immersed in ice-cold RPMI medium. Mucosal tissue specimens weighing ~0.1 g were excised with a scalpel and placed on metal grids in organ culture dishes, to which 1 mL of pre-warmed RPMI medium was added. The dishes were placed in an incubator kept at 37 °C, and after 15 min of preincubation, reagents were added to the RPMI medium at the following concentrations: NaC and DDM (2 mM or 10 mM), LY (0.5 mg/mL), FM dye (10 μg/mL), and TRD (50 μg/mL). The explants were cultured in the presence of the reagents for 1 h in the dark, and after culture they were carefully rinsed in fresh RPMI medium and immersed in a fixative overnight at 4 °C.

2.4. *Fluorescence Microscopy*

Explants were fixed at 4 °C overnight in 4% paraformaldehyde in 0.1 M sodium phosphate, pH 7.2 (buffer A). Following fixation and a quick rinse in buffer A, the explants were immersed overnight in 25% sucrose in buffer A before they were mounted in Tissue-Tek and sectioned (~7 μm thick sections cut parallel to the crypt-villus axis) at −19 °C in a Leica CM1850 cryostat. For immunolabeling, the sections were incubated for 1 h at room temperature with antibodies to EEA-1 (diluted 1: 100), Na^+/K^+-ATPase (diluted 1:100) or aminopeptidase N (diluted 1:5000) in 50 mM Tris-HCl, 150 mM NaCl, 0.5% ovalbumin, 0.1% gelatin, 0.2% teleostan gelatin, 0.05% Tween 20, 0.05% Triton X-100, pH 7.2 (buffer B). Incubation with Alexa-conjugated secondary antibodies (diluted 1:200 in buffer B) was for 1 h at room temperature. Controls with omission of primary antibodies were routinely included in the labeling experiments.

All sections were finally mounted in antifade mounting medium containing DAPI, and examined in a Leica DM 4000B microscope (Leica, Wetzlar, Germany) fitted with a Leica DFC495 digital camera. Images were obtained using Leica HCX PL Fluotar objectives with the following magnification/numerical aperture: 20×/0.40, 40×/0.65, 63×/0.90, and 100×/1.30. The following filter cubes were used: I3 (band pass filter, excitation 450–490 nm), TX2 (band pass filter, excitation 560/40 nm), and A4 (band pass filter, excitation 360/40 nm).

Hematoxylin-eosin (HE) staining of fixed tissue sections was performed according to a standard protocol.

2.5. *Transmission Electron Microscopy*

For transmission electron microscopy, cultured explants were fixed in 3% glutaraldehyde (*v*/*v*), 2% (*w*/*v*) paraformaldehyde in buffer A overnight at 4 °C. After a rinse in buffer A, the explants were post-fixed in 1% osmium tetroxide in buffer A for 1 h at 4 °C, dehydrated in acetone and finally embedded in Epon (an epoxy resin). Ultrathin sections were cut in a Pharmacia LKB Ultrotome III, and stained with 1% (*w*/*v*) uranyl acetate in H_2O and lead citrate. All sections were finally examined in a Zeiss EM 900 electron microscope (Zeiss, Oberkochen, Germany) equipped with a Mega View II camera.

2.6. *Preparation of Microvillus Membrane Vesicles and Treatment with NaC and DDM*

Brush border microvillus membrane vesicles were prepared from pig jejunal mucosa by the divalent cation precipitation method [22]. Briefly, the mucosa was scraped from the gut and homogenized in 10 volumes of 2 mM Tris-HCl, 50 mM mannitol, pH 7.1, containing 10 μg/mL aprotinin and leupeptin. After centrifugation at 500× *g*, 5 min, $MgCl_2$ was added to the supernatant (final concentration: 10 mM), and after 10 min on ice, the preparation was centrifuged at 1.500× *g*, 10 min. The resulting supernatant was collected and centrifuged at 48.000× *g*, 30 min, to yield a pellet of microvillus membrane vesicles (stored at −20 °C until use).

For subsequent treatments with NaC or DDM, microvillus vesicles (~1 mg/mL) were resuspended in 25 mM HEPES-HCl, 150 mM NaCl, pH 7.1, and samples of 75 μL were mixed with 25 μL of NaC or DDM to obtain a final concentration in the range of 0–10 mM. After 15 min incubation at 37 °C and rapid cooling on ice, the membrane suspensions were centrifuged at 20.000× g, 20 min, to yield a membrane pellet and a supernatant of solubilized protein. Both fractions were collected and subjected to SDS/PAGE in 10% gels, electrotransfered onto Immobilon membranes and stained for protein with Coomassie brilliant blue, as described in Section 2.8.

2.7. Detergent Resistant Membrane (DRM) Analysis of Microvillus Membranes by Sucrose Gradient Ultracentrifugation

One milliliter of microvillus membrane vesicles, prepared as described above, was resuspended in HEPES-buffer, pH 7.2. The membranes were then treated with NaC, DDM or Triton X-100 (all at a concentration of 1%) for 10 min on ice. A DRM analysis of the microvillus membranes was performed by sucrose density gradient ultracentrifugation by a method previously described [23,24]. Briefly, centrifugation was performed in a SW40 Ti rotor (Beckman Instruments, Palo Alto, CA) for 20–22 h at 35.000 rpm (g_{max} = 217.000× g), and after centrifugation, the gradient was fractionated into a pellet and 12 fractions of 1 mL. Protein from each of the soluble fractions was isolated by acetone precipitation before analysis by SDS/PAGE.

2.8. SDS/PAGE and Immunoblotting

Samples were denatured by boiling for 3 min in the presence of 1% SDS and 10 mM dithiothreitol, and subjected to SDS/PAGE in 10% gels as described [25]. After electrophoresis and electrotransfer of proteins onto Immobilon PVDF membranes, immunoblotting was performed with antibodies to IAP (1: 1000 dilution), followed by horseradish peroxidase-coupled secondary antibodies (1: 2000 dilution). An electrochemiluminescence (ecl) reagent was used according to the manufacturers (GE Healthcare, www.gehealthcare.com) protocol to develop the blots. After immunoblotting, total protein was stained with Coomassie brilliant blue R250 (0.2% dissolved in an ethanol/H_2O/acetic acid mixture (50:43:7).

3. Results

3.1. Microvillus Membrane-Solubilizing Effects of NaC and DDM

Chemically, NaC and DDM belong to the large class of surfactant PEs of which the main common functional characteristic is the ability to adsorb to cell membranes, and thereby, to modify their physical and biological properties (Figure 1). In order to evaluate the membrane solubilizing effect on the intestinal brush border and to select optimal working concentrations of NaC and DDM for subsequent culture experiments, the concentration-dependency of their ability to release proteins from microvillus vesicles was first established. As shown in Figure 2, NaC had hardly any solubilizing effect above background levels at concentrations up to 2 mM, but at 5 and 10 mM, an increasing release of microvillus proteins was achieved. Both integral membrane proteins, such as the 150 kDa ApN, and the major microvillus cytoskeleton protein actin (42 kDa) appeared in the supernatant, indicating both membrane disruption and leakage. For DDM, microvillus solubilization was detectable already at 1 mM, consistent with the comparatively lower CMC-value for this PE (Figure 2).

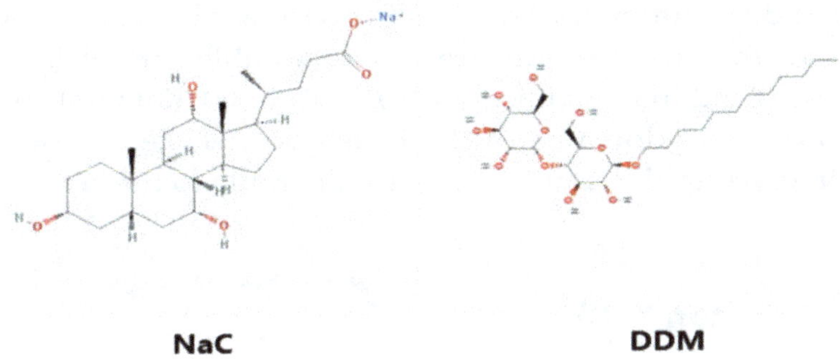

Figure 1. The chemical structure of NaC and DDM. (The images were downloaded from the PubMed Open Chemistry Data Base (https://www.ncbi.nlm.nih.gov/Structure/pdb/2MLT)).

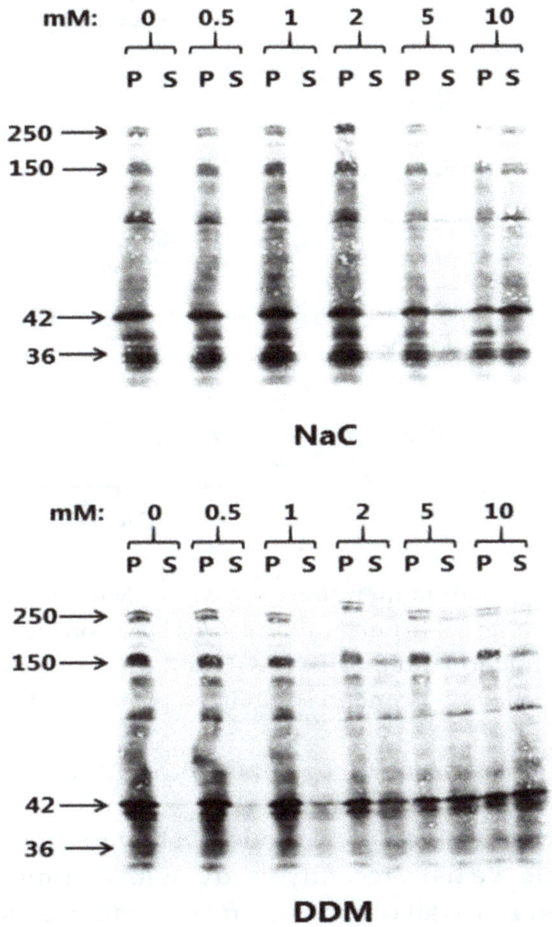

Figure 2. Solubilization of microvillus membrane vesicles with NaC or DDM at concentrations ranging from 0–10 mM as described in Methods. After centrifugation, the pellet (P) and supernatant (S) fractions were subjected to SDS/PAGE and proteins visualized by staining with Coomassie brilliant blue. Arrows indicate the molecular mass-values of the brush border proteins sucrase-isomaltase (250 kDa), ApN (150 kDa), actin (42 kDa), and annexin A2 (36 kDa).

The ability to resist solubilization by detergents/surfactants at low temperature is the biochemical hallmark of liquid-ordered membrane domains (i.e., lipid rafts) [5,26]. Thus, in the glycolipid-rich intestinal brush border, many of the major digestive hydrolases resist solubilization by the detergent Triton X-100, which is indicative that they reside in lipid rafts [24]. The 67-kDa IAP, linked to the extracellular leaflet of the membrane by a glycolipid anchor, is a well-known lipid raft marker [23], and as shown in Figure 3, this protein predominantly partitions in the floating DRM fractions of the sucrose gradient when using the "classical" detergent Triton X-100 for solubilization. An essentially similar DRM distribution for IAP was likewise observed for NaC, as well as for DDM, although relatively more of the enzyme appeared to be soluble. In addition, the profile of total microvillus protein also resembled that obtained with Triton X-100 (data not shown). This experiment thus indicates that the "non raft" domains of the brush border, i.e., those relatively enriched in phospholipids and poor in glycolipids, are those most vulnerable to the action of both PEs.

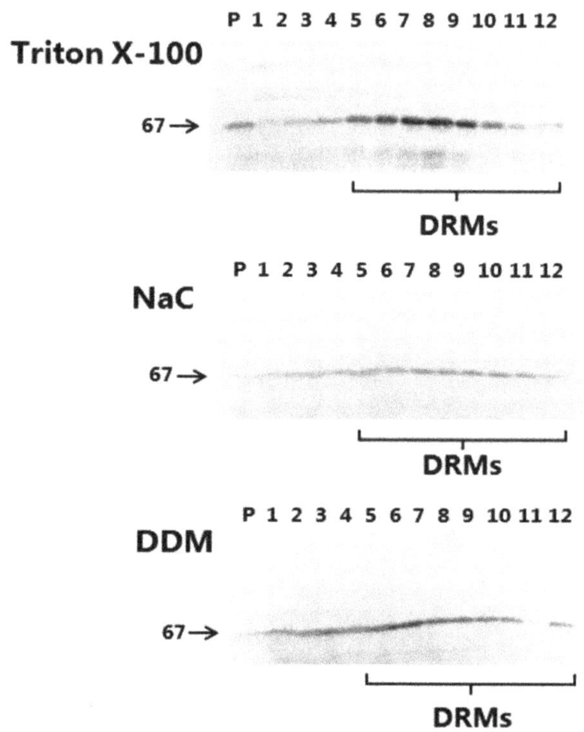

Figure 3. DRM analysis of microvillus membrane vesicles. Microvillus membrane vesicles were prepared and solubilized with either 1% Triton X-100, NaC or DDM on ice, followed by sucrose gradient ultracentrifugation, gradient fractionation, SDS/PAGE and immunoblotting for IAP (67 kDa). "P" indicates the pellet fraction, fractions 1-2 contain solubilized protein and fractions 4–12 contain DRMs.

3.2. Effects of NaC and DDM on Mucosal Morphology in Cultured Mucosal Explants

Organ culture of mucosal explants is an ideal model system for investigating the direct, short-term effects of luminal compounds, and we have recently used it with a number of other types of permeation enhancers [17–19]. In subsequent mucosal organ culture experiments, NaC and DDM were both used at 2 and 10 mM in order to study cell-permeating effects under relative mild, as well as under more membrane damaging, conditions. Both concentrations (corresponding to 0.86% and 4.3% for NaC, and 1.0% and 5.1% for DDM, respectively) are well within the range of concentrations previously used by other investigators [6].

As shown in Figure 4, exposure to either NaC or DDM at a concentration of 2 mM for 1 h caused no gross overall deterioration of the mucosal morphology. Villus height was preserved and the integrity of the epithelium generally upheld; only occasionally could foci of exfoliation be detected, typically at the tip of the villi. In contrast, at a concentration of 10 mM, both PEs caused extensive denudation at the tip of the villi, which are the most exposed and sensitive areas of the mucosal epithelium. Further down along the sides of the villi and in the generative crypts, the epithelium was generally well preserved.

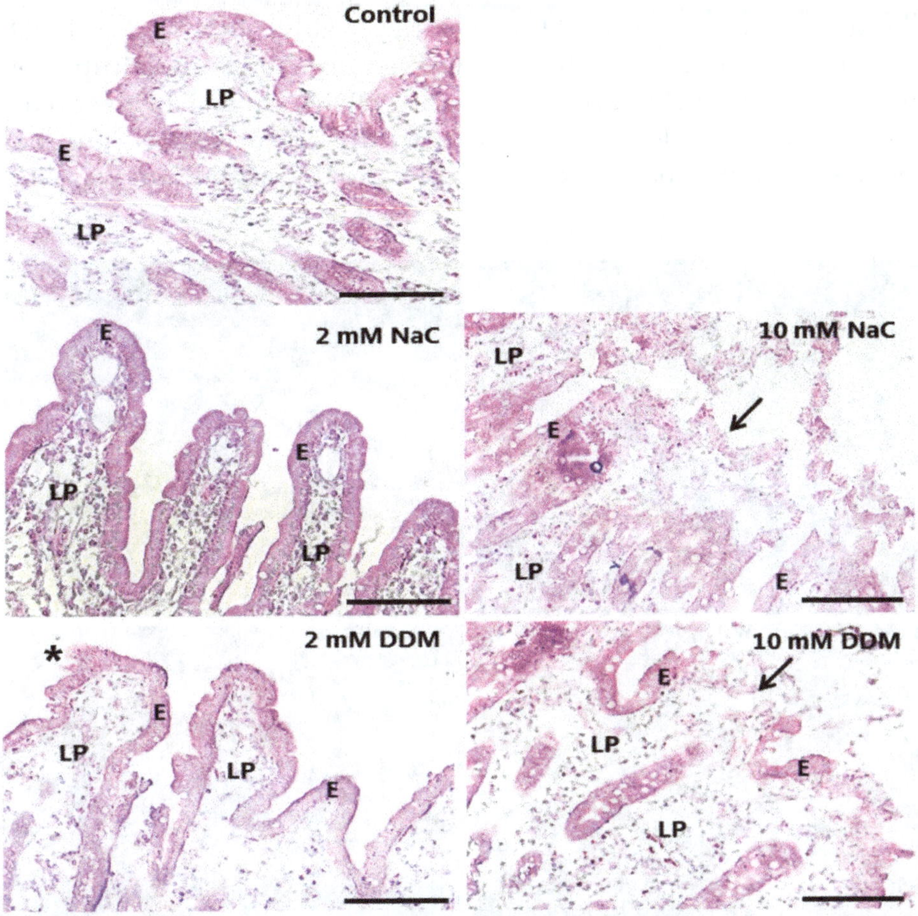

Figure 4. HE-stained sections of mucosal explants cultured for 1 h in the absence (control) or presence of 2 mM or 10 mM of NaC/DDM, as described in Methods. The villus organization and epithelium were generally well preserved at 2 mM of both surfactants, although foci of exfoliation was occasionally observed (asterisk). At 10 mM, both NaC and DDM caused extensive denudation, particularly near the tips of the villi (arrows), whereas the epithelium along the sides of the villi and in the crypts were generally better preserved. Enterocytes (E) and lamina propria (LP) are indicated. Bars: 100 μm.

3.3. *Effects of NaC and DDM on Permeability of Lucifer Yellow*

LY is a small fluorescent polar tracer (MW 444 Da) with little or no permeability through normal cell membranes. It has previously been used to assess paracellular permeability in Caco-2 monolayers [27], and we have used it in the mucosal organ culture system for studying damage to epithelial cell integrity under various conditions [18,19,28]. As shown in Figure 5, little or no staining of the cytosol was seen in enterocytes of control explants, indicating well-preserved membrane integrity with little or no leakage through the cell membrane. Likewise, the brush border was devoid of staining by LY. However, an array of distinct subapical punctae was indicative of an uptake by constitutive endocytosis from the brush border. These punctae were EEA-1-positive, thus representing a subpopulation of early endosomes in the terminal web region of the enterocytes that we have previously termed "TWEEs" (Terminal Web Early Endosomes) [29]. The underlying lamina propria was strongly stained by LY in the control, and widespread stripy lateral staining along the enterocytes was indicative of a paracellular passage across the epithelium. Both NaC and DDM caused a diffuse staining of the enterocyte cytosol, indicating a leakage through the cell membrane. However, only some enterocytes appeared to be thus affected, resulting in a characteristic mosaic staining pattern of the epithelium; occasionally, single exfoliating cells were detected as well (Figure 5). The brush border marker ApN was confined to the apical surface in the presence of both PEs, indicating that no gross membrane disruption had occurred. However, noticeably, both NaC and DDM prevented the appearance of the LY-positive TWEEs, implying a blocked uptake via constitutive endocytosis.

At a concentration of 10 mM, both NaC and DDM caused widespread leakage of LY into all enterocytes, although the localization of both the apical (ApN) -and basolateral marker (Na^+/K^+-ATPase) was seemingly unaffected in areas where the epithelium was still intact (Figure 6).

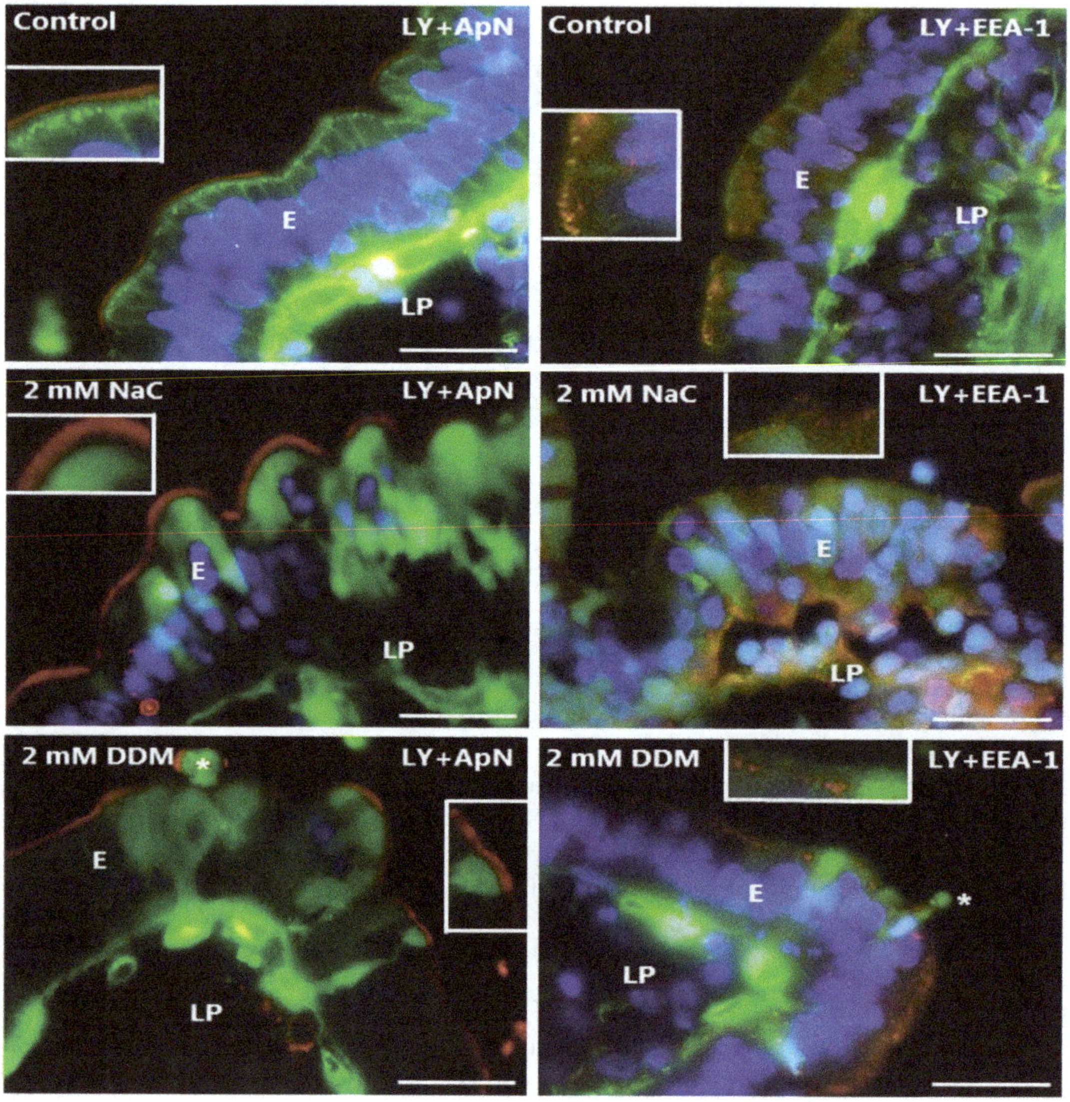

Figure 5. Permeability of the mucosal epithelium probed with LY at 2 mM concentration of PEs. Sections of mucosal explants cultured for 1 h with LY in the absence or presence of 2 mM NaC or DDM, respectively. In addition, the sections were immunolabeled for ApN, a brush border enzyme, or for EEA-1, a marker for early endosomes. In the controls, a string of EEA-1-positive subapical punctae shows uptake of LY into apical early endosomes of the enterocytes, whereas the cytosol is only weakly labeled. Lateral labeling and strong staining of the lamina propria are also seen, indicating a paracellular passage of LY through the tight junctions. At 2 mM, both NaC and DDM frequently caused LY to enter the enterocyte cytosol, indicating a leakage through the cell membrane, but endocytic uptake was not observed. Asterisks indicate enterocytes in the process of exfoliation. Inserts show enlarged image details. Bars: 20 µm.

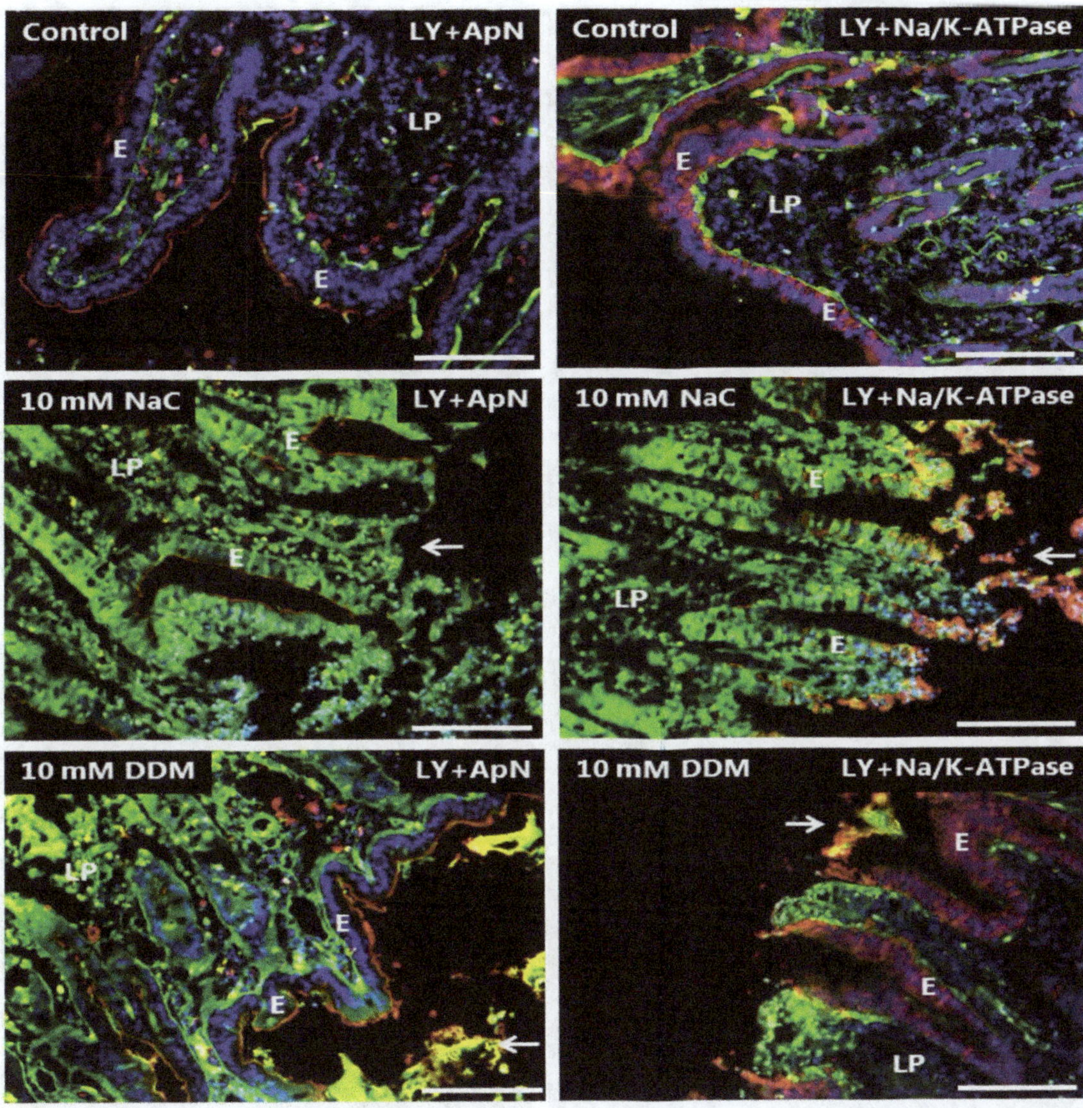

Figure 6. Permeability of the mucosal epithelium probed with LY at 10 mM concentration of PEs. Sections of mucosal explants cultured for 1 h with LY in the absence or presence of 10 mM NaC or DDM, respectively. In addition, the sections were immunolabeled for ApN, or Na^+/K^+-ATPase, a basolateral cell membrane marker. Both NaC and DDM caused extensive denudation at the tips of the villi (arrows), but epithelial integrity with preservation of cell membrane polarity was maintained along the sides of the villi. However, all enterocytes had taken up LY into the cytosol. Bars: 20 μm.

3.4. Effects of NaC and DDM on Permeability of Texas Red Dextran and FM 1-43 FX

The TRD used in this study is polar like LY, but of higher MW (3000 Da), and is a commonly used probe for cellular uptake studies [30]. Unlike LY, it labeled the brush border of control enterocytes, but was only taken up sparsely into TWEEs in comparison with LY, implying a poor accessibility to the bottom part of the microvilli from where endocytosis occurs (Figure 7). TRD stained the lamina propria, but only weakly compared with LY, and a lateral staining along the enterocytes was barely visible, which was indicative of limited paracellular diffusion through the tight junctions. Binding to the brush border was unaffected by NaC and DDM, but no or little uptake into TWEEs was detected (Figure 7). However, both PEs greatly increased the staining of the lamina propria, and a stripy lateral labeling along the enterocytes was now clearly visible, implying a higher paracellular permeability of TRD.

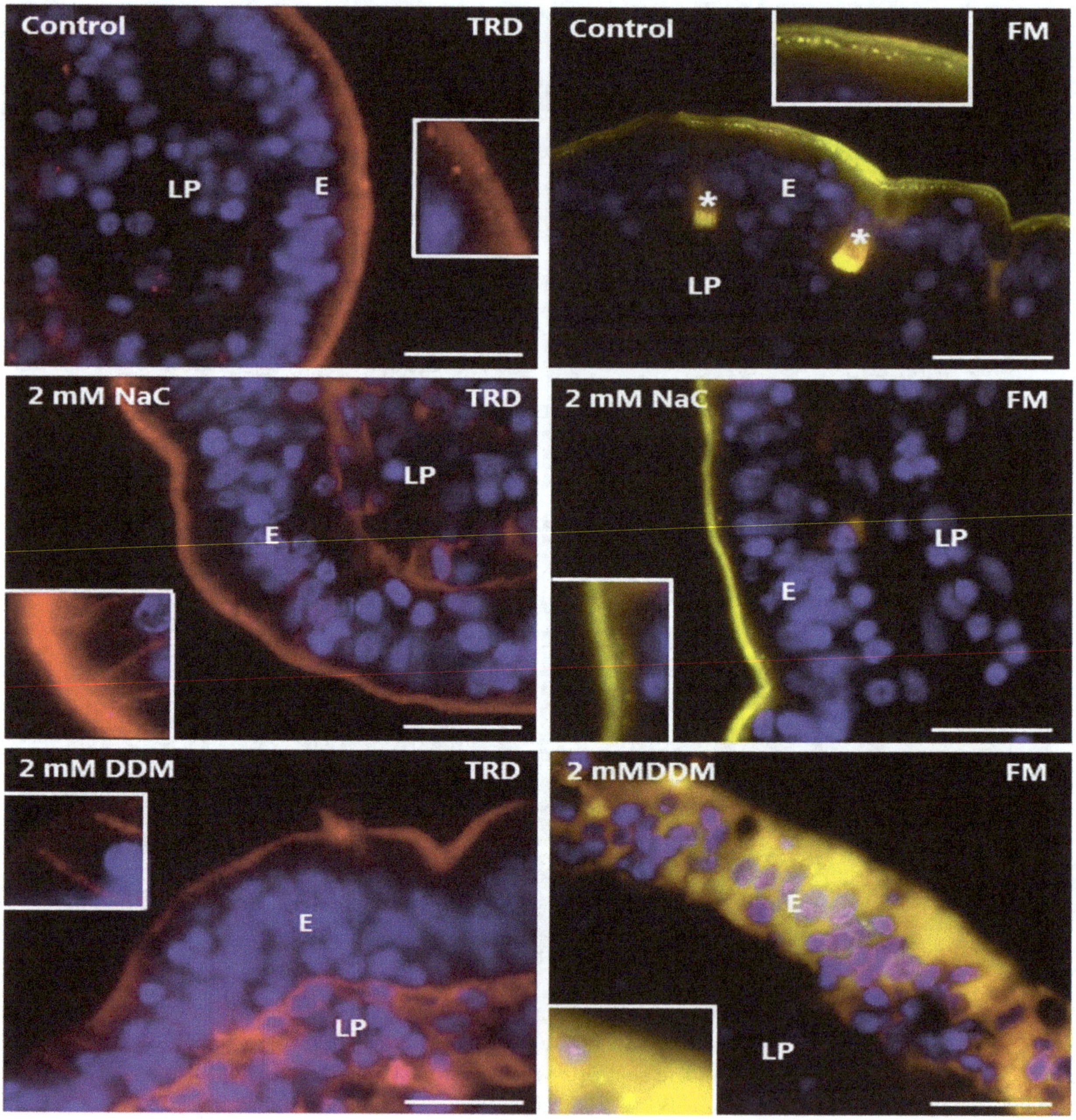

Figure 7. Permeability of the mucosal epithelium probed with TRD and FM. Sections of mucosal explants cultured for 1 h with TRD or FM in the absence or presence of 2 mM NaC or DDM, respectively. In the control, TRD bound to the enterocyte brush border, but only few and weakly-stained TRD-positive supapical punctae were observed. In addition, a faint labeling of the lamina propria was detectable. NaC and DDM both greatly increased the lateral TRD-labeling and accumulation of the probe in the lamina propria without affecting TRD-binding at the brush border, but little if any leakage was seen into the cytosol of the enterocytes. Like TRD, FM strongly labeled the enterocyte brush border, and also appeared in bright subapical punctae in the control. The brush border labeling was generally unaffected by both surfactants, but subapical punctae were sparse. Occasionally, FM was absent from the brush border, but leaked into the cytosol of enterocytes, as shown for DDM, but no staining of the lamina propria was observed. (Asterisks show goblet cells labeled by FM and inserts show enlarged image details.) Bars: 20 μm.

FM is a non-toxic, water-soluble and lipophilic probe (MW 560 Da) that only becomes fluorescent when incorporated into cell membranes [31], and as shown in Figure 7, it strongly labeled the entire brush border of control enterocytes together with goblet cells. In addition, it was efficiently taken up into TWEEs like LY, as earlier reported [29]. However, in contrast to LY, FM did not stain the lamina propria or the basolateral sides of the enterocytes, indicating that this lipophilic probe, despite its small size, is incapable of paracellular passage through the tight junctions. FM labeling of the brush border was generally not affected by NaC or DDM, but the uptake into TWEEs was greatly diminished (Figure 7). Lamina propria and lateral staining with FM was not detected in the presence of the PEs; however, as seen with LY, leakage into the cytosol of enterocytes was occasionally observed.

In summary, the results obtained with LY, TRD and FM documented both paracellular and transcellular mechanisms of action of both NaC and DDM. The data are consistent with the PEs interacting with/inserting into the brush border membrane, resulting in functional leaks in the bilayer that allow passage of both small polar (LY) and lipophilic (FM) compounds. In addition, the ability of the apical cell membrane to engage in endocytosis was largely abolished by both PEs. This effectively excludes the possibility that they act as PEs by stimulating luminal endocytotic uptake.

3.5. Effects of NaC and DDM on the Ultrastructure of the Enterocyte Brush Border

Transmission electron microscopy was employed to study in closer detail the direct action of NaC and DDM on the morphology of the enterocytes. As shown in Figure 8A, the brush border of enterocytes from control explants in longitudinal sections from the mid-villus area consisted of a regular array of uniform microvilli of about 1.2–1.3 μm in length with actin rootlets extending into the subapical terminal web region. Microvillus length gradually increases in enterocytes along the villi as enterocytes move towards the extrusion zone at the tip, but microvillus diameter normally remains unchanged at ~0.1 μm throughout the crypt-villus migration, as shown in cross sections (Figure 8D). NaC (2 mM) did not affect the overall columnar shape of enterocytes or microvillus length in the brush border (Figure 8B). However, in cross sections, the normally ordered, hexagonal alignment of microvilli was less dense and frequently disrupted, and microvilli of smaller diameter were scattered amongst seemingly normal microvilli (Figure 8E). In addition, bulbous protrusions were occasionally observed at the tip of the microvilli (Figure 9A). Membrane-enveloped spherical bodies containing electron-dense material and with a diameter of about 0.3 μM were frequently observed interspaced between the microvilli, and in some cases they were surrounded by small (~50 nm) vesicles seemingly attached to their surface. (Figure 9B,C).

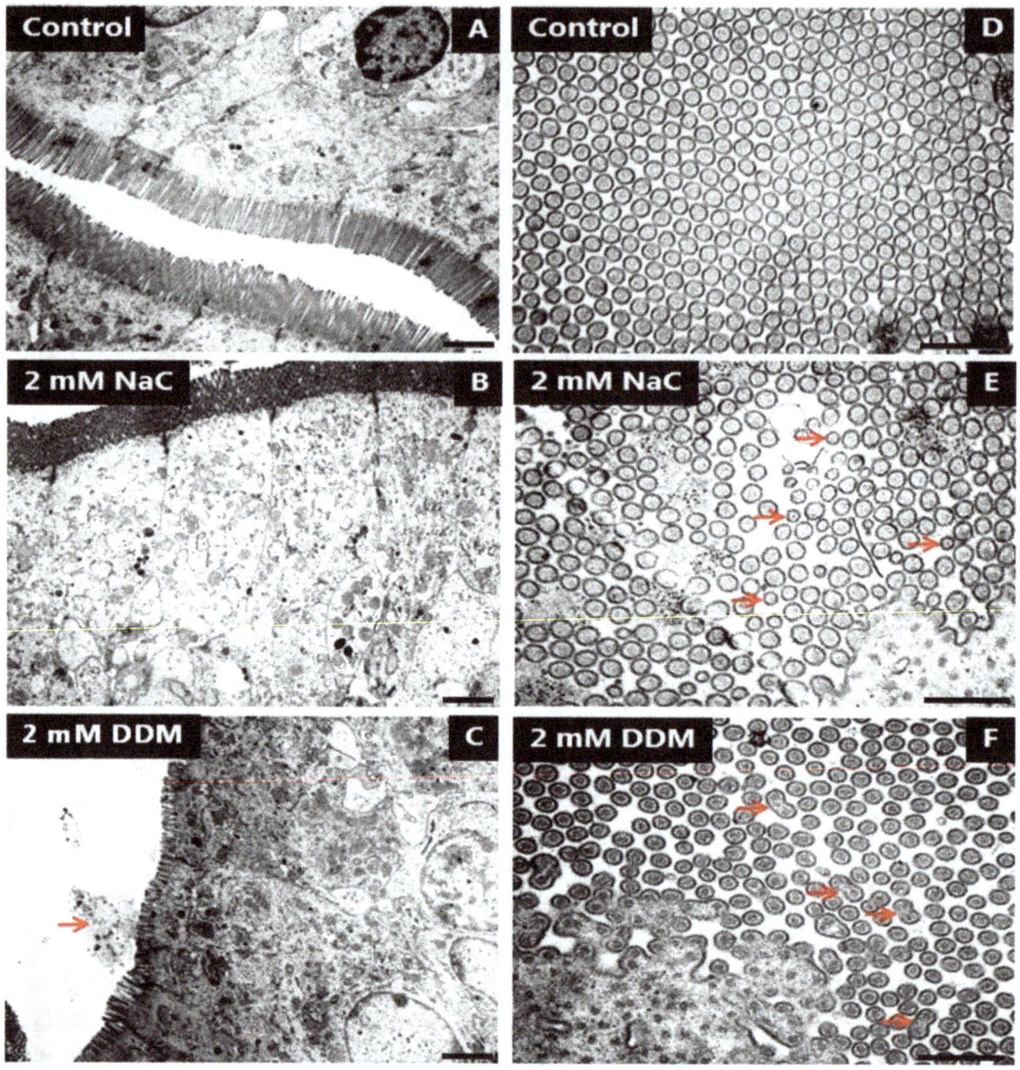

Figure 8. Effects of NaC and DDM on brush border ultrastructure. Electron micrographs showing longitudinal (**A–C**) and cross sections (**D–F**) of the brush border. (Arrows indicate apparent leakage into the lumen of cellular debris from the brush border in (**C**), microvilli with diminished diameter in (**E**) and fused microvilli in (**F**).) Bars: 1 μm (**A–C**); 0.5 μm (**D–F**).

Enterocytes were also generally well preserved after exposure to DDM (2 mM), but in contrast to NaC, DDM caused a marked shortening of the microvilli of villus enterocytes (Figure 8C). The effect was variable, but frequently cells with microvilli as short as 0.5 μm were observed. Although one must be cautious interpreting such data because, as mentioned above, microvillus length generally increases as enterocytes move along the crypt-villus axis, stunted microvilli like those seen with DDM are normally found only at the bottom of the crypts. In cross sections, the microvilli were of normal diameter, but as with NaC, the hexagonal alignment was less dense and organized than in the control. However, longitudinal fusion of pairs of microvilli was occasionally observed (Figure 8F). Noticeably, variation in microvillus length sometimes even occurred between neighboring cells (Figure 9D). At high magnification, microvesiculation of single microvilli was evident, and the tips of the microvilli often appeared flat instead of the normal rounded shape of a cap (Figure 9E). In areas near the bottom of the villi, vesicle-like structures and amorphous material, probably leaking through the brush border (Figure 8C), accumulated in the narrow cleft between opposing villi (Figure 9F). This phenomenon was observed both with NaC and DDM.

In contrast to the brush border, the tight junctions and meandering lateral cell membranes were seemingly unaffected by both PEs at 2 mM (data not shown). Taken together, the electron microscopy data therefore strongly indicate that the brush border is the primary target of both NaC and DDM. The lesions induced by NaC and DDM were similar, but not identical, implying that the two PEs cause disruption of the membrane organization by different mechanisms.

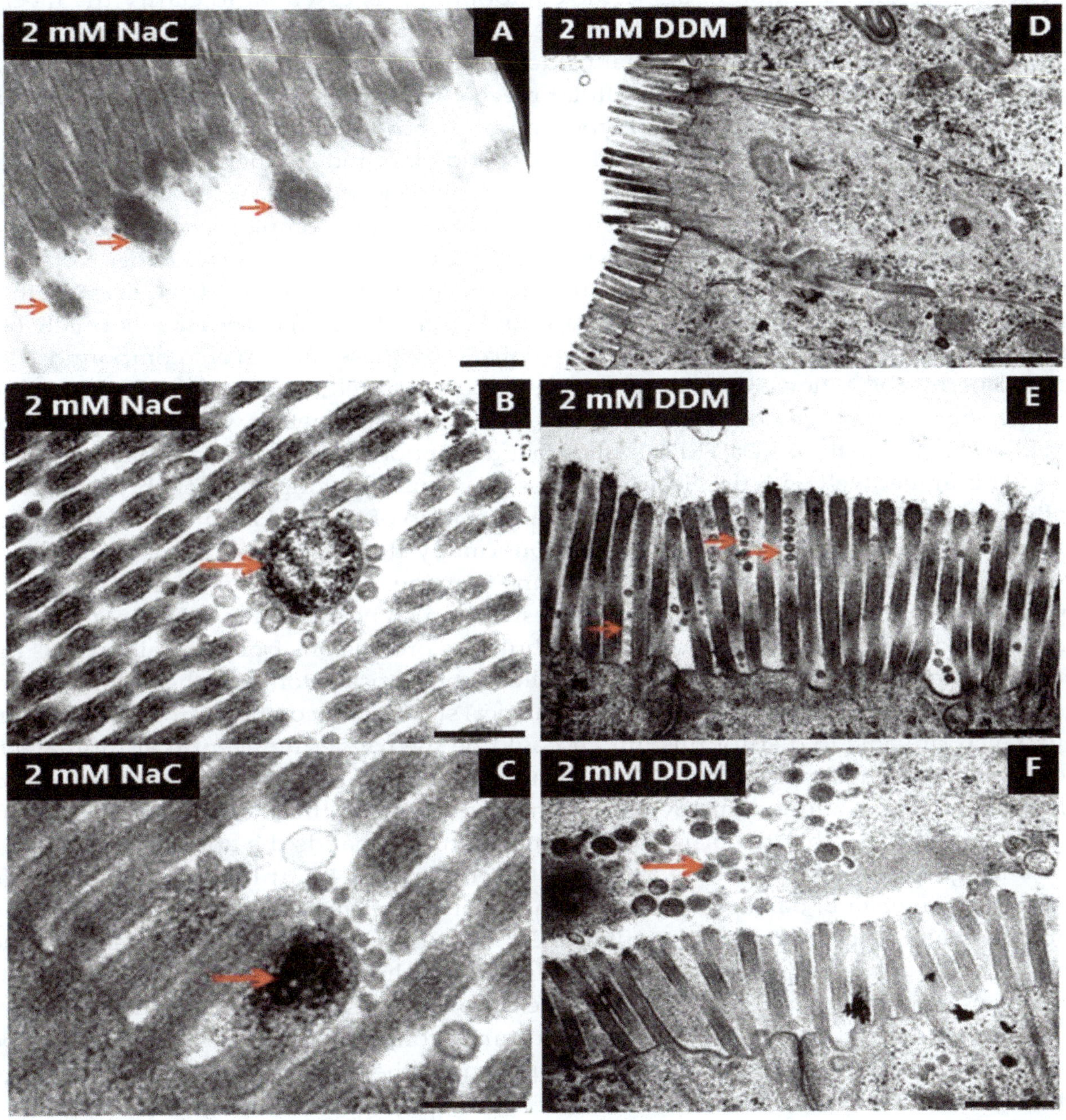

Figure 9. Effects of NaC and DDM on brush border ultrastructure. Electron micrographs showing different lesions in the brush border induced by NaC or DDM. Arrows indicate bulbous protrusions from single microvilli in (**A**), electron dense bodies with small vesicles attached in (**B**) and (**C**), microvesiculated, single microvilli in (**E**) and accumulated cellular debris in the lumen in (**F**). Bars: 0.2 μm (**A–C**); 1 μm (**D**); 0.5 μm (**E**,**F**).

4. Discussion

Surfactants belonging to the bile salt or alkyl maltoside classes of compounds all have a long history as PEs, but with regard to the intestinal permeation enhancement, they have so far been tested mainly either in epithelial cell models, most often Caco-2 cells, or in colonic tissue [6,32,33]. For this reason, we thought it worthwhile to reinvestigate the PE action of NaC and DDM in a jejunal mucosal explant system. The jejunum is the region of the intestine where endogeneous bile salts normally aid assimilation of poorly-soluble dietary constituents and where the brush border membrane presumably is optimally equipped to withstand the action of luminal surfactants under physiological conditions.

In elucidating the PE action of a specific compound, it is essential to clarify the mechanism whereby epithelial permeabilization is achieved, i.e., whether a paracellular and/or transcellular route is facilitated [34,35]. Bile salts and alkyl maltosides are commonly classified as multimodal in their action, i.e., acting both via para and transcellular mechanism(s) [6,36], and the results of the present work agree well with this classification. Hypothetically, transcellular permeabilization may occur by endocytosis by one or more of several clathrin-dependent or independent molecular mechanisms known to internalize cell membrane and cargo to the cellular endosomal system. In enterocytes, apical endocytosis of cargo might be succeeded by trancytosis, leading to a complete crossing of the epithelial barrier [9,37,38]. In this context, the main conclusion of the present work is that neither NaC nor DDM achieved transcellular permeability by stimulating apical endocytotic uptake. In contrast, both largely abolished the constitutive endocytosis of polar (LY) and lipophilic (FM) probes that normally operates at the brush border and which can be readily visualized by these fluorescent compounds. Instead, transcellular permeabilization occurred by rendering the apical cell membrane leaky. The sometimes mosaic appearance of leaky enterocytes adjacent to unaffected cells together with the selective leakiness to the 444 Da LY, but not the 3-kDa TRD, implies that disruption of the membrane bilayer was not too extensive. This agrees well with the electron microscopy data, showing a reasonably well-preserved microvillus ultrastructure. Nevertheless, the partial break-up of the uniform hexagonal organization of microvilli and the appearance of scattered, abnormally thin (NaC) or fused (DDM) microvilli are direct visual evidence of PE-induced membrane damage. Some of the lesions observed in this study resemble those previously reported for intestinal brush borders of myosin-1a gene knockout mice, including disorganization of microvilli and bulbous protrusions from the microvillus tips [39]. Myosin-1a is a motor protein that links the microvillus actin cytoskeleton with the cell membrane and, amongst other functions, is responsible for the mechanical stabilization of the microvillus structure [1,2]. If PEs like NaC are able to disrupt this link, it could be the triggering event that ultimately leads to the observed morphological changes of the brush border. This suggests a stochastic process of disruption where single, affected microvilli form microvesicles and break up, followed by membrane resealing. Given the fact that the brush border architecture expands the apical surface area of the enterocyte roughly ten times compared to a "flat" cell surface [40], it harbors a large membrane reservoir for use in repair of damaged microvilli. Interestingly, microvillus microvesiculation in the rat and mouse has been proposed to be the result of a Ca^{2+}-induced, villin-dependent severing of the actin filaments [41], and the subsequent release of vesicles into the lumen as a physiological process in the gut host defense aimed to deploy catalytic activities into the intestinal lumen [39,42,43]. Microvillus microvesiculation was very rarely observed in cultured control explants in this study on porcine jejunum, but the induction of this process by DDM may nevertheless reflect an uncontrolled triggering of a natural process.

In recent studies, other types of surfactant PEs (lauroyl-carnitine, monocaprin and the ethoxylate $C_{12}E_9$) were found to permeabilize the brush border mainly by inducing microvillus microvesiculation and/or longitudinal fusion of microvilli [18], and the amphipathic cell penetrating peptide melittin caused a marked elongation both of microvilli and their actin rootlets [19]. Nevertheless, despite apparent differences in modes of microvillus disruption, these different types of PE agents all resulted in membrane leakage of LY as well as inhibition of apical endocytosis. Collectively, we infer from these observations that although the mechanism of action of the different types of membrane-interacting agents seems to vary, they possess a similar functionality as PEs. The common endocytosis-inhibiting effect may seem intriguing, and we are not certain of its cause. It could be ascribed simply to energy depletion by leakage of ATP or loss of essential other small molecules/ions, but local changes in membrane fluidity and lipid raft structure might also be sufficient to interfere with endocytosis even in areas where the microvillus architecture remains intact. The latter explanation is supported by the DRM analysis showing that "non raft" areas of the microvillus membrane are preferentially targeted by NaC and DDM.

5. Conclusions

In the present work, we studied the action of a bile salt (NaC) and an alkyl maltoside (DDM) on the different luminal uptake pathways across the intestinal epithelium, using a jejunal mucosal organ culture model. Both PEs increased the paracellular and transcellular pathways for polar fluorescent probes, but of note, one common uptake mechanism, endocytosis, was virtually blocked. Instead, leakage through the brush border membrane occurred. Ultrastructurally, lesions of the brush border included microvillus microvesiculation, shortening, longitudinal fusion of microvilli, and the formation and extrusion of dense bodies. A DRM analysis of microvillus membrane vesicles indicated that both NaC and DDM, like the nonionic detergent Triton X-100, preferentially extract the "non-raft" domains of the lipid bilayer, thereby decreasing the fluidity of the remaining membrane.

Author Contributions: Conceptualization, E.M.D.; Methodology, E.M.D., G.H.H.; Investigation, E.M.D.; G.H.H.; Writing-Original Draft Preparation, E.M.D.; Writing-Review & Editing, E.M.D., G.H.H.; Project Administration, E.M.D.; Funding Acquisition, E.M.D.

Acknowledgments: Karina Rasmussen is thanked for excellent technical assistance.

References

1. Crawley, S.W.; Mooseker, M.S.; Tyska, M.J. Shaping the intestinal brush border. *J. Cell Biol.* **2014**, *207*, 441–451. [CrossRef] [PubMed]
2. Delacour, D.; Salomon, J.; Robine, S.; Louvard, D. Plasticity of the brush border—The yin and yang of intestinal homeostasis. *Nat. Rev. Gastroenterol. Hepatol.* **2016**, *13*, 161–174. [CrossRef] [PubMed]
3. Christiansen, K.; Carlsen, J. Microvillus membrane vesicles from pig small intestine. Purity and lipid composition. *Biochim. Biophys. Acta* **1981**, *647*, 188–195. [CrossRef]
4. Danielsen, E.M.; Hansen, G.H. Lipid rafts in epithelial brush borders: Atypical membrane microdomains with specialized functions. *Biochim. Biophys. Acta* **2003**, *1617*, 1–9. [CrossRef] [PubMed]
5. Simons, K.; Ikonen, E. Functional rafts in cell membranes. *Nature* **1997**, *387*, 569–572. [CrossRef] [PubMed]
6. Maher, S.; Mrsny, R.J.; Brayden, D.J. Intestinal permeation enhancers for oral peptide delivery. *Adv. Drug Deliv. Rev.* **2016**, *106*, 277–319. [CrossRef] [PubMed]
7. Lichtenberg, D.; Robson, R.J.; Dennis, E.A. Solubilization of phospholipids by detergents. Structural and kinetic aspects. *Biochim. Biophys. Acta* **1983**, *737*, 285–304. [CrossRef]
8. McCartney, F.; Gleeson, J.P.; Brayden, D.J. Safety concerns over the use of intestinal permeation enhancers: A mini-review. *Tissue Barriers* **2016**, *4*, e1176822. [CrossRef] [PubMed]
9. Lundquist, P.; Artursson, P. Oral absorption of peptides and nanoparticles across the human intestine: Opportunities, limitations and studies in human tissues. *Adv. Drug Deliv. Rev.* **2016**, *106*, 256–276. [CrossRef] [PubMed]
10. Sanchez-Navarro, M.; Garcia, J.; Giralt, E.; Teixido, M. Using peptides to increase transport across the intestinal barrier. *Adv. Drug Deliv. Rev.* **2016**, *106*, 355–366. [CrossRef] [PubMed]
11. Shiau, Y.F. Mechanisms of intestinal fat absorption. *Am. J. Physiol.* **1981**, *240*, G1–G9. [CrossRef] [PubMed]
12. Aungst, B.J. Absorption enhancers: Applications and advances. *AAPS J.* **2012**, *14*, 10–18. [CrossRef] [PubMed]
13. Fasinu, P.; Pillay, V.; Ndesendo, V.M.; du Toit, L.C.; Choonara, Y.E. Diverse approaches for the enhancement of oral drug bioavailability. *Biopharm. Drug Dispos.* **2011**, *32*, 185–209. [CrossRef] [PubMed]
14. Yewale, C.; Patil, S.; Kolate, A.; Kore, G.; Misra, A. Oral Absorption Promoters: Opportunities, Issues, and Challenges. *Crit. Rev. Ther. Drug Carr. Syst.* **2015**, *32*, 363–387. [CrossRef]
15. Petersen, S.B.; Nolan, G.; Maher, S.; Rahbek, U.L.; Guldbrandt, M.; Brayden, D.J. Evaluation of alkylmaltosides as intestinal permeation enhancers: Comparison between rat intestinal mucosal sheets and Caco-2 monolayers. *Eur. J. Pharm. Sci.* **2012**, *47*, 701–712. [CrossRef] [PubMed]

16. Lorenzen, U.S.; Hansen, G.H.; Danielsen, E.M. Organ Culture as a Model System for Studies on Enterotoxin Interactions with the Intestinal Epithelium. *Methods Mol. Biol.* **2016**, *1396*, 159–166. [PubMed]
17. Danielsen, E.T.; Danielsen, E.M. Glycol chitosan: A stabilizer of lipid rafts in the intestinal brush border. *Biochim. Biophys. Acta* **2017**, *1859*, 360–367. [CrossRef] [PubMed]
18. Danielsen, E.M.; Hansen, G.H. Intestinal surfactant permeation enhancers and their interaction with enterocyte cell membranes in a mucosal explant system. *Tissue Barriers* **2017**, *5*, e1361900. [CrossRef] [PubMed]
19. Danielsen, E.M.; Hansen, G.H. Impact of cell-penetrating peptides (CPPs) melittin and Hiv-1 Tat on the enterocyte brush border using a mucosal explant system. *Biochim. Biophys. Acta* **2018**, *1860*, 1589–1599. [CrossRef] [PubMed]
20. Hansen, G.H.; Sjostrom, H.; Noren, O.; Dabelsteen, E. Immunomicroscopic localization of aminopeptidase N in the pig enterocyte. Implications for the route of intracellular transport. *Eur. J. Cell Biol.* **1987**, *43*, 253–259. [PubMed]
21. Danielsen, E.M.; Sjostrom, H.; Noren, O.; Bro, B.; Dabelsteen, E. Biosynthesis of intestinal microvillar proteins. Characterization of intestinal explants in organ culture and evidence for the existence of pro-forms of the microvillar enzymes. *Biochem. J.* **1982**, *202*, 647–654. [CrossRef] [PubMed]
22. Booth, A.G.; Kenny, A.J. A rapid method for the preparation of microvilli from rabbit kidney. *Biochem. J.* **1974**, *142*, 575–581. [CrossRef] [PubMed]
23. Brown, D.A.; Rose, J.K. Sorting of GPI-anchored proteins to glycolipid-enriched membrane subdomains during transport to the apical cell surface. *Cell* **1992**, *68*, 533–544. [CrossRef]
24. Danielsen, E.M. Involvement of detergent-insoluble complexes in the intracellular transport of intestinal brush border enzymes. *Biochemistry* **1995**, *34*, 1596–1605. [CrossRef] [PubMed]
25. Laemmli, U.K. Cleavage of structural proteins during the assembly of the head of bacteriophage T4. *Nature* **1970**, *227*, 680–685. [CrossRef] [PubMed]
26. Brown, D.A. Lipid rafts, detergent-resistant membranes, and raft targeting signals. *Physiology* **2006**, *21*, 430–439. [CrossRef] [PubMed]
27. Hanani, M. Lucifer yellow—An angel rather than the devil. *J. Cell. Mol. Med.* **2012**, *16*, 22–31. [CrossRef] [PubMed]
28. Danielsen, E.M.; Hansen, G.H.; Rasmussen, K.; Niels-Christiansen, L.L. Permeabilization of enterocytes induced by absorption of dietary fat. *Mol. Membr. Biol.* **2013**, *30*, 261–272. [CrossRef] [PubMed]
29. Hansen, G.H.; Rasmussen, K.; Niels-Christiansen, L.L.; Danielsen, E.M. Endocytic trafficking from the small intestinal brush border probed with FM dye. *Am. J. Physiol. Gastrointest. Liver Physiol.* **2009**, *297*, G708–G715. [CrossRef] [PubMed]
30. Woodcroft, B.J.; Hammond, L.; Stow, J.L.; Hamilton, N.A. Automated organelle-based colocalization in whole-cell imaging. *Cytom. A* **2009**, *75*, 941–950. [CrossRef] [PubMed]
31. Bolte, S.; Talbot, C.; Boutte, Y.; Catrice, O.; Read, N.D.; Satiat-Jeunemaitre, B. FM-dyes as experimental probes for dissecting vesicle trafficking in living plant cells. *J. Microsc.* **2004**, *214*, 159–173. [CrossRef] [PubMed]
32. Lucarini, S.; Fagioli, L.; Cavanagh, R.; Liang, W.; Perinelli, D.R.; Campana, M.; Stolnik, S.; Lam, J.K.W.; Casettari, L.; Duranti, A. Synthesis, Structure(-)Activity Relationships and In Vitro Toxicity Profile of Lactose-Based Fatty Acid Monoesters as Possible Drug Permeability Enhancers. *Pharmaceutics* **2018**, *10*, 81. [CrossRef] [PubMed]
33. Lucarini, S.; Fagioli, L.; Campana, R.; Cole, H.; Duranti, A.; Baffone, W.; Vllasaliu, D.; Casettari, L. Unsaturated fatty acids lactose esters: Cytotoxicity, permeability enhancement and antimicrobial activity. *Eur. J. Pharm. Biopharm.* **2016**, *107*, 88–96. [CrossRef] [PubMed]
34. Blikslager, A.T.; Moeser, A.J.; Gookin, J.L.; Jones, S.L.; Odle, J. Restoration of barrier function in injured intestinal mucosa. *Physiol. Rev.* **2007**, *87*, 545–564. [CrossRef] [PubMed]
35. Odenwald, M.A.; Turner, J.R. The intestinal epithelial barrier: A therapeutic target? *Nat. Rev. Gastroenterol. Hepatol.* **2017**, *14*, 9–21. [CrossRef] [PubMed]
36. Moghimipour, E.; Ameri, A.; Handali, S. Absorption-Enhancing Effects of Bile Salts. *Molecules* **2015**, *20*, 14451–14473. [CrossRef] [PubMed]
37. Doherty, G.J.; McMahon, H.T. Mechanisms of endocytosis. *Annu. Rev. Biochem.* **2009**, *78*, 857–902. [CrossRef] [PubMed]

38. Mrsny, R.J. Strategies for targeting protein therapeutics to selected tissues and cells. *Expert Opin. Biol. Ther.* **2004**, *4*, 65–73. [CrossRef] [PubMed]
39. Tyska, M.J.; Mackey, A.T.; Huang, J.D.; Copeland, N.G.; Jenkins, N.A.; Mooseker, M.S. Myosin-1a is critical for normal brush border structure and composition. *Mol. Biol. Cell* **2005**, *16*, 2443–2457. [CrossRef] [PubMed]
40. Helander, H.F.; Fandriks, L. Surface area of the digestive tract—Revisited. *Scand. J. Gastroenterol.* **2014**, *49*, 681–689. [CrossRef] [PubMed]
41. Mooseker, M.S.; Graves, T.A.; Wharton, K.A.; Falco, N.; Howe, C.L. Regulation of microvillus structure: Calcium-dependent solation and cross-linking of actin filaments in the microvilli of intestinal epithelial cells. *J. Cell Biol.* **1980**, *87*, 809–822. [CrossRef] [PubMed]
42. McConnell, R.E.; Higginbotham, J.N.; Shifrin, D.A., Jr.; Tabb, D.L.; Coffey, R.J.; Tyska, M.J. The enterocyte microvillus is a vesicle-generating organelle. *J. Cell Biol.* **2009**, *185*, 1285–1298. [CrossRef] [PubMed]
43. Shifrin, D.A., Jr.; Tyska, M.J. Ready ... aim ... fire into the lumen: A new role for enterocyte microvilli in gut host defense. *Gut Microbes* **2012**, *3*, 460–462. [CrossRef] [PubMed]

Permissions

All chapters in this book were first published by MDPI; hereby published with permission under the Creative Commons Attribution License or equivalent. Every chapter published in this book has been scrutinized by our experts. Their significance has been extensively debated. The topics covered herein carry significant findings which will fuel the growth of the discipline. They may even be implemented as practical applications or may be referred to as a beginning point for another development.

The contributors of this book come from diverse backgrounds, making this book a truly international effort. This book will bring forth new frontiers with its revolutionizing research information and detailed analysis of the nascent developments around the world.

We would like to thank all the contributing authors for lending their expertise to make the book truly unique. They have played a crucial role in the development of this book. Without their invaluable contributions this book wouldn't have been possible. They have made vital efforts to compile up to date information on the varied aspects of this subject to make this book a valuable addition to the collection of many professionals and students.

This book was conceptualized with the vision of imparting up-to-date information and advanced data in this field. To ensure the same, a matchless editorial board was set up. Every individual on the board went through rigorous rounds of assessment to prove their worth. After which they invested a large part of their time researching and compiling the most relevant data for our readers.

The editorial board has been involved in producing this book since its inception. They have spent rigorous hours researching and exploring the diverse topics which have resulted in the successful publishing of this book. They have passed on their knowledge of decades through this book. To expedite this challenging task, the publisher supported the team at every step. A small team of assistant editors was also appointed to further simplify the editing procedure and attain best results for the readers.

Apart from the editorial board, the designing team has also invested a significant amount of their time in understanding the subject and creating the most relevant covers. They scrutinized every image to scout for the most suitable representation of the subject and create an appropriate cover for the book.

The publishing team has been an ardent support to the editorial, designing and production team. Their endless efforts to recruit the best for this project, has resulted in the accomplishment of this book. They are a veteran in the field of academics and their pool of knowledge is as vast as their experience in printing. Their expertise and guidance has proved useful at every step. Their uncompromising quality standards have made this book an exceptional effort. Their encouragement from time to time has been an inspiration for everyone.

The publisher and the editorial board hope that this book will prove to be a valuable piece of knowledge for researchers, students, practitioners and scholars across the globe.

List of Contributors

Minmin Chang, Xinxin Liu, Ling Meng, Xiaohui Wang and Junli Ren
State Key Laboratory of Pulp and Paper Engineering, South China University of Technology, 510640 Guangzhou, China

Simone Lucarini, Laura Fagioli, Luca Casettari and Andrea Duranti
Department of Biomolecular Sciences, School of Pharmacy, University of Urbino, 61029 Urbino (PU), Italy

Snjezana Stolnik and Robert Cavanagh
Drug Delivery and Tissue Engineering Division, School of Pharmacy, University of Nottingham, Nottingham NG7 2RD, UK

Jenny K. W. Lam and Wanling Liang
Department of Pharmacology & Pharmacy, The University of Hong Kong, 21 Sassoon Road, Pokfulam, Hong Kong, China

Diego Romano Perinelli
School of Pharmacy, University of Camerino, 62032 Camerino (MC), Italy

Mario Campana
Science and Technology Facilities Council (STFC), ISIS Neutron and Muon Source, Rutherford Appleton Laboratory, Didcot OX11 0QX, UK

Gergő Fülöp
Gedeon Richter Plc., Formulation R&D, Gyömrői Street 19-21, H-1103 Budapest, Hungary
Department of Organic Chemistry and Technology, Budapest University of Technology and Economics, Budafoki út 8. 3, H-1103 Budapest, Hungary

Attila Balogh, Balazs Farkas, Attila Farkas, Bence Szabó, Balázs Démuth, Enikő Borbás, Zsombor Kristóf Nagy and György Marosi
Department of Organic Chemistry and Technology, Budapest University of Technology and Economics, Budafoki út 8. 3, H-1103 Budapest, Hungary

Sonia Trombino, Camilla Servidio, Federica Curcio and Roberta Cassano
Department of Pharmacy, Health and Nutritional Science, University of Calabria, Arcavacata, 87036 Rende, Italy

Ilona Gróf
Institute of Biophysics, Biological Research Centre, Hungarian Academy of Sciences, H-6726 Szeged, Hungary
Doctoral School in Biology, Faculty of Science and Informatics, University of Szeged, H-6726 Szeged, Hungary

Alexandra Bocsik and Mária A. Deli
Institute of Biophysics, Biological Research Centre, Hungarian Academy of Sciences, H-6726 Szeged, Hungary

Lóránd Kiss
Institute of Biophysics, Biological Research Centre, Hungarian Academy of Sciences, H-6726 Szeged, Hungary
Department of Pathophysiology, University of Szeged, H-6701 Szeged, Hungary

Ferenc Ötvös
Institute of Biochemistry, Biological Research Centre, Hungarian Academy of Sciences, H-6726 Szeged, Hungary

Ottó Zsíros
Plant Biology, Biological Research Centre, Hungarian Academy of Sciences, H-6726 Szeged, Hungary

Lejla Daruka
Doctoral School in Biology, Faculty of Science and Informatics, University of Szeged, H-6726 Szeged, Hungary
Synthetic and Systems Biology Unit, Institute of Biochemistry, Biological Research Centre, Hungarian Academy of Sciences, H-6726 Szeged, Hungary

Csaba Pál
Synthetic and Systems Biology Unit, Institute of Biochemistry, Biological Research Centre, Hungarian Academy of Sciences, H-6726 Szeged, Hungary

Lívia Fülöp, Norbert Imre and Tamás A. Martinek
Department of Medical Chemistry, University of Szeged, H-6720 Szeged, Hungary

Monika Vastag
Division of Pharmacology and Drug Safety Research, Gedeon Richter Plc., H-1103 Budapest, Hungary

Ágnes Kittel
Institute of Experimental Medicine, Hungarian Academy of Sciences, H-1450 Budapest, Hungary

Piroska Szabó-Révész
Department of Pharmaceutical Technology, University of Szeged, H-6720 Szeged, Hungary

Adele Faralli, Elhamalsadat Shekarforoush, Ana C. Mendes and Ioannis S. Chronakis
Nano-BioScience Research Group, DTU-Food, Technical University of Denmark, Kemitorvet, B202, 2800 Kgs. Lyngby, Denmark

Eleonora Russo and Carla Villa
Department of Pharmacy, University of Genoa, Viale Benedetto XV, 16132 Genova, Italy

Tammam Alama, Masaki Morishita, Hidemasa Katsumi and Akira Yamamoto
Department of Biopharmaceutics, Kyoto Pharmaceutical University, Misasagi, Yamashina-Ku, Kyoto 607-8414, Japan

Kosuke Kusamori
Laboratory of Biopharmaceutics, Faculty of Pharmaceutical Sciences, Tokyo University of Science, 2641 Yamazaki, Noda, Chiba 278-8510, Japan

Toshiyasu Sakane
Department of Pharmaceutical Technology, Kobe Pharmaceutical University, Higashinada-ku, Kobe 658-8558, Japan

Maria Cristina Cardia, Pierluigi Caboni, Anna Maria Maccioni, Sara Erbì, Maria Cristina Meloni, Francesco Lai and Chiara Sinico
Department of Life and Environmental Sciences, Unit of Drug Sciences, University of Cagliari, 09124 Cagliari, Italy

Anna Rosa Carta and Laura Boi
Department of Biomedical Sciences, University of Cagliari, 09124 Cagliari, Italy

Caroline Twarog, Sarinj Fattah, Joanne Heade and David J. Brayden
UCD School of Veterinary Medicine and UCD Conway Institute, University College Dublin, Belfield, Dublin 4, Ireland

Sam Maher
School of Pharmacy, Royal College of Surgeons in Ireland, St. Stephen's Green, Dublin 2, Ireland

Elias Fattal
School of Pharmacy, Institut Galien, CNRS, Univ. Paris-Sud, Univ. Paris-Saclay, 92290 Châtenay-Malabry, France

Jing M. Yong, Julia Mantaj, Yiyi Cheng and Driton Vllasaliu
School of Cancer and Pharmaceutical Sciences, Faculty of Life Sciences & Medicine, King's College London, London SE1 9NH, UK

Franklin Afinjuomo, Paris Fouladian, Ankit Parikh, Thomas G. Barclay, Yunmei Song and Sanjay Garg
School of Pharmacy and Medical Sciences, University of South Australia, Adelaide, South Australia 5001, Australia

Daniella S. Silva, Leonardo Marchiori and Sidney J. L. Ribeiro
Institute of Chemistry, São Paulo State University—UNESP, Araraquara 4800-900, Brazil

Danilo M. dos Santos
Embrapa Instrumentação, Rua XV de Novembro 1452, São Carlos 13560-970, Brazil

Bruno Sarmento and Andreia Almeida
Institute for Research and Innovation in Health (i3S), Rua Alfredo Allen, 208, 4200-393 Porto, Portugal
ICBAS—Institute of Biomedical Sciences Abel Salazar, University of Porto, Rua de Jorge Viterbo Ferreira, 228, 4050-313 Porto, Portugal
CESPU—Institute for Research and Advanced Training in Health Sciences and Technologies, Rua Central de Gandra, 1317, 4585-116 Gandra, Portugal

Sérgio P. Campana-Filho
Sao Carlos Institute of Chemistry, University of Sao Paulo—USP, Av. Trabalhador São-Carlense, 400, São Carlos 13566-590, Brazil

E. Michael Danielsen and Gert H. Hansen
Department of Cellular and Molecular Medicine, The Panum Institute, Faculty of Health Sciences, University of Copenhagen, 2200 Copenhagen, Denmark

Index

www.ingramcontent.com/pod-product-compliance
Lightning Source LLC
LaVergne TN
LVHW082200200926
848484LV00008B/2191